MIRACLES ARE MADE

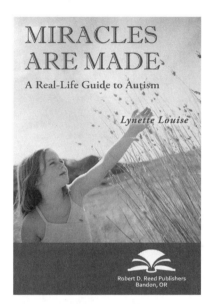

Miracles Are Made is a real-life guide written from the happenings of real life. It is a ***How To*** on living with and healing autism.

Lynette Louise began life's journey first as an individual, then as a mother, and eventually as a grandmother reaching into the heart of this disorder and helping first herself and then her children to become independent. Lynette's journey, challenging as it was, taught her many lessons on the very real possibilities and limitations buried within the diagnosis.

At present Lynette Louise holds a Masters in Social and Behavioral Science, a degree in Main Frame Computer Languages as well as counseling and neurofeedback certifications. What Lynette is proudest of, however, is her PhD in M.O.M. Lynette is a globally respected neurofeedback/play professional specializing in autism.

In ***Miracles Are Made*** Lynette not only shares stories from her personal and professional life but also illuminates the whys and the wherefores of the social climate parents find themselves in when coping with autism. She does this by educating us on the history of science and social awareness in relation to this disorder. She then teaches us how to make the best of what is possible and recreate the healings she has been fortunate enough to facilitate. You will come away understanding how to understand autism.

You will come away knowing what to do.

I have had the privilege of working, as a mental health provider and medical consultant, with Ms. Louise with her neurofeedback training work for almost five years. She has always been professional, courteous, and respectful in her behavior and attitude with the specified clients and their families.

Ms. Louise has a superb grasp of the neuro-anatomy, neuro-physiology especially as related to neurofeedback. She always tries to reason why or how a treatment is working, to have a theoretical framework for her choices of modalities. In addition to the excellent intellectual grasp and knowledge of her varied areas of training, she has an uncommon gift of a "sixth sense" that allows her to be "tuned into" the clients, their needs, and what approaches will be helpful in the given situation. Her people sensitivity has allowed her to be effective in some very difficult situations. Her approach to working with the client is flexibility in response to the situation and yet deliberately chosen—not just happenstance—to work for optimal effectiveness.

I have no hesitation in recommending Ms. Louise as a fully competent, trained, empathetic professional in her varied areas of expertise.

— Rebecca M Argo, MD
Diplomat, American Board of Psychiatry and Neurology

*Lynette Louise is rather unique and remarkable in the field of professionals working with individuals with ASD in that she combines at least four modalities (i.e., behavior therapy, neurofeedback, family therapy, education of patient and family) into an integrated individualized treatment that utilizes the best of each. Moreover, she seems to have a great gift in her ability to help the patient and family re-conceptualize what it means to **have** ASD but **not to be** ASD. That is, she appears to "connect" with patients in such a way that they come to realize at an intellectual and emotional level that they are unique and special, with strengths, weaknesses, and the possibility of change. This is no mere technique that Lynette has simply learned from formal training. Rather, in Lynette's case, it represents the culmination of years of study about ASD, living with ASD, and having a "special gift" for building rapport with individuals with ASD. Indeed, such a gift and Lynette's ability and passion for helping patients and their families change for the better are clearly reflected in* **MIRACLES ARE MADE: The Real Life Guide To Autism.**

— Harold Burke, PhD, ABMP
Board Certified in Medical Psychology
Board Certified in Neurofeedback
Clinical Neuropsychologist
DBH Associate, Arizona State University
Clinical Director, The Brain Therapy Center
Chief Science Advisor, EEG Spectrum International, Inc.
Licensed Psychologist, PSY12879

*The book **MIRACLES ARE MADE** describes a mother's journey to improve and heal her children with autism. Lynette Louise explains the benefits of neurofeedback, details the neuroanatomy of the brain and how it works along with an extensive description of autism spectrum disorder. She shares her experiences of being a mother of several children with autism and also her professional experiences working with other families. She stresses the importance of parents guiding their child into healing and the hard work they must sustain with a positive and loving attitude. With this book in their hands parents are empowered to teach their child, to learn from doing, and that learning is fun. Parents know their child better than anyone else.*

— **Lynne Gillis, O.T.**
Co-author of ***Autism Recovery Manual of Skills and Drills***

***MIRACLES ARE MADE** is for parents of children on the autistic spectrum. Parents have been on the forefront of progress in dealing with autism ever since they were first blamed for the problem. Few have as much relevant experience as Lynette Louise, having raised four adopted children on the spectrum while the professionals were of very little help. Three of the four are no longer considered autistic. The grounds for hope now include neurofeedback for training brain behavior directly. Here Lynette is passionate in calling for affected parents to take advantage of this new technique.*

Everything that parents can do directly points in the same direction: to labor lovingly and persistently within the comfort zone and the capacities of the child. All the while neurofeedback enhances that comfort zone and builds mental competences. Neurofeedback shows the brain where good function lies, one incremental step at a time. This is symbolic also of the parental role, that of engaging the child enduringly in his nascent competences.

If one looks back on Lynnette's children, one would not have suspected the capacities they would one day exhibit. This, we are finding, is a general truth. Yet Lynette is also still struggling with one child, now a young adult, who still has severe problems. The point is that one cannot judge the child's potential in advance. This obligates us to explore every potential without pre-judging. In that effort, which can indeed be daunting, Lynette's book can be a comforting, motivating, and energizing companion.

Further, the history recounted here gives parents support in interacting with caregivers. There are still no experts on autism. There are only experts on different aspects of the condition. The parent is inevitably left as the final arbiter of what is good for the child, the final judge of what is and isn't helping. This book gives them the necessary background, and backbone, to level the playing field in the face of so many therapeutic options.

— **Siegfried Othmer, Ph.D.**
Chief Scientist of the EEG Institute, President of the Brian Othmer Foundation
Author of ***ADD: The 20-Hour Solution***

MIRACLES ARE MADE: The Real Life Guide To Autism by Lynette Louise is a must read for anyone who has a child with autism, works in the field or simply wants to understand more about the spectrum. Having an eight-year-old son, I have been searching for five years since his diagnosis for an intervention that not only made sense to me psychologically but also actually led to improving the areas in which my son was challenged. Home training with neurofeedback has been the most effective approach by far and continues to move my son in the direction of more normal functioning in all areas. I love how Lynette wrote the book with more comprehensive information about this impressive intervention first, using plenty of detailed examples to demonstrate her discoveries. The second half of the book is loaded with useful information about diagnostic criteria and an overview of many other treatment options. Lynette is knowledgeable and writes with a profound understanding of the entire autistic spectrum, which in my experience has been unparalleled. She is funny and entertaining and brutally honest. I could not put the book down as I fervently kept reading for one more golden nugget of information, of which there were many even up until the very last page. Well-done Lynette. Thank you,

— **Deborah Portnoy**
Producer/Director/Playwright, *MOTHERS AND OTHERS ON AUTISM*

*I am a firm believer that children can significantly improve and in some cases make a full recovery from autism with different forms of intensive intervention. Lynette chose to use neurofeedback to help her own children as well as many others improve their condition of autism. In her book **MIRACLES ARE MADE** she explains how neurofeedback alters a child's brainwaves and teaches the brain how to rebalance itself and process information, curtail negative behaviors, and learn more easily. I enjoyed how she uses humor throughout her book to explain how neurofeedback works to change how you feel, react, and interact with others. Her love, dedication, and commitment to her children are exemplary, and how she explains in detail how effective neurofeedback can be to help improve problems with the central nervous system that afflict children with autism **MIRACLES ARE MADE** shows how a devoted mother made so many miracles come true for her children.*

— **Elizabeth Burton Scott**
Author of ***Raindrops on Roman: Overcoming Autism: A Message of Hope***
and ***Autism Recovery Manual of Skills and Drills***

MIRACLES ARE MADE is an important book. Lynette Louise offers a living example, inspiration, and concrete information about the amazing power of neurofeedback in changing lives. This book is a must for seekers, doubters, parents, educators, healthcare professionals, and scientists.

— **Mark Steinberg, Ph.D.**, Licensed Psychologist
TV Medical Consultant, Author of ***ADD: The 20-Hour Solution***

MIRACLES ARE MADE

A Real-Life Guide to Autism

Lynette Louise

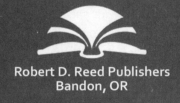

Robert D. Reed Publishers
Bandon, OR

Robert D. Reed Publishers
P.O. Box 1992
Bandon, OR 97411
Phone: 541-347-9882; Fax: -9883
E-mail: 4bobreed@msn.com
Website: www.rdrpublishers.com

Cover Art: Tim Hale
Cover Designer: Cleone Reed
Book Designer: Amy Cole

ISBN 13: 978-1-934759-49-3
ISBN 10: 1-934759-49-X

Library of Congress Control Number: 2010940127

Manufactured, Typeset, and Printed in the United States of America

For Tsara and Brandessa who willingly bathe me in trust, adoration, appreciation and support.

Thank you.

Table of Contents

Introduction

Some people, mental health professionals and parents alike, have been known to feed LSD to autistic children in the hopes that it would make them normal. Some people, parents, grandparents, aunts, and uncles traveled great distances to acquire that drug and the opportunity to hope.

I am not one of these people… though I confess I've considered it… enough to do the research.

Perhaps the first thing any parenting self-help (or child-help) book should start with is what makes the author credible. Why should you take the time to read what any professional—he/she or I—has to say let alone follow our advice on how to change the prognosis of someone with autism? In fact why should you even believe that such a thing is possible? Why shouldn't you? The truth is, my credentials don't include a doctorate or a medical degree, but if there were a PhD in parenting—especially if it were a PhD in being challenged as a parent parenting challenged children—I would have easily completed it by now. This is because I raised eight very special kids—or perhaps it is more accurate to say—eight very special kids raised me. Some of my children were biological, some were adopted, and most were special needs. The four littlest guys were on the spectrum of autism, and all but one now live completely on their own, in lives of joyful independence. The last one? Well he's joyful too, now.

Dar is my twenty-eight-year-old slow-moving miracle. He's the one I am still focused on, the one for whom I even considered LSD… until I did the research.

Real-life research is the real reason that, whether you are an individual, a parent, or a professional dealing with autism, I see my lived experience as useful to you. Because I am all of those: a previously afflicted individual, a parent, and a professional. I understand autism from the vantage points of living with it on a twenty-four-hour-a-day basis and from working with it eight hours a day for weeks on end. I've been, and am, aspects of you. I share some or all of your situation and have armed myself with twenty-five years of acquired knowledge that you may not yet have had the time to learn. I am blessed. My clients are improving and most of my kids have grown healthy as well as independent.

While traveling my path I trained in various therapies in order to help my own family. I created an individualized plan for each and every child. Learning to understand them helped me to understand myself and so we healed, each of us in our own way. As a result of that learning I also ended up helping not only our family but also many, many more. At first I was just self-educating as I read and gulped and followed up on every autism clue. Eventually I embraced more formalized training and received certifications in the Son-Rise® method (a form of play therapy aimed at improving autism) and in Option Process Mentor counseling. I trained in and apprenticed under some of the top clinicians in the field of neurofeedback (AKA biofeedback for the brain), which as it turns out is the easiest and most excitingly impactful therapy I have ever used. I then branched out on my own using family dynamics counseling, play therapy, and neurofeedback to heal children and their families around the globe. Eventually I ended up with a Masters in Social and Behavioral Science. I study neuroanatomy to be better equipped when working with neurofeedback and align myself with the minds of as many highly respected professionals as I can attract. For that and many other reasons I continue to learn about all brain-related subjects like pharmaceuticals and supplements, genetics and toxins, physiology, and psychology. I do this on an ongoing basis. And then, believe it or not, I make jokes about it, on stage.

Looking back, it sometimes seems as if my entire life has been dedicated to walking two different paths: One of learning in order to improve mental health and happiness and the other of light-hearted endeavors in performance and creative arts. I raised my kids in part on the meager wages of a Canadian actress who was a sometimes journalist, children's entertainer, karaoke singer, and standup comedian with very big dreams. But as I examine these lifelong interests it becomes clear that they are not actually parallel paths, that they are in fact the same, one and only path, for me. It turns out that my entire life has been about sharing in order to make a difference intended to help us all feel good about ourselves. And it also turns out that my idea on what will help us feel good about ourselves is a scientific understanding of the brain, those internal bits and pieces that make people tick. I suppose that's why, whenever I have control of the project, the subject matter in my performance art and standup comedy is generally about learning from behavior in order to improve mental health and happiness. Of course like any good playwright I do my best to disguise the lessons as entertainment because being entertained is an emotional experience, and emotional experiences are more easily recalled. It is for that reason that even in this fact-heavy book about autism I will do my best to keep your interest, to joke and tease, teach and please, frighten and relieve you. I hope to share stories that bring tears, laughter, and hope —and then leave you with enough knowledge and understanding to change your own story, if you so wish. If you're going to take the time to read what I write, then it's my job to help you remember what I said. This way you are more equipped to use the gifts within.

In fact you should be more equipped to use these gifts than I was. This is because I gained the gifts I will share via the benefit of hindsight and of having the majority of my life behind me. But that's OK because sharing gifts with you is a gift to me, since in order to tell you about it I have to know what it is I want to say. In order to describe my life, I have to look at it. And because of that exercise I am able to stop thinking of myself as a part-performer, part-parent person with too many interests and get to realize that I have been consistently congruent all along. What a gift. Thank you! Because of that exercise I finally understand that I have always taught others in order to learn, even if I had to adopt them to do so. However, I have to admit, when in the midst of it all, when living my life, things seemed anything but congruent.

Time and again I thought of myself as living in a mess of confusion. This feeling of being lost while trying to still make choices is common to parents of autism. It is a feeling worth getting adjusted to. Be comfortable with it. We aren't always able to see where a choice will lead us, but we can still pick. This is because it is our intention that separates the possibilities and chooses the path. As long as we hold on to our intention and keep that clear, we will gather our choices along a continuum that makes it make sense—even if we can't see it until we have the benefit of hindsight and even when the choices we see ourselves making seem irrelevant to our goals.

For example, before I even dreamed of embarking on a career dedicated to changing brain function, I was educating myself in ways that would later become useful; in my early twenties I got an honors degree in the seemingly unrelated field of main-frame computer languages. Given that I work with computers to fix brain-wave activity, part of that training came in handy while also enhancing my understanding of the activity of the brain. Most notably, understanding the bits and bytes of the basic machine language of computers crystallized for me the concept of how the excitatory and inhibitory behavior of neurons could create a binary code for the brain and build an enormously complex system from a simple two-signal starting point. Big deal—oh sure—ho hum—so what?

Truth is none of this fancy-sounding jargon has anything to do with why I think you will benefit from reading this book. I believe we will benefit (me from the giving, you from the receiving) not because of the knowledge I will share as a result of my training (though these things are plentiful and infinitely valuable) but because of the learnings I will share as a result of my life. It is from my story of trying to raise children and grandchildren out of autism that the treasures come and the mysteries are unraveled.

It is because…

Most of the children I am referring to are no longer diagnosable as autistic.

And these children grew miraculously normal, despite me, and because of me, even though when it comes to modeling relationships for ones' relationship-challenged autistic children… I was about as stable as nitroglycerine.

And speaking of the levity I just used while discussing the subject of husbands, I've had quite a few of them. In fact I got married five times. Five times so far (wink wink nudge nudge). Now, now don't close the book just yet; let me explain. Truth is I only really felt married twice, and in fact I seldom and sometimes never even lived with my other three husbands. It's not so much an excuse as a fact that I was socially challenged and physically and mentally abused as a child. In my case the reason for having a sensory disordered brain is hard to chicken or egg. Was it my family's genetics or my family's behavior? Likely both. I do know I loved my first husband immensely and we had children together, but as broken people are wont to do, I picked a broken man. The stories of my search for romance are long and involved and not the purpose of this book; but suffice to say that after twenty years of disconnection, my first husband and I re-found each other. At that point I lifted him from a deep depression by giving him the opportunity to help me help my son and in the process, we found neurofeedback, which helped us all.

When I first began writing this book the following five sentences came next: *And so nowadays whenever one of us needs a little help getting things done we get together and do it. Fortunately this is made easier by the fact that Brent and I usually cohabitate (in fact more often now than when we were married). My marriage tree is an interesting one. According to my mother I got it right the first time. According to me, it was impossible to know that I had gotten it right the first time until the first time was over because I didn't have anything to compare it to until I did "You don't know what you've got until it's gone."* Fortunately gone doesn't always mean forever. Those five sentences used to come next but now, as I enter into rewrites, I find myself sitting in a hospital room watching my first husband sleep off the effects of his cancer therapy: a therapy that isn't working. I find myself remembering who we used to be and how much I've healed in the past few years of brain biofeedback. This man that I have known since I was sixteen years old is about to die. He has been awful and he has been beautiful. We were lucky enough to find our way into healing and happiness and cooperative parenting before the end of our story. But still it is the end of our story and he is about to die. I have loved him since the day we met.

This is a heavy truth that I will speak of lightly. I believe that in order to be a great help to you, my reader, I must become a good friend first. I believe a good friend speaks plainly about plain truth and then cares enough to help you find the humor. It's through that insider's-joke approach that we are able to connect as people in the know. If you are here to learn about autism it is likely that you already know and understand difficulty. I will occasionally nudge you with a wink and a smile because humor gets you through and rearranges your perspective so that you can see and learn and grow and be… happy with autism… even as you try to change it. Thus I speak lightly of myself with my harem of husbands because I have gained the ability to laugh. I've healed enough to move beyond the need to cry for my faulty judgment and myself. Moving beyond is a wonderful skill I hope to empower you with. Brent and I became something new at the end. We were lucky. We found our way back and then we used Neurofeedback to heal the family. Everybody dies. All stories end. At least ours ended with forgiveness and love.

His breathing is thick with tumors and his face ashen. Our children are scared. I am resigned. He will die having learned how to love and I will live having done the same. So perhaps that's the *romantic* end of it for me, or perhaps it is the beginning. I have no idea whether or not the word romantic will cease to be in my dictionary of ideas. However, if, after this, I do still believe in it I will believe in it differently. If after this I ever reenter the world of dating I will enter it differently because I am different, a different woman than I was the last time I stepped onto that field. This time I am a healthy one.

Fortunately my past is not only good for learning, it is also good for a laugh. So I have compiled a cohabitation husband history collage.

Lynette Louise Marriage/Cohabitation Collage

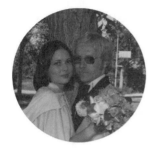

 # 1. James Brent Leach
Married 7/12/75 – 2/22/79

Lived together 2/1/74 – 11/16/77
and again
9/01/03 - 4/9/10

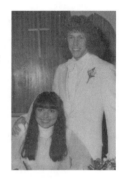

 # 2. Matthew David Webster
Married 8/18/79 – 8/19/83

Lived together 2.5 months
8/18/79 – 10/31/79

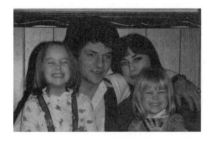

 # 3. James Rodney Shelton
Married 9/2/83 – 7/10/93

Lived together 1981 – 1989

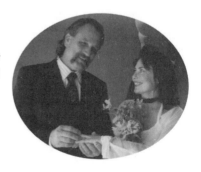

 # 4. James Thomas Sawyer
Married 3/31/95 – 12/9/96

Lived together 2 weeks
4/15/95 – 4/30/95

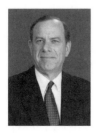

 # 5. Timothy David McMillin
Married 8/6/00 – 9/30/08

Never lived together

However, fun as it is, this husband cohabitation collage is somewhat misleading. For example: I cohabitated with Brent for less time when we were married (four years off and on) than when we were not (seven years… sort of). As you may have guessed, my life is never quite what it seems on the surface. Another example of appearances being misleading is that, despite all the marriages, if you do the math and line up the dates you will discover that I was mostly a single mom. Because most of my live-in-helper-type marriages were short lived. I believe this is because, for me, children are the priority. For my husbands that was never the case.

Young people are and always have been my life's calling to the point that I have even helped co-parent four of my eight grandchildren—two of whom showed definite signs of autism until we all worked together to change the picture. As a mother my friends often called me the "young lady in the shoe" because I was raising eight children, though truth be told I only birthed three. A few years after my son was born dead I began adopting. My eyes were wide open about the challenges of adoption because my own brother was adopted at age seven. And I remembered clearly the difficulties my parents had dealing with his transition into our family, a transition that was never quite complete: My brother moved to the streets at around sixteen years of age and was murdered at twenty-two. I was determined to do a better job than my parents had. I began with two healthy biological daughters. Then I gathered four kiddos on the spectrum of autism as well as another two who were beset by emotional traumas and learning challenges. Raising special-needs children is hard on relationships so whenever I was forced to choose, I chose to keep my children. This meant that I lost some husbands instead.

Thus it was that I spent most of my time as sole matriarch and single parent.

In this book I will bounce around without historical chronology in order to underscore the point I am making so, in order for this not to be too confusing, here is my relevant life history in a nutshell:

1974 *biological daughter, Tsara*
1975 *married her dad, James*
1976 *stillborn son, Christopher*
1977 *second biological daughter, Brandessa*
1978 *divorced James*
1979 *married again*
1981 *divorced again*
1982 *remarried*

1984 *adopted first child with autism, son, Dar*
1986 *adopted three male siblings with autism, oldest to youngest Cash, Chance, Rye*
1989 *separated from husband*
1990 *custody of teenage runaway daughter with a learning disability, Jady 1991 custody of homeless teenage girl, eighth and last child Khiya.*

Lynette Louise Family Tree

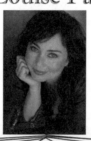

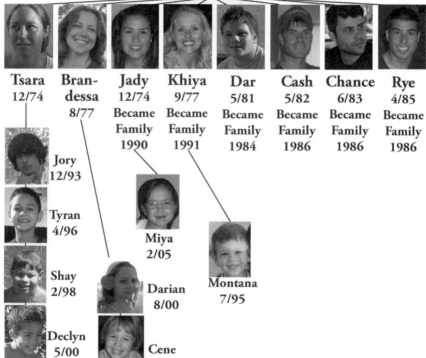

Tsara	Bran-	Jady	Khiya	Dar	Cash	Chance	Rye
12/74	dessa	12/74	9/77	5/81	5/82	6/83	4/85
	8/77	Became	Became	Became	Became	Became	Became
		Family	Family	Family	Family	Family	Family
		1990	1991	1984	1986	1986	1986

Jory
12/93

Tyran
4/96

Miya
2/05

Shay
2/98

Darian
8/00

Montana
7/95

Declyn
5/00

Cene
8/03

As previously stated I spent most of my time as a single mom raising eight children. My grandkids began arriving in 1994 and at present, I have eight of them. Though we are soon expecting an identical set of twins, for the moment we are a balanced set of eight plus eight. And once the twins arrive a new type of balance will be struck: five girls and five boys in the grandchild zone. I am relatively attracted to balance so this makes me happy. As you shall discover within the pages of this book, I come by my attraction to balance naturally.

I know that to be true because my main and most-used therapy is neurofeedback: it will be referred to often. It is a means of reading brain wave activity and then giving the brain information about how to balance that activity. Balance, as it turns out, is the secret to mental and physical health and all life is endowed with the desire to achieve it. Sometimes we call that desire for balance "the pursuit of happiness."

Doing neurofeedback is not unlike having a practitioner listen to your heart with a stethoscope and then, having found it running at too fast a pace, put it up for you to observe on an EKG screen. If he then taps a rhythm on your wrist and instructs you to match your heart to this rhythm, your heart will slow accordingly. With neurofeedback we don't tap a beat on your wrist; instead we speak to the brain through the use of beeps. We entertain and train the brain by having the person attempt to run a video game simply by shifting his focus and changing his brain-wave activity. With the heart example we listen through a stethoscope and display the visible rhythm on an EKG screen; with the brain example we use sensors on the head and display the activity on an EEG screen. In both cases the task the patient is being asked to accomplish sounds impossible but is in fact simple and easy to do. So much so that I teach parents worldwide to use this approach at home in order to relieve their and their children's symptoms of cognitive challenges and emotional discomfort.

Initially I used this therapy at home with my own children with remarkable results. I want to thank them for their trust and willingness to be at my hands throughout their entire lives. Had they not lent me their heads to learn on and heal, I would have no happy-ending journey to share. It is because they were so open to me and my crazy ideas that so many others will now be helped. I want to make a special note of the constant help with regard to this project (and my everyday life) from two of my children, Tsara Shelton and Brandessa Shelton. Tsara has been my right hand in all things related to the home front since she came out of my womb. She is an ever-present source of support and love that has taken me from teenage mom to competent grandmom. Brandessa is my right hand in all visionary things related to today's need to work within the technical landscape. She is brilliant and overflowing with impossible ideas that land on their feet. She is a great neurofeedback technician and has worked with me as I work to help families of autism. It was as a direct result of observing me teach parents that Brandessa literally pestered me into writing this book. Thus it is fair to say that the existence of this written guide into the world of autism is because of my children and all their support.

The other approach that I use alongside neurofeedback is an operant conditioning play approach. This combines several present-day Cognitive Behavioral Therapies with the Son-Rise® Program and Family Dynamics Counseling and is designed according to the physiological functioning of the brain. In this way we create an individualized program that is designed from the needs of each child and respective family. The thinking behind this approach will be fully explained. These are my ideas about how to implement already existing theories and therapies. They are based on my experience and intuition.

EXPLANATIONS AND DEDICATIONS
How This Book Works

Embrace this book as your best friend and then throw in a grain of salt to account for the fact that all the opinions contained within are based on my own personal and professional experience and as such do not necessarily reflect the views of the majority of professionals specializing in autism. (Autism is a whole-brain disorder that has as its main features difficulty with social situations, communication, and a need to engage in repetitive behaviors). This book is presented in two sections. If you are just finding out about autism then it is written backwards. Section Two is a less reader-friendly, fact-heavy resource of what is available, diagnostic criteria, and treatment options. It can be used as a reference section while you read the first portion, or you can begin by informing yourself first and then flipping back to the beginning.

A DIAGNOSIS WITHOUT DIRECTIONS: this is what it is to be told your child has autism. It is my intention to help you understand why that is and then to change that reality by teaching you what to do to improve the prognosis.

Section One

As a mom my greatest frustration was being treated as if I had sole responsibility for my children's mental health while simultaneously being considered ill equipped to make a difference in their developmental IQ. So I grew a chip between the specialist and me: the very specialist from whom I was seeking the answers. In this section I explain the phenomenon that creates this cross firing of professional and parental snobbery and give you a taste of the damage that was (and is) levied as a result. To do this I share openly my own personal, fraught with errors, journey of trying to heal the autism within my family and myself. There were people who helped and people who stood in the way. I will show you both. For the most part I write by putting the microscope on me and mine because ours is the story I have the right to share. That is not a limitation but a liberation giving me the freedom to tell all that I know with no concern for confidentiality. I will share what we came to know. Then in order to help you generalize these lessons rather than see them as unique to me and mine, I will be culling similar examples from the journeys of the clients I work with globally. Working with them has taught me much: like that my story is not as unique as I had previously thought. As it turns out our story is just a variation on all the other stories being lived out over and over again worldwide. (The number of children being diagnosed with autism today is one in a hundred and ten. This is so astronomically high that it is considered a global epidemic.) I am certain that sharing its happy ending and the road we traveled will facilitate a similarly fantastic fate for others.

In Chapter One, I will introduce you to the boy who introduced me to autism. I experimented, educated, and problem solved in search of an understanding on how to help this boy. That was a good thing because it was attempting to understand Dar that taught me to understand autism.

I spent all my exhausted mommy hours wishing I could fix him (and eventually his brothers as well) with a pill or a diet or a magical potion. Inevitably I was to discover that I was in good company—most of the amazing parents I've worked with did the same. So in this next chapter we ponder the Achilles heal of parents—their (and my) desire for a miracle cure and the problems that leaves us vulnerable. Most professionals in the field of autism try to say it's impossible to change the autistic child's prognosis by much more than a skill or two; some say it can be done but only if the child is young and only if the road is extremely unpleasant to travel; a few of the charlatans say not only can it be done but its easy. Fact is it's both none and all of those: You can make a curative difference and yes it's hard but it's also fun. It does however take loads of time and effort. And that's why I've called this book *Miracles Are Made* because in fact they are. That's what makes neurofeedback so great. Though you still do the work and make the miracles yourself, neurofeedback makes it quicker, which makes it possible to move farther or move on to a new kind of fun.

In this chapter I explain why speed matters. Though it's possible to heal some children via responding techniques with or without neurofeedback, it's not possible to heal all. In fact the number of children that can be healed this way is small. Since the amount of healing enabled is increased by the speed with which the reward (aka positive feedback) is delivered to the brain, by using the faster processing of a computer it becomes possible to heal not only more quickly but also more completely. Understand that: Responding to behavior in a noticeable manner whether it comes from the computer, the sensory system, or the parent IS feedback. Brains use feedback to direct their growth patterns. Responding faster cures quicker.

Personally I raised most of my kids the old-fashioned way, *feedback from my own frantic desires*. I used words, rewards, and punishments with a lot of natural consequences thrown in because autistic children learn more through experience than verbal or visual teaching. I also used natural consequences as much as possible because I didn't always want to be the *enforcer*. Besides I had eight kids. I was too busy to see everything. I tried to guide my children's interpretation of these experiences and then follow the feedback they gave me via their (very often non-verbal) reaction to the feedback I had given them. This information mixed with my goals and wishes for them created my next bit of feedback in their direction. And so we leap-frogged as I taught them to listen to me by telling them how great they were at listening. In other words I raised the bar, constantly. I redesigned the next feedback from me to fit the new child I was hoping to find. This making of miracles is a lot of work. And, for those of my children who were either normal or close enough to the edge of the spectrum to be nudged off, this huge amount of work was enough.

However, for the others, even all that constant feeding back wasn't sufficient because those others had so much farther to go. I needed a better way… something that could take them farther, faster. The something I found was neurofeedback. At this point all of my children were adults and I'd been a parent for twenty-nine years. According to the present-day beliefs about autism, it was too late to help them. I tried anyway.

When I first started using neurofeedback I found myself looking at all those years of parental feedback, then at these young men changing before my eyes, and I realized that had I found this therapy sooner, in the length of time it had taken to heal my high-functioning children I could have healed the whole group. That's why I want to share it with you, so you don't have to wait, because speed of change matters if you want to watch your children live without the sensory stress of autism, sooner.

Since neurofeedback supports the feedback you give as a parent and increases the speed of healing, then it stands to reason that if the feedback of the environment the child lives in is congruent with the feedback of the parents, the resultant constantly reinforced lessons will be learned even quicker. This kind of supportive seeding into the garden of the mind makes desired change grow even faster than using neurofeedback and parental feedback alone ever could. Thus it is possible to cast the net wider reaching an older, much more damaged brain than was previously thought possible. To do this a parent needs to be more than I was when I started the journey. Thus I share what I had to learn in order for me to be strong enough and clear enough to be able to create this collective congruence.

In the beginning social workers and well-meaning teachers would listen to me explaining what I was doing for my children and end up saying things like "Yes, but what are you doing for yourself?" For my part I always thought the same thing: "Helping my children, goofus!" (OK, maybe it wasn't goofus; I was a little less refined back then!) In fact back then no matter how many times I had the concept explained to me, I couldn't understand the degree to which I wouldn't be able to help my kids before I helped myself. Actually I didn't even understand what that meant. I raised myself on movies of martyrs making miracles happen. I recognized the heroes I wanted to emulate by the degree of their self-denial. I recognized them because they were always dirty, sweaty, and sadly smiling. I wanted to be just like that: too busy choosing the business of saving the world to choose the business of taking a shower. I wanted to put my needs aside as they seemed so able to do and beat myself for the betterment of others. I was certain such a life would feel heavenly (pun intended).

In Chapters Three and Four, I do my best to hold hands with most of the mothers I've had the privilege to meet. I try to walk through the pages with them, learning again, that martyrdom never heals anyone: Martyring requires suffering in the same way that being a hero requires the existence of a victim. Thus heroes are codependent on villains just as nurses are codependent on sick people and parents who want to put themselves second to their child are codependent on keeping their child under their wing. Beating oneself for the betterment of others is a very selfish act that only accidentally, if ever, benefits anyone. It is an act committed by people using feedback that is caught in a loop.

When I was one of those people I remember checking on myself to make sure I was doing it right. Being an audience to my own self-denial became a habit meant to reassure me that I was a good person. But instead that habit led to overwhelming bouts of depression. This is because I couldn't see if anyone else was noticing just how much I was giving up for my children so I ended up feeling taken for granted and abused. I couldn't see the onlookers, not because they weren't there but because a person can only focus on one thing at a time and I was focusing on me. Not only could I not see any appreciators, I couldn't see anyone. I was way too busy martyring to see the person (child, husband, friend) I was trying to help, let alone what they needed. In other words I was too busy helping people according to my need to help them, to help them according to theirs. And since my own personal need was to help others and not myself, nobody was helped. And that is the conundrum of common ground that this chapter solves via the stories of my life.

I spent most of my children's lives peeling away layer upon layer of this aspect of me. When I found neurofeedback it fell away in bunches. I dropped my need to suffer in silence. I learned to embrace with great gluttony my joy for life. I was energized, focused, and became actually useful. I finally got the concept that doing something for myself actually made it more possible to do something for my children. I used neurofeedback on my own brain and cured my own attention, sensory, and perception issues. Then, because I had successfully treated myself, followed the changes in my own symptoms, and stepped myself toward a state of balance and mental health the way Hansel and Gretel followed the pebbles out of the forest, I came to understand how to do the same for others. Happily, because I then had sensory symptoms common to autism, I was especially equipped to understand how to help the autism still left in my children. My goal in Chapter Three is to teach you how to be well enough to want wellness for your child, and then to tell you how to go about getting that because I think autism should come with directions.

Chapter Five comes before Chapter Six because that's how most people count (wink) and because, before providing an overview of neurofeedback and how it works, I sincerely want to set you up for success in hopes you choose to use it.

In my opinion the children who travel the farthest in their healing journey are the ones whose entire families participate in the therapy with the intention of healing the whole group. This works so much better than seeing only the "autistic child" as the broken one. When groups think like that they focus only on the child in question and by so focusing reinforce his state. This happens whenever they look his way to see if he is still broken. Questions create answers. It is much more useful to ask, "What is our next step towards becoming even more comfortable and happy both individually and as a group?" than to ask, "Why can't he stop screaming?" Questions create answers!

So ask yourself, "What do I want?" But be specific when you answer because vague answers stop most of us from acting and lead to sweepingly ineffective responses. For example, "I want to feel lighter in my body" is more useful than "I want to be happy." This is because your happiness comes from too many possibilities and so it is overwhelming trying to figure out what to do next. However, "lighter in my body" is more specific, and since it is also how you feel when you are happy such an answer could lead to solutions like "take yoga to stretch my muscles and become more flexible" which would also oxygenate your body and release endorphins effectively making you more happy. Thus when you answer in specificity, it is easier to come up with ways to achieve your goal. Then since very often parts of your child are like parts of you, you may come up with an answer that applies to others in your family. In this way seeing the sameness in you and your autistic child is much better than looking at him or her as an alien living in an unknown world that you can't comprehend. If you want desirable change you have to act toward it, and since all change is incremental the important thing is to begin and then spread the learning around the house. This vaster improvement for your child by learning from yourself is what we do anyway. I am just saying it can be applied purposefully to create wanted neuronal change, for the whole family, especially once you learn how to be specific about what kind of neuronal change you want.

The therapeutic effect that can be attained by mass creating change is especially desirable in genetically connected families of autism wherein, for the most part, the entire group has some sort of mild to moderate brain dysfunction. That is one of the reasons I believe the best use of neurofeedback is when it is done in the home: Parents treat themselves, learn about brain behavior and, under the guidance of an expert, combine their subjective knowledge with the therapist's objective knowledge and proceed toward healing themselves and their loved ones.

- Be aware that the majority of Mental Health and neurofeedback professionals would disagree with me on the above point. They would argue that the very presence of dysregulation in the parent's brain means that the parent is destined to be an unreliable, poorly prepared therapist. They are wrong. In fact sometimes the dysregulated parent is more aware of their limitations, more motivated to feel better and thus a better student than the regulated one. It's quite a funny argument anyway, since most of the neurofeedback therapists I've had the good fortune to meet were drawn to the field because they were looking to help themselves. In other words, they, the good ones and bad ones alike, are themselves dysregulated in some way. I am certain that, just as it is for the parents, the therapists who treat themselves and gain the knowledge that only the personal experience of "doing it" can give are often the ones who end up more gifted as healers.

- Regardless, the world of medicine is always fraught with argument due to differing opinions. So there are those in the field who think that neurofeedback is so strong it is too dangerous to be used in the home. But there are also many medical professionals who believe that there is no hard science backing up the efficacy of neurofeedback having any effect whatsoever and certainly not enough to be considered as a brain rehabilitation tool. They too are wrong. There is plenty of hard science and many well-designed studies on the subject. There are, however, no well-paid drug representatives offering free samples to make prescribing easier, spread the word, and gain cooperation from doctors. However, that fact alone is not reason enough to explain why neurofeedback has taken so long to hit mainstream medicine.

In this very raw chapter I examine social responsibility related to autism by illuminating various aspects of social culpability. This is not because I have a political bent and want to point fingers of blame at the authority figures and organizations in our society, but because understanding the world around you helps you to understand the world within. And in my experience understanding the world around you is best done by understanding how the past became the present. Coming to comprehend why the field of medicine, even in the face of indisput-able evidence, moves so slowly to change its collective mind and accept new truths eases the frustration and the judgment one normally feels when dealing with that reality. Thus you can problem solve from within the reality instead of wasting energy wishing it were different. This enables you to get about the business of actually making it different in your home. In order for you to understand how we (my family and the present-day global community of parents and professionals) got where we are, I indoctrinate you into the climate of the times and the reasons for resistance to change. I stay true to life by telling most of these stories from my own back yard. Though the term "autistic" was thrown my way as early as 1961, my search for answers didn't begin until 1982 because that is when the problem included my children. I was not only willing to look, I was compelled to act on what I found. And because I took action with what I found, what I found turned into answers. These answers led to great improvements in cognitive functioning for my entire family. Throughout this journey called my life I have to admit that for me, the biggest challenge was not teaching my children, but teaching the world to believe that my children could be taught, and that I, the unstable relationship model, could be the one to teach them. This is a big chapter sharing very personal parts of my family history with the kind of honesty that leaves me at risk of being treated with disdain. I risk it anyway.

These self-revealing stories of being misunderstood by society help distill what did and what didn't work from all the preconceived ideas of the time on what would and what wouldn't. It was difficult because the "woulds" and the "dids" were diametrically different. True, we managed it anyway. I helped my children grow strong, healthy, and independent. But it would have been a more pleasant journey had we not had the issue of opposition. That's why I try to shine light on the subject of how not working together to help the child can undermine the process of anything working at all. I explore the need for educators, mental health professionals, social workers, and parents to become informed enough to create congruence in order to globally or even individually heal. Because opinions are feedback and feedback results in behaviors and emotions like pain or pleasure, pride or shame, truth or lies. We create people, out of chaotic noise or harmonious ideas. We create people depending on how and what we do and say, together or apart.

Call it by its name: THE BRAIN

Learning about your brain and how its physiology affects your behavior can make understanding tangible. It can also help to eradicate the guilt, judgment, and victimization that a primarily psychological approach spews upon social situations.

In Chapter Six, I will explain neurofeedback in detail and then follow with a chapter on how to apply it while using neuroanatomy as a guide. I invite you into my brain and use my own mental challenges to teach this subject. I use me, not only in part to walk my talk and model healing oneself in order to learn enough to heal others, but also because I am more intimately connected with my own journey than with anyone else's. I am the subject I know best.

Chapter Seven and even to some degree Chapter Six are technically deep chapters because if you are going to do therapy on your family you have to learn how. These chapters are invaluable even if you never intend to use neurofeedback. They teach the very necessary yet seldom-taught skill of following behavior in order to understand how to create a next-step plan of action that helps you get to your goal: help your child off the spectrum. By the end of these chapters you will have been taught *how* to choose from inside the chaos. This is a more valuable tool than being told *what* to choose because *what* to choose changes minute-to-minute, child-to-child, and environment-to-environment. A true understanding of this concept frees up your creative ability to think out of the box and find solutions. Having the ability to think like a brain detective clears away the confusion created by that mosaic of behaviors your autistic child is presenting you with and can be applied to improve the results of any therapy you may be using. Understanding the brain helps you to understand the details and gives you the energy to continue. For example, if you know why motivation matters and/or why happiness improves memory, you are more likely to use them both. So you see understanding the brain helps you to understand to what you should attribute a behavior, which helps you to understand how to follow and consequently affect symptoms that show up as behaviors. In addition, understanding the brain helps you to appreciate and comprehend the unbelievable degree to which your behavior can and does affect someone else's brain. This is empowering as it helps you focus on how to behave in order to properly address the symptoms in the person you are trying to help: most likely your child. Thus by learning how to follow, you come to understand what to do in order to make a positive difference with the knowledge you have. And suddenly autism is no longer a diagnosis without directions.

Add to that an understanding of neurofeedback which, as you may recall, is merely site-specific brainwave information being fed back very quickly to the brain, causing changes in emotions and behavior to be experienced almost immediately, and you become more convinced of the value of feedback itself. Knowing how feedback works and seeing such obvious change being achieved by a method similar to your own feedback via reaction behavior helps you analyze and intentionalize the feedback you use at home. It also helps you understand the degree to which you, your relatives, your neighbors, and your child's teacher can and will affect your babies brain.

In addition since I want to help parents AND professionals to reach children AND adults in need of help I have chosen to share at a level that interests and informs us all. There are as many approaches to making protocol choices for neurofeedback as there are neurofeedback therapists making them. As I am to share what I have learned I want to ensure that the reasons for my choices are clear. That way anyone wanting to choose similarly will know how. Finally these chapters are information heavy because I want to make available to parents information that was not made available to me. Back in the eighties I reached for books in my search for answers. I never got any—unless one thinks being told "take him to the doctor'" is an answer. If you have ever taken an autistic child to the doctor for help, you know how completely lacking in helpfulness that response really is. I wanted something beyond diagnosis followed by warnings that I should seek professional help and not do it myself. I remember looking at one doctor and saying, "'I did seek professional help. I'm here." He didn't seem to understand what I meant by that anymore than the "autism experts" knew what my son meant when he growled and spun in circles.

I wanted more than a Catch 22. I wanted the kind of answers that would make me a better mom by telling ME what to do for my autistic child to help him become more like a regular kid. I wanted permission to hope. I also wanted something more flexible and uniquely designed than the answers that came later in our journey, like those "do this or else" books on diet or homeopathy or vitamin therapy. I wanted the kind of concepts and understanding that would help me to help them myself. After all, even if others could assist in teaching and healing my children, their time with them was limited. I was the one who would be with my boys every single day, connected to them forever and ever, amen. I wanted to be treated with the respect that responsibility brings; these were my children and I was responsible for them. I wanted to be equipped with the information so I could add to their answers and find my own. When I was a child my teachers were often frustrated with me because I couldn't remember any facts unless I knew the reason why what I was trying to remember was considered a fact. This turned out to be a fortunate personality trait: The books didn't help me but my need to understand did. I found or rather "invented" the answers out of understanding the mindsets around me. It worked. However, if I had it to do over again, I'd like to have known more of what is available yet hidden away. I'd like to know more because I'd like it to not take so long. In case there are others like me, this chapter teaches the details in depth, with respect for your intelligence, and your role of parent expert in search of education.

To repeatedly make the kind of difference that is actually possible for the autistic child, we need a global paradigm shift of believing that parents are the people to teach. Thus I hope to help us embrace the widespread use of home training for autism.

The secret to life: DON'T RESIST; CHOOSE!

(Oh dear, I've already told you the secret. Lousy marketing on my part, especially since you could be standing in the bookstore perusing the introduction and now you think you've no need to buy this book. However, even though I just told you the secret, you may still need my help to understand it fully.)

Many people resist experiencing the very happiness they seek. The problem with feeling better for these folks is that very often they view happiness as a delusion; and so they fear being happy, lest they be deluded into believing it is so. I meet many clients caught in this circle of self-infliction. Obsessive behavior is a good example of that. I treat the compulsiveness and obsessive thinking. When I leave their home they feel clear, happy, healed. Then something (like the very fact that they are suspicious of feeling good) or someone (who believes in preparing them for the worst) brings to mind the idea that happiness is scary. Thus my clients find themselves asking, "What if something bad is happening and I am too busy being happy to see it?" Then in order to be vigilant they stop themselves from feeling good and attend to the conundrum. They bring to mind anything that might possibly be going wrong for themselves, their loved ones, the world, their pets, their property, etc. Now they have plenty to think about. And so they have opened the door to misery and drunk its poison. Sometimes even caretakers, teachers, and entertainers do this for the children they are trying to help: they point out the pitfalls instead of the prize.

Resisting happiness in order to ensure that your happiness is both authentic and well protected just creates stress and prevents the health and happiness you are trying to attain. These next two chapters weave that truth together and help you understand how to move forward and away from such a cycle. It is here that I explain how the two approaches of behavior responding techniques and neurofeedback work together in order to achieve whatever long-lasting results you are seeking to create. Hopefully the long-lasting results you are seeking to create include health and happiness.

The science of shaping minds began the minute that man met woman and they started raising children. It cannot be dated, though it can be assumed, that in one form or another it has always been in evidence: brainwashing, preaching, parenting, teaching, grooming, enlisting, coaching, convincing, persuasion, coercion, etc. Each of these is both potentially poisonous and life enriching. The poison is not in the words or the techniques employed so much as the reason behind the stories told. Life is full of choices. When we overly examine in search of absolute knowing, we run the risk of senility arriving before we are ready to act. I suggest trusting yourself, seek to know, and then choose. Take a breath and a minute to examine why you did what you did, and then if the answer feels right, continue on down the road. Do the same when others give you advice: examine why they said it. If it was to brainwash you into being on their team, make sure it's a team you want to be on. If it is to slow you down in order to get ahead of you in the race, make sure it is a race you want to run… and then lose. Some people who come to therapy in order to feel better, then go back home and re-infect themselves with whatever was wrong before they went to therapy, do it for reasons other than fear of happiness. Some people do it because they want to go back to therapy and repeat the cycle. Because the emotion they want to feel is dependent upon the misery, because the emotion they want to feel is relief. Some parents and professionals engage in a similar co-dependence with the autistic child. Because if he/she gets all the way better, then they themselves would have to find a new calling. Poor environment, doubt, therapy jumping, self pity, over researching, waiting until it's perfect, diet flipping, and more can all be like taking an antidote and then drinking the poison, taking an antidote and then drinking the poison, taking an antidote and then drinking the poison… We choose how we spend our lives, going back and forth and getting nowhere or learning through resources like this book in order to succeed, and going for it.

It's easier to heal your child into feeling something new when you learn to feel something new too. Therefore…

Don't resist; choose: joy, pride, love, motivation, acceptance, commitment and daily fulfillment. Then…

KICK the habit of "I don't want to do it."

Of all the avoidance techniques I employed, "wishing someone else would do the work and save my child" was the most debilitating. And here we are, at the gift the last chapter brings: I finally figured out what it was about my parenting techniques that was different from so many of the families I meet who are still sinking in the struggle. Finally I was able to put all the learning together and understand what it was that worked even before the inclusion of neurofeedback into my home. Amazingly enough, what I came to realize is that ultimately my children were helped the most by me, Lynette, the mom who "let them learn through natural consequences." I followed these bumps and bruises, wins and losses, with explanations, approval, and guidance." As I said earlier this was my parenting style, possibly because there were too many kids to stay on top of anyway. And as it turned out we were fortunate that I parented in this way because with the imagination challenges of autism, experiential learning is the most learnable kind of lesson for the autistic mind. And since the lessons of natural consequences are born in the experience of the present moment, which is accompanied by emotion, by making the experience and its pursuant lessons more memorable, the learning becomes easier to generalize. Instead of overprotecting my children I let them learn. At first I tried to find teachers and social agencies to help me help my children, but then we argued my style over theirs, my belief that the kids could learn safety rules over their belief that they could not. The arguing stopped the learning and "in the end nothing worked until I rolled up my sleeves and did it myself." Then since I was the one doing the teaching, I was the one in control of the environment my children found themselves immersed in, which meant I could give them consistent feedback that was congruent with their experiences and my beliefs. Thus I learned how important feedback is and that's why I was able to recognize the potential value of neurofeedback the minute I read about it. That was the last step: I learned how to speed the process by adding machines that could speak to my children's neurons while I spoke to their brains.

I did it myself, with the help of others who were willing to see me as the expert in my child's development, and so can you.

After the last chapter is a summary. The summary summarizes. (wink) This book covers so much about autism from so many vantage points that I felt the need to pull it all together and consolidate the points (at the beginning in this introduction and at the end in the summary). Since so much of the book contains the stories from my life and many of those stories have me standing in opposition to the experts of the time, I wanted to ensure that I closed on a very necessary point. This book is not meant to fuel the war between therapies but to bring parents and professionals together to cease the crossfire that kills the children's hopes for mental health. Its intention is to inform and equip you, the parent or professional, with techniques and brain information.

This book's intention is to bring respect and value to the role of "parent of a special needs child." Because when parents become the educated expert for their children, the children then hold the greatest likelihood of reaching their potential for success.

Section Two is the resource section. It is there to help you with things like diagnostic criteria, available therapies, causal theories, and as such is self explanatory by chapter title. Good Luck and Good Reading.

Teachers, Helpers, and Angels

I would like to express admiration and intense appreciation to the Chief Science Officer of EEG Spectrum International, Inc.: Harold L. Burke PhD. Dr. Burke took time from his busy schedule as Director/Founder of The Brain Therapy Center and Advisor to the Foundation for Neurofeedback and Applied Neuroscience to ever so carefully examine the pages of this book. Having such an amazing mind to help me ensure that I found clear methods with which to explain the science behind the success and/or failure of various therapies was a great gift and I am indebted to his friendship. The book you will read is of more value because of his input. I would also like to express my indebtedness and deep abiding respect for friend and colleague Psychiatrist Rebecca M. White Argo, MD, for making my career as an in-home specialist possible. It is because of her trust and association in business that I have been able to help so many people and will help so many more. She is truly my angel.

I am eternally grateful to Brent Leach, my previously mentioned first husband and forever friend. Often having Brent back in my life turned out to be lucky for me. For example, he went through this text in less than forty-eight hours because I wanted to get it into the hands of potential agents and publishers sooner rather than later. Brent did this despite the fact that it was Obama's historical election night and despite the fact that he wanted very much to be glued to the tube watching that history unfold. Brent chose instead to stay with the project of this book and help me unfold, or rather refold, the history of autism into one blessed with a more useful perspective than was generally embraced. It makes sense that he should assist me in this way given that we have both been blessed by refolding our own history in order to see through the more useful eyes of love, acceptance, and healing. Still, impacting on the world is my personal life path—not his. I was surprised and amazed at Brent's dedication to helping me help you. And now as I watch his life slip away, I can only hope he is happy to have walked my path with me. I will forever live in gratitude for his having been willing to push aside his own preoccupations and pay attention to the things I personally deem as important. I'm sure his willingness to miss the vote counting had nothing to do with the fact that we didn't have a T.V. (wink wink nudge nudge)

SECTION ONE

BY, FOR, AND BECAUSE OF MY CHILDREN, I CAME TO UNDERSTAND THAT EXPERIENCE ONLY TEACHES THE ONE WHO LEARNS

The road to wisdom?
Well, it's plain and simple to express:
Err
and err
and err again
but less
and less
and less.

—Piet Hein
"The Road to Wisdom," *Grooks,* 1966

CHAPTER ONE

Sharing the Magic

I began this journey in 1983 when I met my oldest soon-to-be son, a three- year-old boy with autism named Dar. He came to me as a child who was slated for an institution but whose bed wouldn't be ready for another two months. Originally he was diagnosed as blind, deaf, and mentally retarded. He arrived malnourished. On occasion we nicknamed him "Stop and Go" because with Dar there was no transitional state between the two. Visually, he was interesting to watch. His body would twist into an upward-looking pretzel whenever he ran—always in circles—dragging his right leg behind him and keeping people at bay by growling in their general direction. If stopped, he would flip his upper body over and become a downward-facing question mark flicking his fingers near his eyes. He was non-verbal with the only thing coming out of his mouth being drool and projectile vomit. In my eyes, he was adorable, though smelly.

The life story that came with Dar was delivered via the gossip chain of social workers and as such cannot be verified. However, I was told that Dar's mom had kept him confined to a small walk-in closet for three out of his now four years. Due to these extenuating circumstances, no one really knew which of his behaviors were psychologically driven and which were based in the reality of his physiology. And since very little was known at that time about the neurological workings of the brain, there was little to do except sit and wait. I was often told that if his condition was psychological, then it would mean he was a feral (wild) child, which would then also mean he'd get better with loving care. But if his condition turned out to be physiological, then there was nothing to do but teach him a few skills like eating with a spoon.

One could assume they said this because the field of mental health at that time did not know the degree to which psychology creates physiology and vice versa. However, there was an incongruence of beliefs afoot like a nonsensical loop that when fed into a computer might crash a hard drive. That circular thinking came in the form of conflicting ideologies. I say this because while I was being taught that the neglected feral child would heal and change once given affection and direction, I was also being taught that an autistic child wouldn't. I was told this even though the predominant belief at the time was that autistic children were created via the psychological damage inflicted by the cold aloofness of the child's unaffectionate mother. In both cases the causal belief was that a lack of exposure to proper love and role modeling had damaged the child. So why the different prognoses? Absolutely no one I asked seemed prepared to answer this question. I believe the myopia of the time was due to a collective desire to construct theories that not only gave answers but also pointed fingers at some easy, downtrodden target—someone for society to blame (which women at the time were). The incongruence came from the simultaneous need to excuse the practitioners any time the child they were helping refused to heal. Thus, children that got better got a different diagnosis.

Dar improved, even learned to use the toilet, but none of his new skills were remarkable enough in the eyes of the psychiatrist to warrant calling him a wild child that was going to normalize. So he was diagnosed as on the spectrum of autism even before they called it a spectrum.

Dar was labeled PDD (Pervasive Developmental Disorder). At four years of age, Dar's IQ was placed at a nine-month-old level leaving him in the extremely retarded range. I began to read about autism at the same time that I applied to adopt him.

Most of the material at that time said that autism was caused by rejection, and Dar certainly fit this criterion. Apparently Dar's behavior was his birth mother's fault. Since I believed the experts and wanted more than anything to keep Dar away from her, I believed the experts even while noticing the incongruence between saying that rejected kids who get feral labels get better fast but rejected kids who get autism labels stay disabled for life.

I began to be more questioning of the so-called "experts" after my first real awakening in regard to the effectiveness (or non-effectiveness) of the system protecting our children happened. It occurred almost immediately. Social services called to say that the judge had insisted Dar have a series of visits with his natural mother before he removed custody from her and gave it to me. I thought this was a bad idea. Since Dar's understanding was so hard to read, I was terrified that he would feel betrayed having one mom hand him off to another. I was afraid he would regress and lose his newly acquired toileting skills. I was afraid he would become distrusting and lose all belief in me just when we were beginning to bond. I was afraid he would stop seeking me out and lose that brand new desire to look in my eyes, as long as I wore sunglasses. So I refused to deliver him to them. Not to be diverted from their mandated goal, a social worker was sent to pick him up. I watched the car roll down the driveway with Dar in a car seat situated behind yet another stranger. He was growling and drooling and rocking his head. Five hours later she brought him back.

Dar—again in the car seat—sat motionless, in a state of catatonia: dry mouthed, barely breathing, and never blinking. I touched his unmoving body and was surprised not to see him recoil. "What did you do to him?" I asked. Even though her perception of Dar was that he was just having a calm moment—sixty-minutes long—she trembled recounting her day. She told me that he had been rocking and looking at his fingers until she turned the corner onto his street. Then all of a sudden he started screaming "NO! NO! GO! CAR! RUN! WAY!", undid his seat belt, and tried to climb out of the window. She said she had never seen his hands work that well, and neither had she nor anyone at the office even known he could talk. She was shaking as she spoke. She extended her hand to show me. "He kept trying to get away from me and I literally had to drag him kicking and screaming up to his house. He kept saying it over and over again 'NO! NO! GO! CAR! RUN! WAY!' His mom acted like she didn't even want him there. It was awful. We have to get him away from her! When I picked him up an hour later he was like this, completely vacant, laying under the coffee table while his mom played cards with her friend." The social worker told me the story and drove away. I had no idea what to do. So I curled Dar up in bed with me and cried myself to sleep. Six hours later he came out of his stupor and using a wooden toy carpenter's bench beat his face black and blue before I could stop him. When I phoned the social worker's supervisor to tell her about the incident she said, "Oh, that's too bad."

Dar never said any of those words that clearly ever again!

While he has made great leaps on many fronts, even today his fine motor skills are still so poor that his pronunciation is difficult to comprehend. At present one must focus on Dar to understand him. Back then, on that day, he was the one who focused, in order to be understood.

That incident was the beginning of what would become my path, singular in nature, often diverting away from the advice of the professionals I would find along the way. Very quickly I began to see a huge disparity between what Dar would be capable of with me and what he was capable of with others. Some professionals applauded me, saying that Dar was better off with me than he would be with them because they couldn't get him to do anything. Others resented me and claimed Dar's successes were due to a symbiotic relationship. They said that I should send him away to a training center.

About a year after officially adopting Dar, the apparently helpful behavior of these social service agencies confused me yet again. An admissions diagnostician and social worker came to see me at home. We lived in Toronto at the time. After observing Dar for at least ten minutes, the "expert" shook his head and told me that Dar couldn't do anything and that he was one of the most disabled kids he'd ever seen. He insisted I put Dar in a program immediately stating that Dar had absolutely no social skills! I was hurt and insulted by the vehemence in the man's voice, especially given that I'd thought Dar was performing beautifully. (He turned his head at an upward angle when I called his name.) "What kind of program?" I asked holding back the tears. He told me that his agency's program would be perfect and assured me that Dar would learn to comply. "Great!" I blurted, "When can he start?" This admissions social worker told me that Dar could not start, ever. He said that there was a year-long waiting list and that once Dar waited a year he'd be too old. He said they didn't take any kids after five because they were too hard to help. He sat, comfortable in the pregnant pause, then turned and looked deep into my eyes. With a Nostradamus finger of indecipherable foreboding he warned that I'd better find something. I was fighting back the tears at this point and barely able to speak through the enormous lump in my throat. "Well, what would you do with him if he was in your program?" The man seemed shocked by my audacity. He refused to tell me indicating that he feared I might try the techniques myself.

And all I could think was, "Yeah! Of course I would."

I was to discover this secretive silliness (like being disallowed from observing and/or helping teachers) time and time again on a regular basis during my son's early years. These stories are only the tip on that icy berg. One reason "the specialists" didn't want to be observed was because they didn't have any answers. They were making it up as they went along just as much as I was because there was little understanding of brain function back then. In fact, most of what we know has been learned in the past fifteen years. The other part was shame and fear (that they might see themselves through my eyes). Because if I did what some of the schools at the time did, it would be considered abuse.

It was common practice at the time for behaviorists to pinch and scream "NO!" whenever the autistic child acted autistic. They tried to eradicate the autism by slapping faces and hands. They would time the children out by placing them in cubicles that made Dar's walk-in closet seem like the Taj Mahal. They zapped them with cattle prods, used straight jackets, and sprayed ammonia jets in the children's faces. They worked very hard to redesign the cover while ignoring the moral of these sweet little life stories. And like the desire to keep from being observed, these punitive control techniques that I have shared with you are merely some examples also from the tip of the icy berg.

So, the method of the day for healing autism back when I began this journey was called Aversion Therapy. (Funny how many of us are willing to try a thing simply because it has been labeled a therapy.) And, like a good student, I tried it too. For Dar it meant I squeezed his shoulder often leaving pinch marks whenever he "pretended" he couldn't tell a fork from a spoon. (I put pretended in quotes because he wasn't pretending. I just thought he was.) The Aversion-Therapy-Concept kind of made sense when you thought about it—as long as you didn't think about it too long. The theory was that no one would choose to pick up a spoon instead of a fork or flick their fingers in front of their eyes if they knew it was going to bring pain. Turns out that that theory is incorrect and that Aversion Therapy doesn't work. Dar still chose the behaviors. And I was EXTREMELY FRUSTRATED WITH HIM! Thus, when I tried aversion I simply found myself averted from loving my son or seeing the possibilities in who he might become.

The theory prevalent at the time implied that if we could get the children to stop using their weird behaviors, they would become normal. I'm embarrassed to admit it was a theory I bought into it even when no one was selling. For example, during Dar's first year as my son, I took him to several diagnosticians. One of them asked me repeatedly whether or not Dar could alternate his feet on the stairs. I said, "Of course." And since Dar's fear of falling prevented him from climbing the fake set of stairs with no handrails or walls to cling to that the diagnostician was presenting him with, I was nestled safe within my lie. The truth was I had no idea. I'd never really looked. When I got home I watched Dar. He dragged his right leg up behind the left, step after step after step. Lo and behold he could not alternate feet. Eureka! I had found the cure for autism. I decided to teach him to exchange feet while ascending, because certainly that would make him normal. Again, as embarrassing as it is, I must admit for a time I actually believed that to be true. Educating his stair-climbing feet didn't change the quality of Dar's life much. He still couldn't talk. Or read or follow simple directives. He did, however, look a lot better whenever the escalator broke down at the mall.

Interestingly it only took Dar six months to learn this new climbing technique. Back then, though, that seemed like a long time because I was worrying over teaching each skill one after another. I wished he were able to multitask and learn a variety of things simultaneously. Fortunately for both of us, I eventually thought about it in a different light. And that's when I came to realize that in many ways Dar was actually smarter than I was. For example, Dar had had the ability to grasp a new way to walk in the world. This was quite impressive and had taken less time for him than it had taken for me to learn my own very similar lesson: I came to understand that if I were going to teach anything to myself and/or my son, I too would have to find a new way to walk. For me this meant changing the way I looked at things. Dar had had to learn to alternate feet whereas I had to learn to alternate my eyes, from seeing only his awkward gait and autistic brain every time I looked at him, to seeing how he jumped for joy whenever he caught sight of me or heard his favorite music or touched the lawnmower.

Slowly, I came to see him as a whole person, who just happened to have dirty blond hair, a flat butt, and autism.

Since then I've gained tankers full of experience. What I now believe happens when we try to expunge the behaviors we don't like in a person, any person, is that the undesirable behavior either pops up in a new undesirable form, grows bigger (especially in our absence), or we succeed and end up expunging the entire personality. Thus it is possible to un-create a child and make them like Dar was when he came home from his other mother's that "NO! NO! GO! CAR! RUN! WAY!" day. In using such techniques we risk ending up with children who are gone.

For those reasons I didn't like Aversion Therapy. So, I tried Holding Therapy (another reputed choice of the time). But no matter how much I hugged and held and loved and sang to him, Dar was still autistic. He was still void of language, still avoiding my eyes, and still fascinated by his fingers.

Every speech therapist and psychologist I told the "NO! NO! GO! CAR! RUN! WAY!" story to labeled his words a coincidence or a lie or a hallucination of approximations experienced by the stressed-out social worker. After a while, it occurred to me that these answers were probably derived from their desire to not have to explain what they didn't understand. Before that, though, I accepted the explanation. After all, I hadn't actually been there. Perhaps it was a lie, I hoped. That would mean it never really happened, this story of his panic being ignored and of him being seen as too unimportant to respond to. But then that would also mean he just beat himself that day because he had a yen to do so. Perhaps it was the truth, I prayed, because I didn't want to think of him as mindlessly self-abusive. Then it happened. I was there. Dar's new sister (my third-born biological child) grabbed his crayons and offered to color a page for him. He grabbed them back and, as I walked by, he said, "I can do it" with perfect enunciation. Dar immediately reverted to looking at the ceiling while rocking his head side to side. The therapists and teachers didn't believe that story either. But I did, because I was there.

The more I diverged from listening to others and trusting what I knew to be true, the more I was able to embrace my son. The more I embraced him, the more I observed him. The more I observed him, the easier it was to understand him. The easier it was to understand him, the easier it was to understand his brain. Those lightening-quick occasions of never-to be-repeated, perfectly enunciated and absolutely appropriate spontaneous words were not lies; they were clues to the mystery that is autism.

I noticed how rare they were and that they only happened if he perceived himself as under attack. "OK," I thought, "so he's in an emergency state and non-self-conscious when he speaks. Maybe that's the secret." Tempting as it was to follow that logic and try keeping him in an emergency state in order to gain language, I knew better (besides I didn't want to live the life of being the person who keeps her son in an emergency state). I was positive that hurting, threatening, or scaring Dar on purpose simply as a technique to teach language wouldn't likely work because it sounded a lot like Aversion Therapy. After all, getting a fork instead of a spoon was the one thing Dar hadn't learned. Love, support, cheers, consistency, repetition, and patience were the only tools that ever paid off. That's why he was toilet trained in less than a week; I was sure of it.

In fact, fear, I suspect, would have made Dar more acutely aware of needing to succeed, and that would be counter productive because it would have added pressure to learning and kept him in a state of low-grade anxiety. This low-grade anxiety would have made the emergency state less "different" from his every other moment, and lessening the relative intensity would therefore make it less and less likely that miracles would be popped out of his mouth. In addition, constant low-grade anxiety eradicates the option for internal calm thus increasing the inability to think. I say this as if it is a fact because I know from experience that it is. Fear freezes. It removes activity from the frontal lobes and drops a brain into limbic-driven reacting. That's why when I'm afraid I cannot think. Thus I am convinced that the real key to anyone's success is being non-self-conscious when attempting to problem solve issues that are driven by one's own desire to do so.

Though I didn't know why back then, it turns out there is some good scientific reasoning in support of my theory. For example, we now know that keeping a person in a state of fear releases copious amounts of cortisol—aka stress hormone—into the system, effectively killing neurons in the hippocampus and irrevocably damaging memory. To say the least, that is not very conducive to skill acquisition. We also know that the effects of adrenaline being released over and over again are internally addictive. This means that we become addicted to our problems and move toward instead of away from things we fear. This effectively ties us to the perceived dangers everyone else wants us to overcome and increases the damage to our memory system.

Adrenaline (flight or fight response) also has a body-wide effect and causes changes to the heart, the stomach, and the genitals. Adrenaline literally flips switches, changing the places in our brain and body that are oxygenated and turned on. And there's more, like the depletion of adrenal glands or the over-activation of the amygdala which is harmful to the sensory system and can cause startle responses that send inaccurate messages about potential danger when they come upon you without warning, etc. Over the course of becoming a trained professional, I learned all that and Whew! I sure am glad that I dropped aversion therapy from my toolbox. (Nice to be right even if for the wrong reasons. That happens in science all the time.)

Back when my theories first began to take shape, I (figuratively) donned a Sherlock Holmes hat and started paying attention. I watched not only what I said around Dar but also how I said it, when I said it, and why I said it. Then I attended to his reaction. I took my recent discovery of his ability to talk at a level beyond my previous expectations as an indication that his ability to understand might also be at a level beyond my previous expectations, or even beyond my previous ability to hope. I decided to believe in his receptive language and assume he understood even when he didn't seem to be listening. I shared my viewpoint with teachers and practitioners. And right away, at the very beginning of the journey, as I spent my first moments with speech therapists, occupational therapists, and diagnosticians, I began to get a glimmer of what lay ahead. It was a path I resisted. I didn't want every aspect of Dar's learning to be up to me. I just wanted to be his mom. However, as I was quick to discover, having every aspect be up to *me* is what it is to be the mom of a special-needs child.

The thing is, a parent or primary caregiver is always irreplaceable. But with mentally challenged children that becomes tangibly true. Since the child may not be able to visualize a past event, teaching to an issue very often means responding at the time of the occurrence. I was the one available in those moments of rarified speaking. So, I was the one who knew he could, and I was the one on whose shoulders the teaching fell. But I felt ill equipped for the job. I believed I would be handicapped as his teacher because I was uninformed. Obviously the speech therapist knew more than I did about speech in general. But then I realized that she was also uninformed, because I knew more about Dar's very unique style of silent speaking than she ever could.

This place of mutual need is why it has been my lifelong goal to help therapists and parents find a common ground of mutual respect and admiration. Such an environment truly is the only way to consistently get the job done, by sharing what we know and staying open to learning what we don't. Once I took on the role of Sherlock Holmes examining things without panic or judgment, Dar's sudden moments of verbal clarity and the constant focus on his wiggling finger didn't seem so mysterious. These things made sense. I found the answer because I didn't judge the answer as a problem: We were bombarding his system with noisy confusion. He was trying to keep things, like us, in his peripheries where we were non-threatening by focusing on his fingers and pushing us into the background. This way he could spontaneously be happy. Unfortunately, it also prevented him from learning how to interact.

I tried to explain this concept to his teachers. They said they were convinced I had misunderstood Dar's behavior. Other than to say he did it because he was autistic, they had no replacement theories of their own. They insisted that autism is just autism and that there was no point in trying to understand it. Our job, I was told, was to control his behaviors and accept his limitations. As proof, they pointed out that my ideas were incongruent with the fact that Dar liked to lean into their shoulders and bury his face in their necks all the while keeping his hands and chest away. They saw this behavior as a sign of affection and insisted that Dar was not trying to keep them in his peripheries. I saw it as a way of hiding his eyes from theirs and keeping them away from making contact. I observed the moments when Dar would do this with them or with me and noticed that it tended to happen when he was being asked for something. It seemed to me that while we were trying to control him into behaving, he was trying to control us into backing off.

Dar's actions reminded me of all the times in my teen years (and possibly beyond) when, feeling nervous about a boy, I would come in close for a kiss because I wanted to avoid eye contact and the possibility that he might see me as unworthy. I learned at a very young age that being in charge of an interaction with someone allowed me to hide inside his or her need to "deal with my behavior." Like Dar, I too had a way of wall flowering to keep folks in my peripheries or taking the limelight to keep them at bay. I believed that Dar and I were enough the same for me to understand what he was doing. I assured his teachers that these seemingly opposite behaviors were two halves of the same whole. Whether you push the people away or bring them in close, you are still seeking a way to control their ability to see you. Thus, whenever they forced Dar to give them eye contact, he would disappear before them and himself by coming in too close to be looked at.

I believed understanding Dar was the key to figuring out how to teach him. But either I wasn't any good at explaining it or they just didn't understand the concept of hiding in a crowd as intrinsically as I did, because every one of them just looked at me and walked away. Maybe that's because they weren't like the part of me that was so like Dar. After all, I was also trying to find ways to avoid eye contact and social situations, also using focus shifting to avoid interacting with the people around me, also bothered by depth perception issues and pixilated vision. I understood him—just a little bit more—because of the parts of me that were the same.

That's when I became first the person, then the parent, and then the clinician who followed the clues and applied the solutions that matched the need to herself, her children, and her clients. That's when I decided to figure this disorder out, change the course of my own children's lives, and share the magic with whoever else wished to know what I had learned.

Chapter Two

Neurofeedback to the Rescue

or How to Heal a Family

The father of a young autistic boy named DW was driving me to the airport. Neurofeedback (biofeedback for the brain) was not why they had hired me, but neurofeedback was what I wanted to give them.

It was late summer 2006. I had begun working professionally with this family as a result of my Son-Rise® play therapy training. (Son-Rise® was founded by parents who—back in the seventies—worked with their autistic son until he was no longer challenged enough to be considered autistic. This was an amazing feat at the time and was the reason behind creating a teaching center for people working with autism.). The family I was working with wanted to be able to tell a similar "saved their son" story. They wanted a new way to teach because they were burnt out from listening to their son scream as he resisted being taught by their ABA (Applied Behavior Analysis) therapists. They had decided to give Son-Rise® a try. Uncertain whether this was the right approach for them, DW's father arbitrarily allocated a six-month trial period within which to assess the decision. The six months were up. DW had changed a little but he was still very challenged in the usual areas of speech, social skills, and repetitive play. I had managed to convince them to try neurofeedback on two separate occasions, but the mom and dad had been so nervous about "messing with their baby's brain" that whenever I tried using it on their son, DW picked up on their nervousness as they oversaw the procedure. DW resisted having the wires on his head. I let it go, for now.

DW's dad spent our half-hour drive to the airport sharing his disappointment over their Son-Rise® Program and his son's lack of progress. He coughed a little as we pulled up to the terminal and whispered, "I just wanted the miracle." I touched his hand, "I know, but you wanted it too quickly." I checked my purse for ID. "The truth is *Miracles Are Made* out of sweat and hard work. When you approach them with the need for time-lapse photography, you make the miracle into a lie," I told him, adding, "You read a story that an editor edited in order to fit it into a book. The truth, however, took thousands of hours more to live out than it did to read. That family's story spanned years. You gave it six months."

Amidst the action of pulling out bags and tipping baggage handlers I reiterated, "Miracles happen when you make the impossible possible and are, usually, the result of good old-fashioned hard work. Those parents just taught their child, over and over again. Most miracle stories are like that. At some point somebody did the work. Unfortunately, the minute they decided to try and inspire people by telling them about it, they had to leave out the repetitious details. That's why you feel disillusioned, because it's the details that you're trying to avoid. And it's the details that make the difference. The fact is your son is doing better. He's talking a bit and playing with me more, and I haven't even worked with him much. I've only seen him three times in six months. If I tell that story to a family whose son isn't getting any better, it sounds like a miracle. Look, if you want him to gain skills faster than that and still work with him at the same rate, use the neurofeedback… that's your quicken-the-pace microwave miracle maker." I hugged him, felt for him, promised to always be available, and ran into the terminal to catch my plane home.

Fortunately for DW neurofeedback made its way into his home despite his family's aversion to training their son's brain. The mom had been on meds for years to help her depression, so even though she didn't plan to use the neurofeedback on DW, she did want to use it on herself. She had purchased the home equipment and I was to be overseeing her application and progress via Internet and telephone. I hugged DW's dad goodbye, hoping for another chance to help their totally adorable child.

Six months later they invited me back. While working with her son using a different play approach called Floortime, she had continued to use the neurofeedback on herself, according to my protocol advice, and had cured her anxiety disorder. She was a believer. Her husband was amazed. And I was happy. I winked at the dad and said, "Told you this was your miracle." It was time to do the same for their son. So we talked about the mom creating a combined play approach using bits and pieces of all the therapies she had studied. I encouraged her to trust herself as the primary expert in her son's journey and to trust me as the neurofeedback/play professional that would guide her expertise. Since the mom was now comfortable with neurofeedback the son was comfortable too. And so we began. I say "we" but in truth once I get the family started I am just a guide—the families do the work that I've already done.

As a mother I raised eight children. They came to me through a variety of ways. I birthed two (I actually gave birth to three children but my boy child died in the same moment that he was born), adopted four, and took custody of a couple more. The four that I adopted were on the spectrum of autism. Much like DW's parents I tried many things while attempting to heal my children's brains. For the most part—and until neurofeedback—only constant vigilance as a parent worked in any notable way. While I had managed to teach three of them what they would need to make it on their own in the "world of normal," two still didn't have sufficient enough control of their temper to not be arrested. And one, my darling Dar, had barely changed at all. Thus, I was still looking for answers.

I had already tried utilizing different therapies and nutritional approaches, but they had made little difference, maybe because they were half-baked ideas based on my half-baked understanding of them and the disorder in the children I was trying to heal. After all, I, and the rest of the world, were just learning about autism. So though it felt at the time like I was trying everything there was to try, compared to the parents of today, I tried very little because back then, there was so little to try. There were no Asperger's advertisements shouting out promises in parent magazines, no diets for autism, no care clinics with cures, no inoculation/chelation theories, or hyperbaric for hyperlexia. There was just fumbling your way to a professional who was willing to diagnose, ineffectively drug, and forcefully teach. And, even so, despite all this lack of knowledge and despite all this ineptitude, my kids had improved.

Why?

As is true for many parents today, my distaste for the mainstream methods of the time led me to the alternative choices of the future based on the holistic thinking of the past. I found muscle testing, hair analysis, cranial sacral, blue green algae, garlic cleansing, focus factor, auditory training, vision therapy, and light therapy, to name a few. And still I reiterate that, compared to the parents of today, I barely scratched the surface on the overwhelming vocation of medical investigation into which raising a child with autism indoctrinates families. In contrast to a world wherein one tried to take existing therapies and apply them to their child's disability, as of this writing, parents now have over four hundred therapies geared for autism to choose from. That's a mind-blowing number of choices. Especially since most of these therapies come with their own associated professionals, many who present themselves as more knowledgeable than the rest. Most problematic of all is when said professionals portend to be more knowledgeable than the parents, even when they are not. Such an ego soup of psyches served to the often desperate, often humble pie of parents creates great potential for guilt and fear whenever mom or dad chooses to step away from the table and leave untouched any portion of the possibilities offered. For parents, sometimes it is just easier to choose nothing than to jump into this no-win situation wherein duty deems the need to try everything even as logic says that biting into everything means finishing nothing and helping not at all. When I look at the history of things, I come to see that perhaps my children and I were advantaged by the lack of possibilities: it made the doing easier. On the other hand that advantage was offset by the challenge of searching beyond the childrearing ideas left over from my own inapplicable childhood because back then we couldn't just Google for ideas; we had to create them. Perhaps that's part of the reason for why they improved: I had the freedom to create answers.

I searched the libraries and I observed my sons. I was intent on combining all that knowledge to invent change in the form of improvement. I noticed that Dar seemed less intelligent when he drank milk. I read books about different cultural diets and found that people who were macrobiotic didn't use dairy products. I read that enormous Macrobiotic bible in three days. I educated myself on the concept of medicinal eating using weird foods I'd never heard of. I learned the approach of looking to the east for answers and recreated our table. I was excited to be doing something proactive. Of course, it was hard to get the kids to embrace fermented foods and seaweed salads, but I was determined to make it work. The older ones were told by their counselors that I was putting their health at risk by feeding them sushi instead of sandwiches, and my determination was fueled by fury. I had not expected the world around me to react so viscerally against my choice to change my family's dietary approach to wellness.

Before I knew what happened I found myself fighting everyone. My mother was particularly offended. I listened to her huff and puff about the insult implied in my not believing that the way she fed her children was a good enough way to feed mine. She snuck my delighted darlings boxed foods loaded with dried dairy and preservatives. It was the only time my then husband ever joined forces with her. They side by side yelled at me. He screamed at me for taking any initiative that included eggplant or daikon, quitting cigarettes, or banning beer. He spent years attributing this assertive change in me for the reason that he ended our marriage.

Remarkably I still see this struggle in homes today. Food, it seems, is a very personally held thing. I watch parents debate and argue while sharing reams of anecdotal proof with each other because every dietary approach has reams of anecdotal proof. I watch and try to ease the struggle as the fighting unfolds. I tell them my story explains that food matters but that it wasn't the defining difference in my children's journey into being mentally healthier. Generally speaking, their ears perk up and the fighting stops.

For me, though the diets and supplements did (and still do) help us feel stronger, they didn't "cure" anyone. They did, however, add a constantly applied awe-inspiring drain on my finances. That inescapable pressure of "one has to eat THIS in order to heal" is just another reason why I see neurofeedback as our hero to the rescue. Because I never had the money to afford anything—though I always seemed to find it anyway. If it was going to be this hard I wanted to find something—regardless of cost—that showed enough promise for me to believe that the burden would someday ease. I wanted whatever

I found to work well enough to change the picture. Neurofeedback did. It helped my sleepless child sleep, my mute child talk, my slow-minded retarded ones think quicker, and my twitching, stuttering, violent nineteen-year-old relax. He grew enough to come off the spectrum in two years. It did all that and more. True neurofeedback was expensive at first, but unlike restocking a kitchen to implement dietary changes, neurofeedback was only expensive at first. With food and supplements as the primary biological healing tool, the cost was always rising because the perceived changes in my family were too minor to keep me hoping for a happy ending, thus I remained open to every new and improved infomercial pitch or vitamin-pill-popping promise. Conversely, with neurofeedback the cost didn't grow; it shrank. And VOILA! The burden eased.

The fascinating thing here is that while treating myself with neurofeedback, financial burden didn't manifest as financial stress anyway. This is because I was balanced enough to stop worrying about bills, which meant I could think clearly enough to figure it all out and actually pay them. So, although this therapy required that I spend more money, it turned out OK because ironically, I had more money to spend.

I know it seems as if I am saying neurofeedback is the perfect panacea that heals everything from finances to depression, but that is because brain disorders always present as clusters of symptoms rather than just one singular problem. For example, a child with autism may have sleep issues, depression, or sensory-seeking behavior that is only satisfied by great big deep pressure hugs and tics, while another with the same disorder may have outbursts, periods of despondency, contact avoidance, seizures, and self-abusive behavior. Thus it is true to say that "autism" is a group of symptoms rather than a particular thing. And that these symptoms, these clusters, are connected and reinforced by each other so as you heal one you affect the others: While you heal the autism you smooth out all the behaviors created by the sub-disorders contained within it. I have observed this chaotic clustering to be true with every disorder I've treated. Therefore, it is logical that any brain reparative approach should be able to heal many problems. Since neurofeedback is flexible enough to be applied to any type of brain dysregulation, my children's brains and mine weren't the only thing that improved; our lives did too.

In fact, as a result of neurofeedback our lives still improve, daily. This is because there is no point at which you have gotten all you can get from this therapy (many famous musicians and athletes use it for peak performance work). The ability to be constantly assisting in the evolution of a person's skill sets is one of the reasons I view neurofeedback as the most effective all-around therapy for autism, regardless of the individual's place on the spectrum. How freeing to have access to something that will help everyone in the family get more out of life no matter what they are getting out of life now. Neurofeedback is the only therapy I know of where I would feel comfortable claiming such a thing to be true.

And yet, even though I credit neurofeedback with doing amazing things for my family and for everyone I work with, it is not as if you need a neurofeedback system to give feedback to your children's brains. That's what you do every time you express praise or disappointment. Feedback itself is built into our very reality. Things like temperature, digestive comfort, and fabric texture are all forms of feedback. This cohesive, constant inputting to the brain via every one of our working senses is what binds all the therapies together and makes logical the fact that so many different approaches can help to heal the brains of so many different people. Neurofeedback uses technology to shorten the time span between action and information/feedback, effectively speeding up the rate of change. We live in a time of toxins and technology. Hopefully technology can improve healing enough to offset the illnesses we are creating with our toxins. But whether it does or it doesn't, we are not without resources; we are not empty handed in the face of our children's challenges.

Before computers increased speed of access, virtually everywhere in our society we still taught children. We may have been less effective and over strict with parents and teachers yelling at the child and enabling their future therapists the option of comforting and nurturing them as adults, but however we did it, we did it via feedback. Theoretically, at times, our societally held belief has been that with the right kind of family feedback anyone can feel good about themselves; this is, of course, not true. That theory ignores the reality that when things are broken they very often hurt. And most people don't feel optimally good about themselves when they are in pain. Healing can happen, but simply being kind and encouraging to someone isn't always enough.

The rate of change needed to reach a goal is dependent upon the subject's starting point. When your children are autistic they seldom figure out how to fit into society on their own, and the more autistic they are the more challenging our way of thinking is for them to grasp.

Neurofeedback is fast but even without neurofeedback we can improve the efficiency of our feedback systems at home and in school: Give more compliments. It has been scientifically proven that people learn best when taught with a compliment/criticism ratio of four to one (four "wow nice jobs" to every "this part needs work"). That is one of the reasons I am proud to say that three of my four autistic children came off the spectrum, and most of them got mostly better even without neurofeedback. Hopefully their output was at least partly because of my input.

So if you can give feedback anyway, you ask, "Why the big push on neurofeedback?"

Because it's easier, faster, and you get farther.

Neurofeedback's role in my children's healing was great, even though by the time I heard of it, every one of my special-needs boys was a man. Then, as now, it is many times said that to help an autistic person you must apply the healing therapy when they are younger than five. The fact is that two of my four had already healed and were already independent. However, independent or not, they were still struggling to feel comfortable while fitting in. Of the remaining two, only one had language and a smattering of social skills. At this point in their development, all of my children had done most of their learning via the parental feedback loop of "Do this and don't do that." They had mostly grown better, all without the assistance of computer technology. Most of them had mostly grown abled. But one of the four hadn't seemed to learn a thing—at least nothing that he held onto. This fourth one, who I have already talked to you about, is Dar: my slow-moving miracle. Ever since that forced visit with his birth mother, Dar's changes towards self-sufficiency were so unbearably slow that—except for the occasional burst of brilliance—no progress was apparent, even by the age of twenty-three. He was neither understandable nor comfortable to be around because his toileting skills had again become a challenge and he was self-injurious. In short, Dar was a smelly, scary, mess of a man. That is, until neurofeedback. After that, we could actually watch him learn to calm himself and communicate.

The whole thing was happily surprising. Why had I been able to teach some of my children to perceivably change but not all? And what made neurofeedback strong enough to help even an adult? Why was it not limited to the under five-year-old child? I was so curious to find the answers. I knew neurofeedback must have its limitations, but since it could be applied to all kinds of disorders I didn't know what they were? I decided to find out: After all what better test of a therapy than my own diverse family with its very damaged Dar?

Interestingly, what I had to learn in order to apply this therapy to my family's heads not only helped me understand neurofeedback better but the Autism Spectrum and Feedback itself. I began imagining the spectrum like a road strewn with travelers stretching from the Pacific to the Atlantic. Every vehicle is headed east. The backseat bosses in all the transportation devices on this highway are trying to navigate their drivers off the spectrum analogized by making it to the shore of the Atlantic. Each of these wheeled and non-wheeled people-moving devices starts at different locations along the road. Some begin in California, some in New Mexico, some in Louisiana etc. Some belly crawl, some pogo stick, some sit upon rusty old riding mowers. Still others stylishly speed down the road in their lovely Lamborghini's reaching their goal so quickly that their navigators wonder if they had ever been part of the autism journey at all. Since this is not a race in which the groups have been fairly created, positioned, signed in, or handed ribbons, no one really knows when it starts or ends, and winning has nothing to do with competition. Most people just aim for the shore, and go. Some travel for a while and then u-turn or back up and do it again, and again and again. If and when they get to the end, some decide to turn the wheel and go other places; some just stay and enjoy the edge… of normalcy.

The navigators in this analogy are caregivers, teachers, therapists, and guides. They divide into three types: the ones who think that loving the child means hating that the race isn't fair, the ones who don't think about that so much as that the child's ability and disability is a reflection on them, and the ones who never worried about either of those things in the first place.

The ones who look at their particular set of circumstances and bemoan the brokenness of both their driver and his riding equipment often encourage their racers to just give up and live where they lie. Or (and this is a big OR) they expend so much energy bemoaning the fate of the situation that there is none left with which to pursue the solution.

The second type of navigator thinks that every transporter on this road has the same potential for speed regardless of engine size or body type. This navigator thinks that everyone started at the same location, in this case California, and that they all have an equal chance of making it to Florida. This navigator thinks that the end result is their responsibility. (This analogy reminds me of myself as a brand new parent. My firstborn slept through the night at seven days old. She seldom cried and was always contented by whatever I brought into her world. She could sing at least fifty songs and say her ABC's backwards and forwards by fourteen months of age. I thought I was the cat's meow, the perfect parent, the best baby coach, the woman on the mountain with all the answers, if only someone would ask and even if they didn't. I was seventeen. When my second daughter was born I grew up. She slept when she felt like it and not when I did. I was two months into being her mom when my exhaustion became the catalyst to a brighter day. Just as I thought I wouldn't survive her feisty cries, she quieted of her own accord. Apparently, with this independent, self-motivated child, I was just along for the ride. So I learned to appreciate the role of credit-less guide, which led me to an awesome learning: credit given is credit received.)

I think that without learning to appreciate the individualized potential and operating style of one's child, any of us can become like the self-absorbed navigator. Any of us can find ourselves carrying blow horns and pushing our sweet little autistic drivers to keep up with the other autistic drivers in front. The trick is to catch ourselves and change and become more user friendly, which is akin to kind. Otherwise we are at risk of thinking ourselves to be the creators of our children's skills rather than the conduit through which the opportunity was provided. And if we do become the energy-draining burden sitting on the back of the belly crawler and blindly whipping them to hurry up because we think that their failure is a reflection on us, we force the child not into success but into our fear of failure. And since the child, likely as not, has a different concept of failure and success than we do, he is forced to keep his eyes on us instead of the road ahead. He/she is forced to follow our shifting emotions in search of what makes us disapprove and react. In this co-dependent dance of torment, the child seldom holds the skills she appears to gain. The child can't because the child never understands the reason for running toward this Florida anyway: she is too busy waiting for the whip. And so these navigating participants are doomed to lose the race regardless of the outcome because they don't understand that the whole thing is just a journey.

The third and final type of navigator attends to life's inherent lack of fairness but knows that moving down the road is all there is to do so encourages forging ahead proud and happy for every mile marker they pass. These are the navigators who stay in the moment, support the child, and recognize the miracles they help create, because these navigators know that even miracles are relative to the physical makeup of the body and brain of their vehicle child. I like to think I have become that kind of navigator.

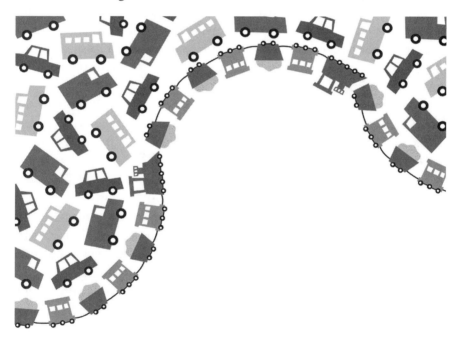

Boys Toys © **Fat Fa Tin from Fotolia.com**

Applying this analogy to my son, Dar I'd have to describe him as barely able to make it to the road let alone start the race. He was submerged by his environment and stuck deep at the bottom of the Pacific Ocean. His vehicle—the equivalent of a one-oared waterlogged boat—would occasionally rise to the surface, at which point he'd paddle in circles or get caught in the weeds. For Dar success might look like making it to dry land and then learning to walk—in the right direction. Had he been my only autistic son I might have given up, seen autism as incurable, and encouraged him to accept his fate while attempting to keep him comfortable. Fortunately for both of us, there were enough autism spectrum participants in my house for me to see and understand the diversity of the disability. This diversity led me to believe there was a different way to help each of them because each of them was different.

For example, next to Dar, my son Chance appeared extremely gifted. I would fit this son into the highway analogy by describing him as an unpredictable teen driving a Kia headed for the coast having starting east from somewhere in the Carolinas. Next to him his navigator (me) barked orders like "Look at the road" or "Stop driving as if you don't have a rear view mirror and can't see the havoc you are leaving behind you." (Eventually I became the other kind of navigator, realized he actually didn't have a rearview mirror and built him one. I did this by describing what was back there, over and over again, until finally he could see it himself.)

To complete the picture of my special boys, I think I would place Rye on a motorized scooter, his hair permanently blown back, his cheeks waving and flapping as he smiled a wind-eating grin. I suspect he began his journey somewhere in New Mexico.

Cash reminded me of the tortoise in *The Tortoise And The Hare*. He was always just putting along in his learning, slow, steady, and consistent. Previous to the creation of the autism spectrum concept, Cash was diagnosed with fetal alcohol syndrome, retardation, and "autistic-like mannerisms". When I remember his journey I imagine him traveling the whole thing on a reliable riding mower, one putt at a time. Considering Cash's motivated personality I would analogize his starting point as mid-Louisiana. And as always I am in the back seat, this time shouting "atta boy" and "you can do it" for all to hear.

OK, yes, I am in the backseat for all my sons… and their sisters, but don't be too impressed. Instead imagine the scene in *The Fast And The Furious* where the stunt woman jumps from one vehicle to the next while it continues to move; only imagine her haggard, frazzled, extremely uncertain if she would make it, and occasionally coveting the comfort of death.

With this visual in mind, and since creating change with neurofeedback covers more ground because it is faster than with parent/ teacher/therapist feedback, you can see why I embraced it. It gave me a break… and the will to live… well. More healing over a cluster of symptoms happens in half an hour of neurofeedback than can be achieved in weeks of twenty-four-hour one-on-one behavioral therapy. It seems like a miracle but it really just makes scientific sense: if you feel more regulated, more balanced, more comfortable in your body, it's easier to learn. Changes in your brain lead to changes in how you experience your body, your ability to attend, and your desire to become more than what you already are. Changes in your brain lead to changes in everything.

Neurofeedback changes brains.

The power of neurofeedback as opposed to everyday feedback or therapy feedback like acupuncture, which gives messages from the peripheries of our nervous system, comes from its speed of delivery to the neuron and the ability to be site specific. In other words, with neurofeedback you give the information to the brain before the peripheries know anything about it. You also give the feedback to the brain before the body turns that brainwave activity into a behavior that is then resistant to change. Even more powerful is the fact that you can give the information to the actual site of greatest neuronal dysregulation by placing the sensor in the spot that is most out of balance and then feeding back to the brain information on how to correct that dysregulation and improve its functioning. Thus it is that neurofeedback has the ability to teach us how to tune up and rebuild our own motherboard to a degree and at a level that was previously unheard of. We do this while simultaneously refining our understanding of the software being inputted by the world around us. Therefore, we reeducate ourselves as the drivers of our own lives. We become our own navigator and learn how to get the most flexibility and efficiency out of our movements, while staying safe, even if we are autistic, even if we are old, even if we don't understand how we are doing it.

Any computer with a glimmer of life, regardless of age, can be rebuilt and so, it turns out, can a person, as long as there is enough time and information to do it with.

So when you hear the miracle story of the child who came off the spectrum, don't compare the Lamborghini in Vegas to the K car in Maryland; compare only that your child's car has gone a little further this year than last. Remember that each brain receiving feedback has a different potential for change and is beginning at a different point. Thus it will take much more feedback for Dar than it took for Rye to get clear communication. In fact, if I were still limited to the normally used speed of feedback looping, it would be impossible to get Dar to that point given the degree of damage in his fine motor system. Fortunately the speed of delivery with neurofeedback makes more feedback possible and thus more change evident. So what if it takes ten times as much feedback to get an equal amount of change from one kid to the other. The sessions are only half an hour, and the amount of feedback possible equals to weeks of lessons and direct trial repetition. My kids learned at their own pace starting from their own place and each of them improved. So can yours—as long as you help them.

You are the most important piece of the puzzle, even if you wish it to not be true. The therapist never replaces the parent. Though, with a little education, the parent can replace the therapist.

However, it is impossible for the parent to replace the therapy itself just as it is impossible for the therapy to replace the parent: they are different things. True, the beauty of neurofeedback is its speed of delivering input to the brain. Thus in a sense it seems to be better at doing what parents and teachers do than they are—precisely because much like the microwave is to cooking, neurofeedback is to brain development—faster—than the old fashioned "do this but don't do that" brain learning way. Still it doesn't replace the old; it simply adds to it some new advantages. This is because, though neurofeedback teaches the brain how to rebalance itself and learn more easily, it doesn't tell it what to learn. That is your job. Brains need parents and teachers to show them what and who they should become. Brains need a reason to heed the "moral fiber of society's feedback" in order to change themselves in that direction. So it's up to us—the parents and professionals—to try and make changing in the direction of responsibility, acceptance, and love desirable. However, even with all the right familial support, employing all the right therapies intent on optimizing the rate of positive change, brain health can remain elusive. This is because even if you can speed up the process and even though if you move faster you get farther (in fact processing speed is almost the definition of IQ), regardless of that fact and the fact that neurofeedback is able to help a brain make the desired changes quickly, even neurofeedback is still limited. It is limited not so much by the person's diagnosis as by the combination of everything: social environment, psychology and the physiology of the person themselves.

But limited or not, it's the best thing I have found for helping people grow, in the right direction.

The thing about neurofeedback is it simply mirrors life. That is why we use the term "natural" when referring to it as a therapy. It is feedback and life is feedback, and this is why so many teaching approaches can have—up to a point—such similar impacts because every teaching therapy gives feedback. Every sensory integration technique, speech and occupational therapy gives feedback. Every moving, breathing, happening, other thing in your world gives feedback. I was no exception. I gave feedback, relentlessly, to my children. I was the autism mommy energizer bunny telling them what to do and how to do it. However, despite the feedback sameness in all these approaches, there are also differences. Two of those differences are extremely noteworthy.

The first difference is that neurofeedback is never judgmental, thus it is never overwhelmed by the job ahead (though its operator may be). The second difference is neurofeedback's site-specific speed of delivery to individual neurons. I know I have mentioned this site specificity before, but now I want to explain it. What does it mean and how does being site specific create an advantage over behavioral cues and biomedical interventions? Simple. It creates an advantage because when talking to a particular part of the brain via neurofeedback, I can do more than just tell someone WHY they shouldn't believe in that fear-creating psychological construct they bought into in order to justify the reason for the emotion they are experiencing. It means I can use the "beeping" (think homing signal) instructions of the neurofeedback computer to tell the actual fear-firing amygdala (small almond-shaped nuclei buried in the limbic system of the brain and responsible for most of your flight or fight reacting) HOW to not fire those feelings of fear in the first place. In easier to understand words, instead of "getting over it" you get to "not have it." Now that's an advantage.

And when I found neurofeedback it was an advantage I needed. Because my son was always afraid (if anything moved too quickly in his peripheries—in a family full of children something is always moving too quickly in your peripheries) and telling him not to be afraid wasn't working. Nor had the antipsychotic, antidepressants, or anticonvulsants I'd tried feeding him helped him to calm.

I wanted so much to find a way to ease his state and make a miracle for him. But, as you already know, until neurofeedback I didn't know how. This was partly because the miracles I was making weren't always visible or obvious to me so they were going unrecognized. And since they were unrecognized, I felt useless and unable and often behaved in desperation. I was stuck in my own blindness wanting a skill I already had. Thus when I behaved badly (frustrated and yelling), I extinguished the very thing I had built when I had been behaving well (persistent yet calm). Perhaps my miracles were unrecognized by me not only because they were hard to perceive but also because back then I didn't even realize the degree to which miracles are made in the first place. In addition, I was so busy trying to help Dar that I took for granted the help I'd already given my other sons. For me the whole "saving them" thing was just a lot of hard work—step by step, day after day, month after month, and year after year. I simply plodded along until my children exited the spectrum, breathed a sigh of relief, and then focused on somebody else.

So in the end I was focused on Dar. (Unless you think the end came when I discovered neurofeedback because then, at the end I was focused on Dar and Rye. However, Rye came off the spectrum from the addition of neurofeedback whereas Dar did not. So in the end I was and am focused on Dar.) Each time I travel to a new family's home, I realize that I have performed obvious miracles with many children. Still, since it is I who makes it happen and I don't really see me as magical, I often discount the unprecedented nature of the success in my journey of helping children. Then I meet another family and am reminded again that with the right tools and techniques, one can do almost anything. Yet I occasionally find myself looking for miracles because the ones I create never happen in the snap of a finger. They happen with intention, education, effort, and attention to detail. Thus, especially where my own kids are concerned, I never saw these happenings as miraculous. I saw them as parenting.

Because I know this lack of self-appreciation and accomplishment acknowledgement is a common problem amongst the many miracle-making parents I work with globally, I will be peppering this book with little stories of the many miracles I see and how they were made.

For example:

THE MIRACLE: Bo was a beautiful black baby only four years old. But when I met him he was a fast enough scratching, biting, leaping little dynamo to have created fear and permanent scarring in all his parents' friends and family. The minute we met (I was not forewarned of his talents) he leapt into my arms and tried to snatch out my eyes and bite off my nose. Cute little guy! Fortunately, I was quicker than he was. I managed to flip him in the air, land his back against my chest, wrap one arm around his torso and one hand on his head to prevent head butting, and while holding him tight, coo sweetly into his ear. I tickled his neck with kisses, snuggled his tummy, and ignored the kicking feet that he aimed at my pubic bone. Left with little else to do, he scratched at my ears. His wide-eyed parents seemed tremblingly afraid I'd refuse to work with him. I told them we'd have him calm by Sunday (three days hence). They laughed... a lot. I understood their apparent disbelief and succeeded anyway. I used the neurofeedback to calm his overactive sensory motor strip, and by Sunday Bo was calm. That morning he ran open armed into my also open arms and was gentle with everyone in the family. He covered us all in big sloppy kisses and ran around dimpling his face with an ear-to-ear grin.

THE FACT: Bo was still very autistic. He was completely mute and wobbled when he ran. We began the job of teaching him that language is more useful than screaming and that swallowing his food didn't have to happen in gulps wherein he put his fists down his throat and made himself vomit. His sensory system was awash with challenges, but by day five he had responded well enough to climb to the top of his newly made, never-before-attempted precarious piles. His parents watched with mouths agape and told me that until that day he had never played with toys, let alone pile them into mountains. While I was there, much learning was begun and progress made. Neurofeedback assisted this speed of change, but when I left to go home I had only proven what was possible and taught what I knew. The parents would now have to continue what I started. They were terrified of failing. Their fear of going it alone (albeit with my Internet guidance and email advice) caused marital issues. Dad had an affair and mom stopped doing the neurofeed-back with her son. Depression led to divorce. Bo stopped making word approximations and requests and the biting returned. Mom, who had been overwhelmed, pulled herself together enough to, after a period of extended silence, get back in touch with me. We began a series of emails and she dusted off the neurofeedback units. There were many more stops and starts along the way, but suffice to say that three years after I first met this sweet four-year-old, he stepped, tentatively at first, then firmly, off the spectrum. Mom remarried and had a daughter.

THE APPEARANCE OF A MIRACLE: Darling Bo made his way through several more disorders before he was eight. For a while he had a tic disorder and then a compulsive need to steal food from garbage cans and pinch his sister's cheeks. He gentled down and settled on ADHD for two years. After that he seemed to have no notable challenges other than a kind of sweet naiveté in regards to social interactions with his peers. He remained a child to be taught and raised, and in many ways mom's job did nothing more than reshape itself from disorder to disorder. (Very soon he'll be developing the disorder of adolescence.) Mom's job was enormous. It was also, I suspect, enormously rewarding, whenever she had the energy to feel it. When asked if she would call her son's journey a miracle, she just smiled and said "No, more like a big undertaking. A miracle is when you take your child to the doctor, he gets an IV or a pill, and he walks out normal. This was just an all consuming life purpose."

I suffered from a similar kind of media-made myopia. Since I didn't have the edited version of my own story but lived out the miracle in its making twenty-four–seven, it never felt like a miracle. So I kept hoping to find one. The disadvantage in that never-to-be-satiated blind pursuit was that when mixed with my own thinking and focus challenges, it left me exhausted. Thus I got sick a lot as I depleted my adrenal glands and lived on caffeine pills. I led my children with feedback, caffeine-fed energizer-bunny parental feedback called "do, do this and don't do that." Fortunately, those of my kids who had a

- 58 -

running start and were only slightly on the spectrum were able to skip their way over the edge and into "normal."

It is clear to see why even without neurofeedback, some of my children changed enough to come off the spectrum, albeit with less self comfort than they would experience with neurofeedback. It is also clear to see why without neurofeedback my other children didn't improve enough to learn to put on their pants or stop carving the number 1985 into every wood surface the neighbors owned. These neurofeedback *needers* had farther to go. So, since these children were so far into the deep end of autism that even their improvement was too underwater to see, they needed more. And, as I eventually understood, what seemed like less was still a miracle. In fact, Dar's learning to point at a desired object (a lesson that required neurofeedback for him to attain) was just as big a miracle as Chance's becoming a helicopter mechanic (a success enabled by my relentless teaching) had been. So, like all parents, whether I knew it or not, I was always changing my children brains. When I found neurofeedback the "always changing" became "always visible" in *all* of my children and in *myself.* Finally things were going fast enough for us to feel the progress. That made living easy (er). And that's I want to share it. And that's why when I say "Neurofeedback to the Rescue," I mean it… from a very personal place.

CHAPTER THREE

MIRACLES ARE MADE
Out of Elbow Grease and Computer Science

THE MIRACLE: Tracy had been through two years of forty-hours-per-week direct trial ABA training. Her weekends were filled with Speech Therapy and Occupational Therapy. She was on a gluten-free casein-free diet for over a year. After all that, Tracy could speak and identify up to twenty-five flash cards on cue, but she was completely unable to spontaneously do more than say the same six words over and over again whenever she stepped away from the training table. Tracy was low-functioning autistic. She walked with a shuffling gate, drooled on her blanket, and seldom smiled. Her parents stopped the ABA program and tried teaching her using the Son-Rise® modality. Tracy loved the non-intrusive approach but was equally as unresponsive to treatment. She spent her daily hours hanging upside down, bouncing on a ball, or masturbating. She would spread feces into the registers and wall cracks and only ate three foods. She was seven when I met her. By the age of nine she had assimilated into school, could speak in eight-word sentences in order to get her needs met, and was happy to engage in five loop conversational exchanges. Her eye contact was low, and she only really held a person's gaze if they were playing and being silly. She was happy and loved to snuggle.

THE FACT: Tracy had crossed these milestones while only occasionally doing neurofeedback. Her father was too busy to help and mom was overwhelmed by fear whenever she imagined tinkering with her child's brain. Fortunately I worked fairly often in their home, so whenever I was there we (mom and I) would first retrain the people and then restructure her program. After that I would do neurofeedback. These visits always leapt Tracy forward into a new functioning level, but it was the constant practice with her mom and her helpers that kept the changes in place. Mom spent millions of hours playing with her daughter and teaching and training all the babysitters and helpers. In my opinion she was creative and consistent and eternally hard on herself. She cried often. She would look at me through teary eyes and berate herself for not being able to implement the use of bio meds or homeopathy, for no longer enforcing a rigid diet, and for fearing to be the one controlling the neurofeedback. She said she knew these were her choices, but that she often hated herself for them anyway. Her crying spells generally happened after some extended family member voiced a negative judgment like telling her repeatedly that if she were a good mom she'd find a way to make Tracy normal. Tracy's grandmother was especially challenging to deal with because regardless of Tracy's milestones Tracy's grandmother says she sees no progress. Tracy's grandmother sees only what's missing. So she tries to spread this perspective to her daughter, Tracy's poor, overwhelmed mom. When Grandma is in the room and for several weeks after she leaves, Tracy keeps her eyes away and Mom flounders into fear. Mom then calls me and we talk. I listen as she builds herself back up by listing all that she does for her daughter and then all that her daughter does in return. Then, possibly in order to feel superior on the backs of others, she conjures up all the other mothers of autism and judges them lazy. She laments the future of all their children and wonders why everyone else doesn't do all the things that she does. At this point little Tracy's mom becomes like little Tracy's grandmom. They are all often life-threateningly sick with worry: All kinds of worry, even now. Tracy's mom, Tracy's grandmom, and Tracy all seem anxious. They wring their hands with work and worry and worry and work. Grandmom reads every story of miracle makers she can get her hands on and then phones her daughter to tell all the ways in which she is ill equipped to make a miracle. Tracy's mom tries even harder to safeguard and protect her daughter by overseeing every moment and keeping her from any unsupervised others. She also stays up night after night searching the Internet for a Miracle Cure while Tracy arranges her room meticulously cleaning the very registers she used to shove feces into. In this family it appears that everyone is looking so closely for the appearance of a miracle that they haven't got the vantage point from which to actually see it.

THE APPEARANCE OF A MIRACLE: At present ten-year-old Tracy can read aloud one word at a time. She can also do simple multiplication. Tracy consistently answers questions about the concepts buried with ten-word sentences, and her facilitator or shadow is now a classroom helper because Tracy operates for the most part independently. Equally as amazing, she can run with an even gait and is potty trained. But wait, there is more! Tracy now eats everything, especially if it comes out of a friend's lunch kit. Yes, I said *friends*. Though she doesn't talk much with her friends, she holds hands and often plays the willing servant to their needs. She still masturbates obsessively but now she does it in private. Her mom has also embraced the miraculous. She still cries a lot, especially after she talks to her mother, but the tears are more easily brushed aside. And yes, she still says she feels less than adequate as a parent, regardless of the fact that hers is an amazing home program. (I have done this journey several times with my children and the children of others, so I believe my opinion here is valid: hers is an amazing home program. At this point in my learning I find no mystery in autism. I simply meet the children and then figure out what the next step should be in order to get to the parent's next goal. But these parents I work with are usually in the middle where the confusion is greatest. Being able to continue at all is a skill worth admiring. This mom had already done five years of home training before I came along. She is a force to be amazed by, despite the moments of desperation, as she picks herself up year after year for the betterment of her child. At this point in her journey, it looks as if Tracy's mom has learned to listen and then take action, to stretch herself and address her issues, to do as much self-help work as she is asking her child to do. Recently I was storytelling with Tracy's mom, hoping to share the reality that no parent does all the therapies that are available and so all the parents I meet seem worried about the therapies they don't do. It's like a global epidemic of fearing that we are selling our children short just in case there's an easier way. So we make our way hard. In this, I assured her, she is no exception. We laughed a bit, and then she asked me about the neurofeedback and if I thought she was abusive for not picking neurofeedback as her main tool. It was an interesting question. This is my answer: All the kids I work with improve at the same rate regardless of what other therapies the families augment with as long as they do neurofeedback (consistently or in bunches when I come over) and as long as their environment is rewarding in all the right places. BUT if the family does neurofeedback without addressing the environment, then the child's changes are unpredictable and occasionally undesirable. Because a more capable brain being rewarded for and taught to act crazy is just better at learning how. I reassured Tracy's mom that if she was limited to only one therapy, then she had picked correctly. In my opinion if, as a parent, you are going to do only one thing, do environment. She took a deep breath and smiled at her daughter who came over to giggle and snuggle on her lap. I pointed out that Tracy would step into the role she gave her. She gave her a role: learner. Tracy's mom continues to teach her daughter seemingly proud of the help she has been in the journey of her child. *And that is the appearance of a miracle.*

Like Tracy's Mom and Bo's Mom and DW's Dad, I wanted the story to be easy and obvious. I wanted to find the therapy that made the difference immediately. I, like all the parents I meet, wanted to find the magic pill or IV solution to my sons' recovery. Reason is, I hoped for the miracle maker teacher so that I didn't have to be. My aversion to accepting that it was my job to do, that it was all just a lot of work by means of feedback slowed our progress and kept me from finding the answer: That there is no miracle pill but that there is a way to improve and often be cured, by using feedback towards the goal… by every means possible.

Now that I think about it, maybe I should have subtitled this section "Feedback to the Rescue" because that's something you can do now, even without a machine. Feedback feeds. It feeds the brain… nourishment… or poison. So choose carefully what you put on the spoon. Affecting your child is up to you… even when it seems like it isn't.

THE MIRACLE: He was such a success story. Within five days his aggression, pinching, screaming, biting, and kicking had stopped. Mom was a neurofeedback advocate for the next year of emerging language and adoring cooperation. All her friends and family were amazed.

THE FACT: Mom had followed my advice and replaced all but one of his tutors, changed his classroom, and changed her way of speaking and rewarding his behavior. She also used neurofeedback religiously. But then she began to think the improvements were due to neurofeedback only and backslid into some of the old habits just as he changed schools and was suddenly being handled in a vague and aggression-rewarding style. Suddenly mom was desperately doing two and three sessions a day of neurofeedback just to keep him reasonably stable. He was fighting again because again he perceived himself as living in an environment wherein he had no control and that would only reward him when he took the stance of fighting back.

THE RE-APPEARANCE OF A MIRACLE: I reminded mom of the "wholeness" in our approach. She pulled him out of that school, reorganized his helpers, and returned to a two-sessions-a-week approach with neurofeedback. Now, all over again, he is a success story; and if I wanted, as my previous editor did, I could leave out the middle and tell you only the sweet, loving, gentle, talking, ball adoring, success story as if it were a miracle unruffled by life. But I don't want to because it creates illusions that hurt by erasing the hard work that heals. Environment matters.

The common denominator between my story and theirs is non-judgmental action, specific feedback, and the similar teacher that aided all of my sons' towards a journey of recovery. It was judgmental feedback that impeded them. Since our family discovered neurofeedback everyone has healed, a lot. Even good old grownup Dar has been snail-pace changing into a capable man since the onset of implementing this therapy. As you know by now, for Dar, a snail's pace is lightening speed. I'm not sure he'll ever be independent. It wouldn't appear so, but he is learning and as such has already exceeded all our expectations. At this point there is no way to foresee how far he's going to get. I do know he has not yet made it to the level of self-care and communication that matches my hopes for him. But at least now I am less confused. I finally know how it is that the other ones learned without neurofeedback while Dar did not appear to because in fact he did. His progress was just too slow to see. However, let's be honest, to the parent and the child; progress that is too slow to see is the same as getting nowhere. Speed matters! To everyone, the watcher and the watched.

As a mom I would have given anything, and I do mean anything, to find a way to help my son stop hitting himself or slamming his furniture around all night. Fortunately I didn't have to sell my soul for that miracle; in fact I found my soul, in the eyes of my sons, when I learned how to help them. I learned how to bring Dar to the computer and sit him down to ease his pain by helping him to communicate through typing. Sure I wanted more, wanted the miracle story wherein the family takes their son to Disneyland and he immediately talks… but those stories are usually lies created by the brevity forced upon the teller of the tale. Many of those children are still hitting themselves. Mine isn't (unless you count behaving like a gorilla to get his teenage nephew to turn off the Xbox and go to sleep). No matter whatever else, he learns nothing will ever top the newfound calmness of Dar's happy hands, because at the end of the day all I really wanted for my children was happiness. Finally, now that I am nearing the end of this journey, I know how to help them be that type of man, the happy type.

Many people ask me how it feels to be me. Well, to me it feels as if my journey was long and arduous, but then I meet other parents whose children are institutionalized or drugged into docility and realize how small my story has grown to be now that it has grown into doable.

THE MIRACLE: His parents loved him no matter what.

THE FACT: Boris was a twenty-year old man who refused to wear clothes, walked back and forth like a caged lion, and inserted string into all his orifices. He was basically calm, spoke only in guttural nonsensical utterances, and attacked himself whenever anyone suggested he wear clothes. Boris' parents were tired of believing in therapies, so they built him a room surrounded by high gates and kept him from view. I saw him only once.

THE APPEARANCE OF A MIRACLE: During that visit he managed to wear clothes long enough to take a forty-minute walk in the yard. I am told he retained this skill and that his parents are happy with this progress: Some miracles are only miracles to the people who know that enormity can be found in small changes. In Boris' parents' world, a walk in the garden was enough change to brighten a life.

Parents and teachers who have lifelong challenging stories like Boris' often ask me how I did it and then discard my explanation of feedback. They tend to fingers-in-their-ears beg for answers, "How did you do it? How? It can't be that simple! You didn't have Brain Computers yet so what made your kids learn? What did you do that was different?" And, realizing they want my story more than my teaching, I search my mind for analogous stories that I think might help them all the while thinking to myself, "Nothing really. All kids learn—unless in their particular case they have a disorder that degenerates." This was something I sometimes wondered about Dar. Sometimes I'd even wonder it while I was being asked to teach. My thoughts would meander for a minute into his childhood, and then I'd shake off the self-absorption and try to share. "Mostly I just believed that they would learn—but only exactly what they wanted to learn: Maybe knowing that was the secret." At this point people generally look at me perplexed and I am unable to fully explain what I mean, though I try, every time a parent asks.

THE MIRACLE: Three days after meeting her, Sam was playing with me, talking to me, and running from one end of the room to the other. Her older brother was doing his homework, and when he said his eyes were displaying an aura and his head started to ache, I hooked him to the neurofeedback and within minutes the migraine was averted.

THE FACT: Sam was a little blond pixie of a Retts girl. Her speech was fairly clear but she spoke mostly about the dolls she was banging on the ground. Her body wobbled precariously when she walked, and though she was five she looked three. Sam was still only able to handle food that had been blended into mush and drunk from a baby bottle. Her brother was twelve and had often been hospitalized for migraines. The last time he was on the ward for over a week. Though the headache eventually stopped, the doctors never did figure it out what had caused it nor found a medication that he would respond to. He was an extremely freckled, extremely ADHD butterball of energy. His mom and dad were trying difficult diets, tutors, ABA instructors, hyperbaric chambers, bio meds, chelation, and homeopathy. They bought the neurofeedback units but became resistant from the moment I explained that when working with me... the parent is the expert and I am the consultant, and that to get the fullness of the approach we would have to change the way they were teaching her. Dad took me for a drive "to chat." He told me that they had never wanted to be the ones responsible for their child's therapy. Yes, they knew before I arrived that after I left it would be up to them to continue, but they had hoped it would be like the hyperbaric chamber they bought. Basically learn what buttons to push and get in. Now that the theory I had explained on the phone and the responsibility it carried was becoming a reality, he said they were afraid. He parked the truck, turned and looked at me. " I just want someone else to fix her. All we want to do is be parents. I just don't think I am any good with kids. To me she is like a china doll and I don't want to be the one making the decisions. I just don't trust us."

THE APPEARANCE OF A MIRACLE: Success comes in many packages. Though this family never embraced the "how-to part of basic responding" and didn't want to partner with me as a co-therapist, they did love the changes they saw in their daughter. So they found another way. They hired a good team of people to reward and celebrate Sam's successes as she learned and researched their area for a clinic that could do the neurofeedback for them. This is an expensive way for a family to treat all its members, but money was not one of their challenges. They made their own miracle by applying what worked to who they were and what they could do. In the end they created the same program we would have implemented together by adding a little more expense and time consumption to the mix. I was thrilled to hear that they had found a solution; after all feedback is feedback and the correct method for dealing with the dynamics is different family to family. I am still thrilled because last I heard Sam has continued to improve, especially in the area of gross motor skills and toileting: A continuous path of improvement is a big deal for a Retts child. And her brother? Well, big brother didn't go to the clinic but that was OK because he hadn't had a migraine since our last treatment session two years before.

Having language fail me in these moments of requested teaching always gets me thinking of the admissions man from Surrey Place who refused to tell me what to do because (I thought at the time) he was afraid I'd steal his edge and copy his school's techniques. The parents ask me for the same reason I asked him, because they want to do exactly that: copy my techniques. And like the man from Surrey Place, I often fall short of a complete answer. So I don't answer. I don't answer, not because my intention is to keep the information to myself but because—like all the people over the years who wouldn't share with me—I don't really know how I helped my children. Though, because of that process, I have come to know how to help other people. You see the thing is I helped my children before I learned how to help. I just sort of stumbled around trying things. This is why I'm not one hundred percent sure which bits worked and which bits didn't. So sometimes, since that is too much to explain, I answer by joking, "Marry lots of men—introduce them to your kids and watch them get the runs." It's a good joke, good for a laugh, but not very informative.

Nowadays I am able to joke about the challenges I had learning what to do because nowadays those challenges are over. Nowadays I've moved so far away from those challenges that I've forgotten... aspects of... what it feels like... to live in a world wherein... because of your children... you feel disconnected from all the other families... who also feel disconnected... from you. I joke about divorcing. But it's not really a joke. After all, I was living in the world of special children wherein the divorce rate is unaccountably high (even though I account for most of them), and I didn't really want to be divorced. Obviously I wanted to be married; otherwise I wouldn't have had so many opportunities to get divorced (wink). So, I joke, even though, maybe, my joke isn't funny. Truth is, there's a good chance that, my being divorced actually was part of my answer, because...

My children were my life. I was focused on them rather than a husband. This is often the reason so many parents of special children get divorced. Divorce has its consequences. Some of them are good. I couldn't afford help. So, since I was married and I hired no help, there was no one to contradict or dilute the consistent nature of my parenting style. In the long run this particular consequence turned out to be a blessing. Especially since for me, at the time, explaining my choices took longer than making them. However, understand that I am NOT suggesting you run out and get divorced. My life is not one to copy (nor desirable for most people I would think). Can't you just imagine the recipe I'd have to write "Well, let's see. I've had five husbands so you'll need five husbands, only one at a time, of course. And don't forget poverty; you have to be poor; otherwise you'll hire folks to help you and then there'll be too many people keeping an eye on your kids." I can't help you figure it out that way because you'd either laugh at me or get my husbands' runs—either way you wouldn't be listening. And if you're not listening you may miss the part when I say, "And besides, affording everything available means trying everything available, and that just diffuses the evidence of what does and doesn't work."

So, I don't advise recreating my story; really, I don't. I'm sure it can be done without all the drama. And besides, not everyone wants to have four adopted mentally challenged kids, two runaway teenagers, a couple of slightly displaced biological children, a series of husbands, and a kind of strange post-abuse-childhood, sensory-integration-disordered, ADHD outlook on life. However, even though you would be ill advised to try and copy my journey, I am certain it is a good idea to try and copy what I learned from it.

I began (when I got Dar) by reading what was available. I tried everything I learned about and then learned to be more discerning. Because—

as the family filled to the rim with autism—I came to realize I'd have to make different choices for different children. Regardless of their matching diagnoses, none of them were the same. Two of them even gained skills like math from going to school. They also made friends and began cooperating in class. Two of them did none of this. My youngest, Rye, went through the typical stages that many of the children with autism go through. First he was mute, and then he was echolalic (repeated the last few words of every sentence you said to him). After that he began to mix what is therapeutically referred to as word salads: bits and pieces of communication all mushed together and making no sense. Rye's combo of word salad ingredients consisted of sound bites from movie previews, teachers' comments, and sound effects. He babbled these audio concoctions incessantly for several years. Eventually his language developed into poorly structured, haltingly spoken sentences. More and more he would look in our eyes as he talked.

However, unlike two of his brothers, none of Rye's communication skills were learned at school, because at school he spent most of his time spitting at the teachers and throwing the chairs. Dar also gained very little from attending class, though *I* got a daytime break from the challenges of teaching him. Thus it was many years before I was willing to roll up my sleeves, take them all out of school, and do it myself. Which was probably a good thing. In the early years I didn't know that patience isn't what is required to teach slowly. For me patience doesn't work; it just leads to impatience. Instead I learned to see each moment as a step in the journey towards success. That mindset merely requires a willingness to work—constantly. Fortunately, working hard is the most fun thing I do. However, since at the time I thought parenting required patience and I defined patience as doing something over and over again that I'd rather not be doing, Dar was the one who could try my patience the most. Dar didn't just move slowly; he stopped!

Dar would freeze into position at the slightest provocation, thus extending the waiting period of task acquisition and of my need to be patient. I believed that Dar was reacting to every request by freezing with fear because of me. This of course eroded my ability to "be patient" which led to anger and filled me with guilt (a truly negative emotion with no redeeming value in proactive parenting). I thought Dar's fear was based in psychology (maybe) and caused by the "get a fork or I'll pinch your shoulder" technique. So my guilt clouded my vision, which led to anger, which added to my guilt and increased my anger. I noticed the cycle and dropped the guilt (because when I just tried to drop the anger, the guilt wouldn't let me). It was then, after clearing my memory of guilt, that I realized Dar had been freezing into position even before I had experimented with aversion. And since I wasn't busying my brain with so much self-condemnation, I was more able to see my own role in this aspect of my son. It occurred to me that Dar had always frozen into position, anytime I asked something of him. This truth was proven by the fact that my first most obvious memory on the subject happened even before the get-a-fork-shoulder-pinching experience.

One time when Dar was about five, he was sitting on the carpet while I helped him complete the task of dressing himself. I bent his knee and raised his foot off the floor. I was putting his leg into position so that he could don his sock. I'd already rolled them up and placed them in his hands for the task. I orchestrated his body so that all Dar had to do was extend his leg two inches in order to begin the process. I played cheerleader and encouraged him for about five minutes; then, needing to cook breakfast and feeling frustrated, I left the room after telling him he could do it alone. Forty-five minutes later I returned to check on him: Not only had he not put his foot in his sock but he had not even moved a hair. Dar had kept his sock-holding arms extended and his leg elevated the entire time. His expression was blank and his body statued. The only evidence of physical discomfort I could find was in his foot: it was blue from a lack of circulation. My buttocks, arms, and legs ached with empathy. I cheered and begged and yelled "PUT ON YOUR SOCK! JUST DO IT!!!" Finally, after an hour, I needed some relief. So I did it for him. Then I sat down and cried, feeling overwhelmed by the life I saw, stretching straight ahead of me.

Nowadays I have a tool to help his apraxia (fancy scientific term for *my brain just went blank and I can't think well enough to continue to the next step*). I use neurofeedback to heal the problem and a gentle nudge to get Dar going. Nowadays I know that this absence of ability is similar in some respects to another aspect of autism, overexcited self-stimulatory behavior (repetitive movement that encapsulates the child's focus as he isolates himself from others). It is almost like a form of excitation (Neurons firing so fast they overload and stop) and similar to the theory of catatonic Parkinson's presented in the movie *Awaken-*

ings. In order to relax the effects of that mental freeze-frame panic position, I often (though certainly not always) use neurofeedback settings and sensor choices that help the left hemispheric pre-motor and motor strip communicate with each other. In fact, I have often had to do this same process on me.

I have healed myself enough to not freeze into frustration when I see my child freeze into fear. Therefore, I find answers and am able to access my own intrinsic understanding of the reason for his behavior: I remember the black hole of thought from my own childhood. I remember many times during math class or math homework time, trying to solve a problem. Initially the answer would instantaneously come to me intact with no steps required (I still experience this instant knowing when doing neurofeedback on clients, but I've also grown and learned enough to verbalize my reasoning after the fact). But then the teacher would require I do the steps and explain my thinking. It was when the teacher slowed me down and asked me to communicate my thought patterns that I would freeze, and fall into a black hole in my head. Eventually that hole grew big enough to completely swallow my ability to do math at all. In fact, the very thought of even being asked to do arithmetic stimulated my fear of the hole and brought the blackness to my peripheries. I always knew when it was coming because my throat would begin closing. I would cry and try to warn people. Then I would disappear, even from myself. No matter who yelled or how hard they hit, the black hole would only evaporate if I was left alone, spoken softly to, or fell asleep. I think, until I had the tools to understand it with, that Dar's fear brought back mine. Fortunately for both of us, once I understood enough brain science to understand that, regardless of what my parents thought and said at the time, those episodes were not proof of my defiance. Therefore, if I had not been being defiant, then neither was Dar. Thus, I was able to stop seeing either of us in this light. And once I didn't see Dar as defiant, I stopped behaving as if he were. And that's what is meant by the term "breaking the cycle."

At present I am more informed and I know that even without neurofeedback, a little nudge would have helped Dar make those connections so that eventually, maybe, he could have done it on his own.

I sometimes wonder where Dar would be if I knew then what I know now. What if I had not seen helping as giving in. What if I had not feared preventing him from learning because I was too weak to not do it for him? What if I had understood the line between standing strongly consistent and bending enough to be flexible, thereby giving him the clues he needed in order to be able to succeed? What if I had not perpetuated the problem by standing strong in my conviction that he should figure it out on his own? But then I remember that regret is also a negative emotion useless in proactive parenting and am consoled by the thought that perhaps Dar's place in life is to lead me to find the answers that I will share with you. I love that image of us—Dar and me—helping you nudge your child into making those connections.

As I mentioned before, when I found neurofeedback, six of my children were already independent. I was still teaching Rye social skills and work ethics, and still trying to get him to stop punching holes in my walls. And Dar, who didn't speak at all, was still struggling to wipe his bottom well enough to keep his anus clean. I was home schooling, which meant hours of training volunteers how to teach twenty-three-year-old Dar through the use of play, even more hours of playing with him myself, and several additional hours of playing with other people's children in an attempt to learn more and make a living.

Blessed with an encyclopedia set of autistic children, plus an additional set of helpful daughters, I was truly the luckiest person I know. Each of them taught me, more than I ever knew I needed to learn. I learned very quickly that they could teach and that they could also learn. I began to show my love to each of them differently, because each of them loved a different thing. So, with Chance I behaved like a drill sergeant, whereas with Cash I used explanations and logic. Both of them seemed to be adapting to the world they lived in. With Rye I simply held on and waited until he stopped screaming long enough to know I was there. And Dar? Well I'm still trying to figure him out.

Dar was always a bit of a tease because every time he gained a skill he also lost it. Every single thing, every new therapy first got me excited because it would work and then later dropped me into disappointment because it would not. We could have nicknamed Dar "The Regressor". From time to time he would come into focus (like the day he played for half an hour trying to do gymnastics with his brothers). He would come into focus just long enough for us to know that we would miss him when he went away. Despite his twenty-three years I wasn't giving up, but I wasn't winning the battle either. I just couldn't figure out how to help him in a continuous manner. We were so road blocked. I wanted something special—the magic key that would unlock Dar's tongue forever. My play methods of *"OK Dar, I'm the store owner and you're the customer. We have pork—hamburger and sausage—oh good, touching the sausage, now say sausage, see you're the customer, and that's how you buy the food—you say the word and I give you the food—good—good opening your mouth, now push air out and make a sound for sausage... sauu— good, good air sound, now sauuuuu——"* weren't working very well. (At that rate Dar was going to be 315 before he could talk). So I was still looking for the answer, still scared that I'd die of old age before my son grew able to communicate clearly enough to deter any potential perpetrators from hurting him. To my way of thinking he'd already had enough being perpetrated upon in his life.

That's when I read about neurofeedback. At first it was just one more thing to try, no different than the millions of other things I'd already tried. At this point no promises fooled me and I bought into no guarantees. But I was still looking, so I would try because that's what parents of autism do. Besides, the science of neurofeedback sounded right to me and completely congruent with everything else I was doing. I decided to add it to my arsenal of attempted cures. As the woman put the sensors on Dar's head, she smiled sweetly, despite her obvious fear of my angry oversized grunting and growling man. Fortunately regard-less of size and strength Dar still listened to "Sit down Dar; watch the screen" from me, his mom. By his third session my son—who had never noticed nature before—was pulling me to touch the snow. It was excit-ing to note but I felt cautious. I'd seen similar changes from treatments like auditory training and vision therapy but no breakthroughs that lasted. In fact, I remember being convinced that the miracle treatment of giving autistic kids IV's filled with the gut hormone Secretin would be Dar's healing remedy. I'd seen him respond well and was excited to continue. But it wasn't ever available. (Eventually I researched its func-tion and realized I might be able to mimic the remedy with baking soda. Baking soda costs ninety-nine cents a box and is easily available. So far it's working. It has partially healed my son's gut. At this point we have been able to reintroduce fifty percent of heretofore reaction-causing foods.). But no matter what I did or how hard I tried, he still remained extremely autistic.

Note to reader: In case you don't already know, many autistic kids have leaky guts. This means their stomach is perforated and minute amounts of food gets into their system and across the blood brain barrier without being properly broken down. When this happens parental directives like "Drink your milk" can cause opium affects in the brain. So kids (or adults) like Dar get totally wasted on what most of us perceive as a healthy choice. I hadn't known about this opioid effect in his early years, but I did suspect that milk was a problem for Dar. However, as I mentioned earlier, keeping it out of his diet was met with great disapproval and so, whenever I wasn't looking, other folks worked on his bones and teeth while effectively harming his brain. Dar was pretty much trippin' most of his life. No wonder he didn't learn to talk. Which brings up a possibility. Perhaps Dar's first mom was doing her best with the knowledge she had. Perhaps she was just feeding him bottles of milk and that's what caused his behavior change and why he was trying to escape. And perhaps all the rest was just gossip and nonsense made up by people trying to make sense of what they saw based on the information they had. This is a common problem for parents of autistic children. I have been known to say (with only ninety-eight percent accuracy), "The definition of an onlooker is an uninformed person." At any rate we've learned a bit since those days. So, if any of you have autistic kids with leaky guts— baking soda ninety-nine cents a box—just the teeniest bit in a glass of water five days a week—try it; it might work for you.

I love the idea of putting the healing in the hands of parents because they are the ones available in the moment of difficulty. That's why I work in homes instead of clinics. I believe in equipping moms and dads with neurofeedback for home training. I believe in sharing information. I believe in enhancing parent power because I believe that making parents into therapists means that therapists won't be spread so thin. I also want to have an impact on increasing the use of neurofeedback worldwide because...

After five days of neurofeedback Dar began moving his tongue to form new sounds—happy sounds—no cries of numbness or headache pain. He stopped punching himself in the face. His shifts in state were mostly subtle but—there were all these little things—like him pointing excitedly to the food in the fridge. Pointing—I'd been trying to teach that since he was four—he'd finally gotten it. He pointed with his whole hand. It was so cute, covered a lot more area too. Smart really; after all, you can get more stuff that way. Dar was twenty-three when he learned to point. That's not what convinced me though. It was something much better: One of the reasons Dar hadn't been able to point was his hands were always in a fisted position, especially if he was touching someone. I remember holding my friend's daughter when Dar first became my son and feeling her melt into my body. That's when I realized that Dar always pulled away from touching his body onto mine, especially his chest and open hands. They were way too sensitive to enjoy contact. But I didn't know that at the time—I thought he was just rejecting me. I wanted him to hug me like that little girl had done. I wanted it so bad. I remember praying for it and promising God that if he ever did, if Dar ever learned to hug me like that, I would never ask for another thing.

You know, I never really kept that promise (it takes a lot of bargaining with the forces of nature to make Dar normal).

This story was pivotal in our lives so I tell it everywhere—and every time I tell it I cry (even now when the telling is done via typing): Because, two weeks into the sessions—a few days after he learned to point—Dar and I were in the foyer. I was taking my coat off when I turned around—and Dar wrapped his arms around my body and melted his chest into mine. And that's the day Dar gave me my first open-palmed hug. I just stood there holding my breath. "Oh my god! Oh my god! He's touching my back" I'd never felt that part of his hand on my body before.

Dar had been my son for nineteen years—before I felt the flat of his hand warm against my back. WOW! You can bet I was a believer.

Two years after starting neurofeedback, despite the countless professionals who insisted he couldn't learn to talk at such a late age, twenty-five-year-old Dar spoke well enough to be understood by some of the neighbors and even the occasional waitress. Best of all, though he occasionally takes rests in his progression of learning, he has never ever again regressed away from what he knows.

As I have said many times already and will likely repeat again, all autism is not the same. So Dar doesn't learn simply through repetition whereas my other son Cash did. In the case of Dar we needed more than elbow grease to help him; we also needed computer science. Fortunately, I understood a little about both. It is my hope that by the end of this book, so will you.

THE APPEARANCE OF A MIRACLE: He was a fourteen-year-old blanket-biting, toe-walking, people-scratching sweetie whose parents had never heard speak. Within five days he was playing interactively and doing neurofeedback (in other words, patiently sitting for half an hour at a time with wires hanging from his head and an amp attached to his shirt) for not only me but his mom as well. For the last two of those five days he had consistently and repeatedly said seven different words.

THE FACT: His parents were both doctors. They wanted the neurofeedback and bio meds and pharmaceuticals to cure their son. They were having serious financial issues due to having outfitted a new plastic surgery clinic just as the drop in the American economy hit. Thus both parents needed to work. There was no money for sitters so the children were left with a very elderly non-English speaking grandma who could barely keep him in his Depends. His mom and dad tried various therapies and teaching programs in addition to the neurofeedback. But they were used to rotating through ideas in their search for a cure, so they quickly jumped ship and though their big guy improved physically (possibly from the neurofeedback or a combination of all) and became very capable at things, like toileting during the day, horse back and bike riding, he still didn't speak (unless I was with him) any words that they could hear. This, I believe, was because their son spoke in word approximations rather than well-pronounced ones (left un-rewarded, word approximations either stagnate and disappear or become unrecognizable gibberish) and, whenever he did talk, he looked away rather than at the person he was talking to. So because it didn't look or sound right, they couldn't hear it. His parents stopped all previous therapies including neurofeedback and tried a lot of new ones in their search for something special. As of this writing they are still looking and he is still not talking well enough for others to hear. So he lives in a world of noisy silence despite all his therapies and despite the fact that he is enrolled in a school surrounded by experts. It is my hope that at some point his mom and dad will circle back to the at-home neurofeedback/family feedback combo that they still haven't fully embraced. The fact that they haven't fully embraced this therapy is not something I write about with any type of judgment against the parents. I know from personal experience how difficult a decision the "it's all up to me so I guess I have to bring the therapy home and do it myself" approach can be. I have no judgment but I do have hope because with no positive feedback for his attempts at communicating coming from the environment he lives in, it will be hard to inspire this child to do the work he needs to do to improve his speech. Fortunately, as long as his parents can "accept and love him the way he is," he doesn't actually need to talk to be happy.

THE ACTUAL MIRACLE: They can, they do and he is.

Pharmaceuticals, supplements, and speech therapy never really worked for my children. Neither did the various repetitive teaching modalities like ABA or Behavior Modification ever work in any tangible way. This was especially true for Dar. In fact, as you know, nothing really worked for Dar in a way I could hold onto—nothing but the neurofeedback/family feedback combo. The truth is, the same goes for me. I was never helped by tranquilizers or antidepressants and never really learned through simple repetition either. After all, though I tried the marriage thing repeatedly, I never did figure it out. (wink) As I mentioned in the introduction, my lack of marital success could be because everyone I married came to be my husband before neurofeedback helped me stay focused. Stay tuned for possible success in this area. (wink again) As you may have noticed I am eternally hopeful. (wink one more time) Besides, the way I figure it, if I'm ancient enough the next time I get married "till death us do part" won't be so insurmountable because it won't require as much longevity of focus. (wink wink double wink no more winking for now I think) I love levity but sometimes its purpose is to hide the hurts. The truth is that I met Brent when I was sixteen, and despite the fact that we separated and tried on other romances in the middle, I am fifty-three now and death is about to bring us to the end. Death will part us for good this time. At the moment that feels insurmountable, even though, much as I tried to pretend it into being, Brent was never my knight in shining armor, save-me-from-misery man. He was just a man, who leaned on me, often. Ironically, after all the marrying I did, searching for a Prince Charming, turns out I was looking for strength in all the wrong places;

my happily-ever-after came to me in the form of two computers, an amplifier, and some brain wave sensors. And finally, I no longer needed to be saved.

Question: How do you heal a child?
Answer: By not seeing them as broken.

Question: Must I be Dr. Lovass or Dr Greenspan or Bears and Samahria Kaufman?
Answer: No! Just be you with their conviction.

Question: Does everyone need a knight in shining monitor?
Answer: No! Not everyone, but, the healing is made easier and, especially if your child is autistic, easier is a good thing. Besides in all likelihood there's something inside you that you can heal too. I mean really, which one of us isn't just a little bit crazy… unusual… weird… awesome… special… unique?

CHAPTER FOUR

Put the Oxygen
Mask on You First

Mary, a lanky nine-year-old, is autistic and has very little language. When I first met her about two years ago, her mom and dad had invited me to teach them how to play with her. They very quickly bought the neurofeedback equipment after hearing of my success with this therapy through another family I was working with. So, given their trust in that friend's recommendation, the many unsuccessful approaches they'd already tried as well as their intense desire to help Mary, they invested thousands of dollars in the equipment, even though up until that moment they had never seen it used on their child.

Like many parents, Mary's were extremely techno-phobic and nervous about working on their daughter's brain. I asked a series of intake questions while assuring them that the therapy was safe. Then I hooked them up to the equipment by placing sensors on their heads, one parent at a time. I watched their brain wave activity generating from various locations and made mini maps of what was going on inside their heads. During the intake both parents said they were suffering from anxiety. Mom admitted to panic attacks that kept her housebound for long periods of time. As often happens with families, alcohol had become part of their support network. For mom it was a

"Phew! I made it through another day!" type of nightly relief. For dad it was more of a weekend retreat into calmness.

This family allowed their daughter to take the lead. While to some outsiders it may have looked as if they were letting their daughter run the house, it was actually one of the more positive things they did for her. Like a Native American medicine woman with a basket full of healing herbs, Mary reached for foods that cleansed, chelated (a means of removing heavy metals), improved her immune system, helped mylinate her axons (think of it as the insulation on the wiring in the brain), and aided her digestion. She ate things like coconut oil, raw onions, anchovies, chives, and garlic cloves. They were an instinctive family, so even though the parents were perplexed they joined their daughter and ate what she ate, all the while searching to understand why. They learned a lot from this exploration. This is one of the gifts of autism. It goes hand in hand with another gift: learning to get comfortable with confusion. Life is confusing. Autistic children are the epitome of confusing, so living with autism requires learning to live within the cacophony. And then make sense of it anyway.

Mary was extremely affected by sensory issues, her vision appeared to have depth oscillations, she loved to tap and throw oversized foam letters, and spent most of her time naked. In fact, one of my favorite memories of this family was when they explained how Mary had spent mealtimes during the first few years often sitting on the table surrounded by unusual foods. They smiled at the memory and called her their naked little centerpiece. We (parents of autism) are a strange brood. I like to think it's because we have been forced by life to assess what is really important, like prioritizing a happy child over a socially appropriate one. Lucky us.

Mary responded well to the neurofeedback becoming happier and easier to play with, though it took me all day to convince her to try it. My visit lasted three days. During that time I trained the family in how to use the equipment, got to know everyone's brains, and designed protocols. As I was getting ready to leave, though, I noticed what appeared to be a look of wide-eye terror cross both parents' faces. To make them feel more comfortable, I instructed them not to do neurofeedback on their daughter but to only treat themselves for the first few months.

They did… tentatively. After some success, however, they quit using the equipment and began trying other therapies. Two years later they called me and said they were ready to try again. Mary had recently become violent after being exposed to nitrous oxide during elective dental surgery. Mary's parents said they had changed a lot during those two years. They were now comfortable with the confusion but tired of not being informed when their child was at risk of a reaction. More importantly, they wanted to have a tool to use to help her whenever things went awry. They were determined to take charge of their daughter's healing. We set a date for my return and I suggested they resume treating themselves.

Note: Chemicals/intrusive situations and autism are touchy combinations so always be careful. It's common in autistic individuals to have extreme reactions to medical events. According to autism specialist Dr. Philip DeMio, children with autism should not be exposed to several common types of anesthesia, with nitrous oxide being one of them. Of course, that doesn't mean the nitrous oxide caused Mary's violence. After all, she was also exposed to fluoride and other drugs and chemicals during her dental surgery. Besides, for Mary (and many autistic individuals) this type of reaction wasn't unique to dental surgery. For example, she didn't receive nitrous oxide when she was in the hospital for ear infections. Instead Mary received a spinal tap, steroids, and antibiotics. She became even more violent after that bout. Hence I repeat chemicals (like medicine), intrusive situations, and autism are touchy combinations.

The first thing I confirmed for myself when I arrived was that Mary's parents were indeed different. They were easy about all their new choices, happy with their employee (a helper-friend for Mary), and familiar enough with the equipment to really learn what I was teaching them. Alcohol was no longer their only respite (possibly due to the effects of their own neurofeedback and/or other positive influences in their life). Whatever the reason, they seemed to be more available to each other and more able to embrace novel ideas as they supported their child.

Mary came down the stairs. She had grown taller, even more beautiful, and still had very little language. Her mom and dad and Mary's new helper-friend were all eager to learn what I had to teach and wanted very much to run the equipment. This time it was easy to get Mary to sit and allow me to put wires on her head. She used the neurofeedback equipment like a pro. It was almost as if she'd been waiting for her parents to help themselves enough so that she could have her turn. And maybe she had been.

Three months after that visit, I received this email:

Hi Lynette,

Mary's doing well! It seems like she's growing up and maturing before our eyes. Good sleep/good mood through most of the days. She will sometimes break down around bedtime, but not too big a deal and brief. This after-noon she helped me wash the car out in the front yard, and we've been playing with water balloons in the front of the house. That's a really big deal since she used to take off to the neighbor's yard and either eat their flowers or climb their trees. She has been great, even when I leave her to come inside to fill up another balloon with instructions to "wait right here." We're very proud of her.

She's up at the neuro computer right now and wants to do a second session. She accidentally pulled the sensor cables from the little shirt-cable unit. Does it attach all the way on the opposite side of the fiber-optic cable? That would be port "A". I think that's right, but I guess I wasn't paying as much attention as I thought!!

Hope you're in good shape and things are going well.

Thanks – Joan

The best part is: I've begun to take emails like this one for granted because I get so many of them, from so many moms. In fact I expect them.

Here is another more recent example:

(This mom is not writing in her mother tongue)

Oh, my dear, Lynette,

Thank you SOOO much. Your email made me cry last night and I really needed that for days, but just couldn't cry. So it was good.

Today I did neurofeedback for Philip in the morning. He was very upset because of his stuffy nose and sat waiting for his brain game through needing to start computers all over again. All with sensors ready and just a promise for the game. His point are f3-f4 and numbers were: 0-4= 28.1, 4-9= 17.9, 9-12= 9.9, 16-38= 24.5

He got upset towards the end of his fifteen minutes (I think because his nose started running more) and then his numbers were: 0-4= 37.3, 4-9= 22.0, 9-12= 11.9, 16-38= 22.7

He was great today!!! We went to two parks and not only he actually left the car, but he ran to the playgrounds, climbed high ladder, etc. He even tried sliding head first on a little slide—something I remember him doing shortly before he started having autistic symptoms and then never again. His looks and non-verbal communication was great. For the first time today afternoon I was just sitting on a bench and watching BOTH my kids happily playing by themselves AND coming to me to share some "news". How lovely.

As for me I planned to do my session in the afternoon, but I always plan for me but never do which is too bad because then I forget how good it works and don't do for Phillip. Well today when I took Philip to the park in the morning, I bumped my head into a metal bar over a big slide. It was quite a bump, because I was sitting under it without noticing it and was about to stand up fast when I felt it on the top of my head. I felt like fainting and a bit nauseated, then a big headache for some time. I also realized it probably messed a lot with my brain waves because I was suddenly not stressed.

Now if you'd ask me, I would say I'd rather do half an hour of beeping than one bump in a head. But who knows if I would do my session without it? Maybe I'd find a reason not to do it again and so God took over and made me hit my head? I was really on the edge with all those stress symptoms I had for weeks. So I hit my head and remember what it feels like to not stress and that that is what the neurofeedback does for me. So when the stress came back I did my session and while now I'm blissfully calm, just with little headache by the bump and some discomfort when I'm outside. But, gosh, maybe if I did my session BEFORE the park I would see that damn metal bar??? :)

Love, XXXXX

P.S. I have to tell you that too: yesterday we were watching with Philip your video and then that little piece on your website of "Learn with Lynette". Shortly after Philip came to me to the kitchen, took my hand, lead me to his room and closed the door, then came to me, hugged and looked at me smiling like saying "Here, I'm ready for the work." I was amazed by how many word approximations he made then during just twenty minutes we were playing!! He even allowed me to open his mouth for making "o" sound. And he was so happy! And all of that after I talked to his speech therapist in the morning about the fact that after two months he doesn't say anything during her sessions and her saying she has no way to teach him words because he doesn't pay attention. So I know that it works, but right now I am stuck since I have no energy to do what I finally KNOW works... Anyway, just wanted to tell you that at least for us you are a pure magic :) Maybe you could think of making a DVD for autistic kids to watch so that they become as eager to learn as Philip does :) It does make a BIG difference for me for sure, as he is so willing to practice. So today with me he talks more than all the days with the speech therapist.

Phillip's mom and Mary's parents are not dissimilar from DW's. In all these cases the real help begins when the parents help themselves. Recently, I was chatting with DW's mom at the end of one of our consults. She mentioned that she and her husband had looked back over all the therapies they had chosen through the years and had concluded that the only two things that had had any real impact were neurofeedback and home schooling. "The best part is when he's too upset to learn I just hook him up and help him balance. Thirty minutes later he's happy enough to try again."

I loved hearing her say that because it was one of my favorite things about neurofeedback for Dar: I could help him in the moments when he needed it most. At present Dar is the reason I stay motivated, the reason I am always trying to learn more about brain and behavior. However, though Dar keeps me motivated now, and was the reason I first sought out neurofeedback, in all honesty, most of my motivation to stay at it during those challengingly steep-learning-curve days of seeking to read brainwaves, came from wanting to help myself:

Around the time Dar was starting neurofeedback, his therapist suggested I might benefit from a little as well. At the time I was popping caffeine pills to the tune of four a day and washing them down with a pot or two of coffee. For me to stay focused and/or come out of my brain to converse required Herculean effort. For years the only way I could pull myself out of whatever daydream I found myself cemented into while my children tugged on my shirt and called "Mom! Mom!

Mom!" was to imagine a little cartoon character running up a long and winding road in my head—when he got to the chimney in my skull he would pop out and I would say "What?" This usually took about a minute from the time my child said "Mom!" to the moment when I would answer the call. My slow responding style had long been the mom joke in the house. My daughters would say "I say 'Mom!' and then I go to the bathroom, get a snack, clean my room—well not that part—I just go to the bathroom, get a snack, return to her side and THEN she says 'What?'" It was funny but it was also true.

I remember one day I was on my way to pick up one of my daughters. I was really struggling with that low-frequency brain wave zoned-out thing. (Brain waves come in a variety of frequencies. Too many of the low ones leave you feeling, well, slow). In many ways it felt as if my neurons were smoking pot. Anyway, I saw my daughter at the corner waiting for me. I would have pulled over to pick her up but my brain kind of went off line for a moment and I drove past her. After mumbling a few expletives, I turned around and headed back in her direction. But, like I said, I was really struggling to stay focused so once again when I got close to the corner where she was impatiently tapping her foot, I fell back into my brain and passed her. At this point my daughter was shouting "ARRGGG!!!" and flailing angrily in my direction, so perhaps avoidance is why I drove past her two more times. Eventually I pulled a u-turn and began to pass her again. BANG! She'd thrown a really big rock at the van. That got my attention, so I hit the brakes. She got in and was just annoyed enough to be snippy. Good news for both of us as her anger kept me alert enough to be safe as I drove away.

OK, suffice to say, I probably shouldn't have been driving before neurofeedback. But what could I do? I had kids to taxi. (wink I think) That kind of negligent thinking is what I mean when I say, "Put the oxygen mask on yourself first." My focus issues put my children in danger. While I thought I was putting their needs before mine by going to get them, the fact is I was too exhausted to drive and treating their safety as secondary.

I have spent my life knowing I was depressed and there was something wrong with me. But whenever I tried to talk to anyone about it, they told me I was being a suck or too sensitive. Thus, it was very validating for me to hear the therapist essentially say, "Yep—it's official—

you're a weirdo." It was a beautiful relief to find out that my quote unquote dissatisfied daydreams were based in something as tangible as my physical being. It was so much better than thinking it was all in my thinking and that I was immoral or thoughtless or stupid—or whatever other kind of *yadayadayada* was in my head to fuel my self-hatred. It was a relief. But it was only a relief because at the same time that I found out I was "officially weird" I was also shown a modality to make it better: A disability without a solution—that's just a handicap. I was lucky. I got to stop avoiding handling life by becoming able to handle the parts of life I had previously avoided. So, I stopped avoiding as I stopped searching… and searching… and searching… for a Prince to save me from my misery—because I was no longer miserable—because I'd found what I'd been looking for: my Prince Charming in the form of video games that change brain waves which allowed me to restructure the very physiology of my mind's CPU. I was lucky.

I remember driving home from my fourth session and Dar's twelfth session of neurofeedback. It occurred to me that the war against the pain of autism was over—I'd found the key—to my children's brains and mine. I was filled with awe. I turned to my son and said, "Dar it gets to be easy." I thought a moment and said, "Now all I have to do is learn neuroanatomy" Dar took my hand, smiled, and said "yef." That was a big deal at the time.

CHAPTER FIVE

The History of Change

or

How Does It Work? Not in a Vacuum!

Before I give you an overview of what neurofeedback is and how it works, let me explain that in my experience the children who travel the farthest in their healing are the ones whose entire families do the therapy. Best-case scenario is when parents treat themselves, learn about brain behavior, and let me guide them in the use of the equipment. There are several reasons for this. I'll cover two. First, since autism is a physiological whole-brain disorder with genetic components to its creation, it's not surprising that family members of autistic children are often riddled with "stuff" seen as smaller, less all-encompassing disorders (possibly subsets contained within the problem of autism itself). Common to the families I've worked with are things like Dyslexia, Attention Deficit Hyperactivity Disorder, Sensory Integration Dysfunction (aka Sensory Processing Disorder), Seizure Disorders, Bipolar Disorder, Cerebral Palsy, Parkinson's, Neuronal Migration Disorder, and Obsessive Compulsive Disorder. (I am focusing here on disorders of the brain only, but it is important to note that it is also common to find physiological issues like—but not limited to—thyroid problems, gastric issues, parasites, yeast overgrowth, toxic overload, asthma, and allergies). Given these far-reaching family challenges and understanding that people see life through the lens of their disorders, it's easy to comprehend why group healing is a good idea. The closer everyone gets to "neuro-typical" (whatever that might be), the more common ground they will have with each other and the world around them. Thus, life will be easier. (Though some would argue against this, I believe easier is better.)

Neurofeedback is a wonderful, non-judgmental way (because it's about brain wave behavior instead of the morality of behavior) to help people bring their brains into balance so that they can enjoy life and all its possibilities through the clearer lens of living in a less overwhelmed state. It is a healing therapy that calls the brain to change the way it functions. And as the family heals, they become more aware of the fact that healing is possible. The sameness of the journey between parent and child is what informs and uniquely separates the parent from the practitioner. I believe it's this special insight that graduates parents into the role of expert. They (not only the parents but the entire family unit) simply know more about each other's idiosyncrasies because they share them. Thus, it is best when they seek outside opinion while willingly walking the path of change together. It puts us professionals in the mental health field where we belong, as consultants for the cause of wellness.

Second is the very real problem-reinforcing issue of "sick person personality" (along with all the roles that are played out in order to uphold it). This is a scenario that evolves in any type of group, professional or otherwise, wherein one person is seen as the problem to solve. Such a viewpoint indicates to the person that he or she is a problem, and being a good listener the brain then continues to make it so for everyone. Once this dance is done enough times, all the people involved begin to define themselves by it. Even if they don't like the dance they are doing, most people do it anyway because at least they know the steps. Breaking up this cat's cradle of dependency is imperative for optimum healing. A common scenario that helps folks to hide from any awareness of being stuck in a repetitious cycle by creating the appearance of movement is what I call the treading-water technique of sabotage. What generally happens in this case is that the progress has a ceiling—a place where no one is comfortable to go beyond. Teachers or family members inadvertently reintroduce an old issue effectively backing the child up and putting everybody back into the dance they already know how to do. Thus it is that they are able to travel the same path, to the same point, over and over again and again.

OK! OK! Sounds like my marrying history (blink blink the two-eyed wink) and my problems with Dar. (wide-eyed serious stare) Dar and I did this dance countless times until I learned to raise the ceiling and expect more from us. Thus it is that I am complicit in his speed of healing. But for now let's look at a different family (Phew! there's only so much confessing a parent/professional—even a foolishly honest one like me—wishes to do).

Sarah was a chubby little loved-to-play-dress-up four-year-old. She had stopped screaming for everything and was doing amazingly well and playing the role of neuro-typical. For example, she was enjoying her ballet class and following directions (except of course during those several moments per class when she just had to spin, leap, or floor writhe because it felt so beautiful she just wanted everyone to see). Her mom knew I was going to suggest growing the possibilities and putting Sarah into other classes. Mom began to lecture Sarah all the way to dance class—"Be good! Stand still! Follow directions and above all else DO NOT DO YOUR OWN THING!" —and Sarah began to scream all the way to ballet. Suddenly I wasn't suggesting that we add more classes but that we go back to the beginning and start again... until I noticed the pattern. Once I explained what was happening, we avoided Mom's knee jerking back into old behaviors by having Dad take Sarah to class. It worked. Sarah calmed down. So we kept it that way until Sarah was well into the next level and going to camp. Of course, there were new problems to solve but at least they were outside the old circle of possibilities.

I've seen this cycle over and over again when working with behavior, speech, bonding, cognitive learning, and repetitive play. (In fact, when you think about it, the cycle itself is like making it so that the child's environment models her own version of circuiting into repetitive play.) When all the members do neurofeedback on themselves, as well as the primary client within the group, these cycles are much more easily broken apart and redefined. This is partly because neurofeedback helps the feelings of stress dissipate making parents and professionals more open to, and able to learn from, new ways of thinking.

Sarah's folks train all four immediate family members and some extended family as well. They are a perfect illustration of that genetic connection point because both children were autistic, Mom had dyslexia, Dad had anxiety just like Grandma, and they all had gastric issues. Mom's dyslexia manifested by having the letters and numbers appear in the wrong order. She had gone through the first years of school being considered retarded and often overprotected her children for fear that their childhood would resemble hers. She had never been able to read a chapter book, and from the way she described her difficulties, I suspect she also had Irlen Syndrome (numbers and letters dancing about and then running off the page). We designed some neurofeedback therapy choices based on neuroanatomy, Mom's cognitive and emotional strengths and weaknesses, and her desires for what she would like to change. We did not make the choices based on her diagnosis.

Six months (of sporadic treatment) later she called babbling with excitement. "I read a whole book! Lord Of the Rings! It's a hard book too. I read it faster than my husband. Oh, I just love you. I couldn't believe it. I could hold the picture in my head and follow the story. I could actually see it. It was so fun. Lynette, if this can fix me and my problems, it'll definitely help the kids. I can't believe it! Hey, lets fix my OCD (Obsessive Compulsive Disorder) next." Interestingly enough, most of her OCD symptoms were already gone; she'd just been so excited by the changes in her dyslexia she hadn't noticed.

Everything was going smoothly for this family: They all responded quickly. Mom stopped checking the locks. Dad stopped yelling. Their son went from wild to well behaved in two months, and Sarah began to speak more understandably. They had changed with such ease that the next time I saw them I suggested they not spend the money on my visits and just use me as a phone resource. That's when they realized that they were in new territory. And that's when (possibly afraid to drop the role of having me as a part of the story) they started to tread water again.

Two months later two things changed (sometimes bringing in the new is a way of bringing in the old behaviors). Insurance covered gastric tests. Since the entire extended clan was cursed by problems in that area, Sarah's parents decided to have their children checked. The reasoning for this, they said, was to feel like good parents, cover all their bases, and basically "do it all" in order to end their story quicker (This "do every therapy in existence" approach is never an action taken with my advice, though many of my families try it anyway). The findings of the tests appeared dramatic. There were pictures of ulcers and pictures of white coatings on the linings of the stomach wall. But, all drama aside, the tests only verified what is already known about what is likely to be found when looking inside the stomach of a child who has autism. Even so, the diagnosticians treated the findings as grave and stated that they'd never seen anything like it before. (Perhaps they weren't used to working with autism.) The parents were terrified. They immediately put their children on the meds that were prescribed and sat back and watched for pain. Their vigilant fear set them on edge. They began to fight daily. The kids shrank back into themselves the minute their parents went back to seeing them as sick. It appears that their parents saw them that way and so they were.

I am not suggesting the emotional climate of the parents was the sole factor in the children's changes—far from it. The new meds, the stress of the trip, and the tests themselves all contributed. But I am suggesting it was a part of the story. Whatever the cause, I do know that their regression was immediate and quite severe. A phone call later, I was back in the story. I came for an outreach, took a deep breath, rolled up my sleeves, and began to mediate the milieu. I convinced Mom and Dad to throw out the new meds and all the new supplements that had been purchased in order to counteract the new side effects the new meds had caused. It was agreed that home remedies and simplicity might be more beneficial. We agreed on regimens of algae (for nutrition and chelation), strong probiotics (for candidas and beneficial stomach bacteria), baking soda and Epsom salt baths (to pull toxins through the skin), a heavily laden with B's multi vitamin that included brain function herbs, flax seed oil (to repair damaged nerves, promote myelination and reduce inflammation) and that's all. I studied everyone's brain-wave patterns, did several sessions a day, and taught behavioral management and family dynamics. Once everyone was on the same page, the children calmed, the parents fighting receded and everyone's stress was eradicated. It had taken three days. (Moral: be careful what you buy into and never buy in out of fear.)

By the way, the children's stomachs stopped hurting within three weeks. However, the parents have decided not to do any more tests for now, so at the time of this writing we don't really know if the problems are gone or just lying dormant. At any rate there is still more to do than spend time worrying about what isn't actually bothering anyone.

Every time I teach a group of people how to stop limiting a child's growth by not playing to the already established roles within that group, I learn how to change a similar thing in my own life. Teaching others teaches me because seeing through someone else's eyes gives me a vantage point I didn't already have. One of the mom's I helped had a way of blurting out every time I said something that she hadn't already thought of: "Oh my God! You don't know what you don't know!" And she was right. You don't! The truth is, for complete healing (especially where major brain disorders are concerned), everyone involved has to change and grow beyond anything they were previously able to conceive. This is because our conceptions come from our vision, which is itself limited by the scope of our disorders. To be specific, for complete healing all members of the group must change their beliefs, their behaviors, and their tool chest of knowledge. Sarah's family is just another example of DW's family, Mary's family, and mine.

So what is neurofeedback? As I said before, it's biofeedback for the brain. There, now you know. (wink) If you are like me you heard of biofeedback long before you ever heard of neurofeedback. But, of course, that doesn't mean you know what it is.

Teaching you everything there is to know about neurofeedback is beyond the scope of this book. Such an endeavor would require volumes upon volumes. And though I love talking about the power and possibilities of this exciting therapy, this section of the book is mainly intended to help you understand first autism and then neurofeedback's applicability in helping with the disorder. However, I do want to at least arm you with a general understanding of the technology.

Let's begin with what it's not. Neurofeedback is not an intrusive therapy wherein electricity or radio waves or magnetic influences are entering the brain and forcing a change. Neurofeedback is just an information system teaching to your neurons in the very moment that they fire. It is operant conditioning for the brain, and its magic comes from the speed of the delivery system: The time lapse between neuronal activity and computer response is only a handful of milliseconds.

This method of giving brain direction was discovered in the early sixties when Barry Sterman was a scientist at the Sepulveda Veteran's ™ Administration Hospital in Los Angeles. Using the basic technique that was first discovered by Joe Kamiya, working at the University of Chicago and the University of California San Francisco, Sterman made a fortuitous discovery. While observing the EEG of several cats, he identified a particular EEG bursting response at a specific frequency whenever the cats were at rest (as in calmly preparing to pounce on a mouse). The rhythm was localized to the sensorimotor cortex; and since they (the cats) tended to generate more of this bursting activity (at least in this particular location) at times of calm alertness than humans did, it appeared worth studying. Given the events that followed I imagine Sterman wondered if the cats could be trained to make an even more robust amount of this brain-wave activity. Most likely he neither knew if that were possible nor what effect such a change would have. Perhaps, because he was a curious man (not historical fact just my assumption given that he was a scientist doing experiments), he decided to try operant conditioning the cats' brains. In order to do that he gave the felines chicken broth mixed with milk whenever they fired more of the desired brain-wave frequency in the area over the sensory motor cortex. The result was: YES! The cats could definitely change their brain waves to get more chicken-milk. (Interestingly, the cats' sleep behavior changed. What later came to be known as a neurofeedback effect had been successfully demonstrated.) Now that the question was answered, the experiment was over. A little curiosity had been satisfied, but it is likely that—for the moment—Sterman had no real concept of the extent to which he had changed the course of those cats (and many people's lives).

Cut to a few months later. The fortuitous event happened when Barry Sterman was asked to test the toxic effects of rocket fuel at very low concentrations. First he chose his test subjects—you guessed it—cats! One of the questions the experiment was attempting to answer was: How toxic can the emissions get before said emissions induce seizures? For a number of reasons some of the same cats that had previously been trained via their EEG were recruited into this study. All the cats behaved similarly after the toxic substance was injected into their gut—at least until about an hour later when some of the cats went into seizure, and others either seized only much later or not at all. The cats were now in two distinct groups rather than one. Why? I imagine that Sterman then examined the lab records in search of what made these cats different from the rest of the population. The answer: All of the cats that had been more resistant to seizure onset had been involved in the original chicken-milk-special-sensory-motor-strip-bursting-brain-wave -frequency-increasing experiment.

So it appeared that neurofeedback could be clinically useful, at least for cats.

Voila! That electrical frequency grouping of 12 – 15 hz (or 13 – 16 hz depending, on whom you ask) was given its own name: SMR AKA (Sensory Motor Rhythm). Actually it is only called SMR if the activity is located in the sensory motor strip; otherwise this frequency group is referred to as low beta. Neurofeedback for the application of creating a stronger more seizure-resistant brain was born.

Since its inception a lot of good studies have been done about the amazing effectiveness of neurofeedback therapy on seizure disorders (many autistic kids have seizures or develop seizure activity in their teens) ADHD, anxiety disorders, and even a few smaller studies are emerging in regards to autism. It is a very exciting and liberating healing therapy that has fought a slowly won, uphill battle in order to be respected by the medical community. This difficulty in gaining acceptance stems from many places and is reflective of the issues I discussed earlier in regards to groups that reinforce problems in order to continue to use the tools they are familiar with. It's understandable since even if your doctor learned about neurofeedback in college and/ or kept abreast through continuing education and science articles in the subsequent years of his practice, in order to use it he would have to seek yet more training and even more equipment than setting up his office had originally required. But he is already able to prescribe medicine (which he probably believes in, otherwise why would he have trained in it) and help you that way. This choosing whether or not to use what is easily available is the same dilemma facing parents as they rummage through the over four hundred therapies touting helpfulness in the world of autism. Sometimes the choice is made by access or popularity rather than efficacy. Like many professionals in the field, your doctor will often rely on the tools he has and knows best. More often than not, out comes the prescription pad.

In addition, the job of keeping up with medical advances is staggering even when keeping within one's own individual specialty. No practitioner (or parent) can actually be expected to understand it all, especially since most MDs trained in the formal school system for medical professionals under the tutelage of professors who trained in the formal school system years before. Keeping textbooks and teachers current is a much-documented problem and is made even more problematic by the amazing speed of scientific discovery as regards the physiology of brain behavior in the past fifteen years. So very often what the young doctor is learning is no longer true. Fortunately, the present-day ability to search for information quickly offsets that a little. However, even if the doctor's training included the most up-to-date knowledge when she was training, if she doesn't constantly seek to embrace new information she can quickly fall behind. In fact, last week my continuing education instructor said that doctors forget eight percent of what they learned in med school. So keep in mind, for the most part, your doctor only knows what he knows based on what he's been able to use.

None of these statements, however, sufficiently excuse the lack of knowing about neurofeedback, especially given that it has been effectively treating brain disorders since the early sixties. That fact alone should make it stand out as valuable enough to remember. Perhaps, in this case, there are other more insidious reasons for the "gaining recognition neurofeedback challenge". Consider mood regulation drugs that help people function and cope. One would think neurofeedback would trump these medicines and be first in the lineup of treatment options since it treats the problem often eliminating the need for medication and/or medical assistance. However, that's not the case. These pharmaceuticals are more popular than ever.

Some of my conspiracy-theorist associates believe that our lack of popularity as practitioners of the brain has been orchestrated by pharmaceutical companies—controlling the industry in order to prevent a foreseeable drop in their profits when several of their products become obsolete in our hands. Perhaps! Even probably! However, all this being (possibly) the case, I still think the stronger resistance comes from a fear of change and extra work. Ironically our brain is set up to resist the position of learner since it wants to be in control of its environment and learners are at the hands of their teachers. Thus, once the studies forced upon us for societal success are complete, most folks want to maintain position and not drop back to the role of student. This is often our want even when we know avoiding learning is not the correct approach since remaining current solidifies success. Hence, ashamed to see ourselves in the light of the shirker, we hide our fear behind a cloak of suspicious nature. And so, basically, for most people, the neurofeedback stories of healing so many diversely different brain disorders seems too good to be true. This is especially relevant to the opinions of much of the medical community who, without training in neurofeedback, are only armed to understand impacting mood regulation through the use of drugs, physical and psychological life changes, or maybe a lottery win!

It's a bit of a Catch 22. To gain mainstream acceptance, neurofeedback therapy needs the professional endorsement of doctors since so many people trust and seek their doctor's approval before buying into mainstream or alternative treatments. Given that our culture lives in a time of commercialism, that's a good thing since we need someone to have some sort of expertise in order to separate the gold from the pyrite or the snake oil from the venom itself. [Of course it is my hope that when attempting to help your autistic child, you will buy neither the snake oil nor the snake venom, as neither is likely to be beneficial. However, in this world of poison versus placebo, at least the snake oil could induce a healing. (wink)]

Fortunately, the expert we must resource is quickly becoming "us." Due to the range of medical information that we can so easily find with one click of the search button on our computer screen, we are realizing that our doctors don't always have all the answers or even the right ones. This is not a flaw in your doctor; it's a sign of the times. We are becoming responsible for our own health and research. This is a learning curve that I believe will ultimately benefit everyone, even though at the moment, it is somewhat confusing and runs the risk of leading us to panic. The truth is we have always been our own best experts because it is we who know how we feel, and it is we who can follow the evidence of our symptoms when presented with the possible causes. It is also we who are our own worst enemy. People can—and often do—manifest every symptom they read about. And since most of us do our research on the Internet, it's important to remember that it's as easy to put things on the Internet as it is to find them. Thus we must also become experts at separating the trash from the treasure even inside what appears like the scientific writings of analysts, doctors, and the like. With no need to satisfy an editor/ publisher team in order to be published culturally, we have contaminated our system of checks and balances. This reality allows many minds to share their thoughts often before they've been fully thought out. Conversely, it also means minds can share fresh new ideas while they are still brilliant and have not yet been watered down by the very system of checks and balances to which I have already referred.

Regardless of the accidental benefits of solitary approaches, more minds seeking to converse on and solve a problem is generally a better, more efficient approach and helps to prevent a constant need to reinvent the wheel. The best-case scenario is when we work as a team with our practitioners because they know what we don't and vice versa. Handled well, our Internet searches and self-education can turn the medical field into a team of consultants instead of God-like representatives of absolute knowledge.

However, be warned, historically we as a people have always resisted change, and the medical community is definitely no exception. A prime example of this happened many years ago (beginning in 1840). A young doctor by the name of Ignaz Semmelweis noticed that women giving birth in the maternity wards of the Vienna hospital he worked in were three times more likely to die if a medical student delivered the baby than if a midwife did. He studied the habits of the student doctors and realized that they were moving between rooms, first performing autopsies, and then delivering babies. Semmelweis realized that something on the hands of the medical students was being transported from the cadaver to the laboring woman and infecting her womb. The result was a case of childbed fever. He came up with an outrageous concept: hand washing. He ordered all personnel to wash their hands, and the mortality rate dropped to a miniscule one percent. Despite this, his story is one of a man challenged beyond his own ability to cope. In following his quest trying to effect change and save lives, his reputation was sullied. He was ridiculed and pushed out of the medical community. The outrage directed at him remained throughout his entire career, even though he proved time and again with verifiable data and good strong hard facts that washing reduced the incidence of illness and death. He saved the lives of hundreds of patients in each hospital that he worked in. Still he was ostracized. Eventually he began speaking out in a brasher and brasher manner. This was perceived as an embarrassment to the field. He was tricked into meeting a trusted colleague at an asylum. He was detained and the guards beat him badly enough to cause an injury, which resulted in an infection. Shortly thereafter he died as a result of Streptococcus Pyogenes (a germ whose spread is prevented by hand washing). Had Semmelweis been a woman giving birth, the cause of his death would have been labeled childbed fever.

Semmelweis wasn't the only doctor in the 1800's struggling to change the germ-spreading habits of his contemporaries. Dr. Lister was also traveling and teaching that hand washing and the spraying of anti-septic solutions would greatly reduce the risks of infection and death in a variety of circumstances. He too was struggling against opposition but eventually—after moving to London in 1877—he began to estab-lish some credibility and in 1883 was knighted by Queen Victoria. This recognition of authority helped Lister's career and the cause of sterilizing operating rooms tremendously. To date it is the more politi-cally savvy Lister, not Semmelweis, who is credited with the science of hand washing. However, Semmelweis did manage to receive a measure of fame, albeit posthumously. A reflex was named after him.

Appropriately, the Semmelweis reflex is not a physiological reflex, but a metaphor for certain types of human behavior character-ized by the reflex-like rejection of new knowledge whenever it contra-dicts entrenched norms, beliefs, or paradigms. Why is human nature designed with such a reflex? And more specifically, why would doctors refuse to do anything as easy as wash their hands? My guess is guilt, aka a negative emotion useless in proactive change. It's actually easy to understand since most of us have done it (avoided knowing some-thing because we didn't want to retroactively become responsible for the actions we've already taken). Imagine being a doctor and finding out that the last ten women who died at your unwashed hands did so simply because you were too shortsighted to notice the connection between the dead you were dissecting and the deaths you were infecting. Imagine facing each of their husbands, parents, and possibly surviving children to admit your mistake and change your ways. Would you do it? Would you want to know that you caused these deaths, deaths that could have been avoided simply by washing your hands? Possibly not!

Now imagine trying to embrace this new concept after you have already rejected it and then—in defense of that denial—dirty handedly delivered another baby who, because of you, will have to live without his mother. Human beings often employ the technique of anger and outrage when trying to avoid experiencing the pain of their complicity in an undesirable situation. We even have a saying for the behavior: the best defense is a good offense. This is the point wherein most people sit, digging and digging a deeper and deeper hole until it's too far to climb out of. Eventually they die. Thus, it takes a generation to effect radical change. This refusal to see is to blame for prejudicial acts, parental abuse, medical blunders, and much, much more. This is the reason for horrific acts that continue way beyond the moment of knowing.

Perhaps we should give ourselves some transitional leeway and understand that changing a lifetime of learning takes repetition and practice. We could consider this transitional period a "several strikes before you're out" approach to re-creation. It's an idea based on scientific thought: apparently it takes seven repetitions to get a new learning to stick in your head. Of course you can reject this concept, but that might mean you are suffering from the Semmelweis reflex! Oh, and since I've decided to embrace the idea, if you find this book redundant on any particular point, count the repetitions to see how important I considered the data to be.

So since, as a general rule, our ability to see or hear the truth of a situation is created by our beliefs about it, we often aren't able to take in any controversial evidence that something different is afoot unless it meets with our preexisting concepts on the subject. Thus different never is. How do we do it then? I believe change comes from growth. Instead of seeing differently in order to change our concepts, we see the same—only bigger. First we hold onto the old ideas and add some new ones, which once ours are at our disposal. We can now compare, blend, keep, or discard the parts that no longer work for us. In this way we are like all life, bringing into ourselves everything once it comes into our awareness. It is at that point that we choose whether to tread in the same water or create our waters anew. A better analogy might be to say it is at that point that we choose whether to live only as a caterpillar or to build a cocoon and transition into the butterfly.

Neither one is better, but in case you haven't noticed, butterflies have wings.

Of course for some people the wings are the problem. Wings effortlessly cover more distance than caterpillar legs do. In fact, being as slow as a caterpillar is no longer an option for the newly evolved butterfly. This fear of flying into new territory wherein one is alone and starting anew is probably why many of the parents I work with occasionally sabotage their children's progress. It's also why doctors sabotage their patients, teachers their students, and pushers their addicts. Each of these roles requires that the other "role players" maintain their place and continue to dance "the same" in order to continue to exist as what they already are. Thus, it is this molting season between caterpillar and butterfly concept that has me loving the moments when families reach for everything new regardless of the momentary results because it is a sign of change preparation.

The relevance to autism in this subject matter is that the inability for many people to see the already existing—or possibly evolving— butterfly within the caterpillar creates a constant challenge for folks with disabilities. This is especially true when, as a result of the disorder, the individual's outside appearance presents as different from the truth about that person's actual capabilities. Cerebral palsy, Huntington's disease, and autism are examples of disorders wherein the body movements and behavioral abilities belie the truth about the person within. An example of a way in which this has and does impact folks with disabilities occurred during the eighties and nineties and involves autism and its relationship with facilitated communication (a method of supporting the arm and applying resistance so that a person with difficulty controlling his body can stabilize the movement and rely on the gross motor system to type, very slowly). Facilitated communication was first introduced to the autism community in the early eighties after Arthur Schawlow, a Nobel-prize-winning physicist, used it with his autistic son.

Schawlow considered it useful. Stanford University took up the cause and became largely responsible for introducing it to the United States. In 1990—when Dar was nine years old—facilitated communication found its way to me. A professional in the field of behavioral sciences who was traveling around Canada, where I lived at the time, introduced me to the method. She was sharing the technique with parents and professionals. Since I purported over and over again that Dar could understand me and on occasion speak, and since he was virtually lacking in any fine-motor control, Dar was considered a prime candidate for the method. I was invited by the local parent relief center to come and try something "brand new" and exciting.

I had no idea what to expect, but if it was going to help my son I was up for it. I went to the center and met the woman. She explained things to me and then sat next to Dar with an alphabet board on the table between them. She explained why she was supporting my child's arm and that she was going to ask him a series of questions to which she already knew the answer. She asked him questions like "What color is this dot?" and then guided his hand to answer, "The dot is blue." The reasoning was that first she wanted him to know how to do it and also to get a sense of his motor functions. She asked about six of these obvious questions. Then as he gained confidence, she asked him something only Dar and I would know the answer to.

The answer she got from Dar via this pointing at letter after letter until they form words answering system was wrong. She asked him, "What did you have for breakfast?" He answered "Toast." The answer should have been "Porridge." And all I thought was, "Well, maybe he wishes it was toast." (Therein lies the difference between people who build capable children and those who do not. The ones who do, do because they chose to... believe... in butterflies.)

It seemed to me that every time she asked a question, the answer Dar gave had an element of possible truth. I figured her not influencing his arm was unlikely and decided they were probably coming up with close approximations to his truth combined with her thoughts. It reminded me of the Ouija board and the way that all the participants at the table always seemed to somehow have an effect on what was answered by the planchette: like a collective creation of communication. This, to me, did not render the experiment invalid, but rather meant that Dar was part of the equation. Oh Happy Day! I could see the possibilities and knew my life had just changed in some very fundamental way. I was AMAZED!

My mind was in a swirl of joyous thought. "What a great idea! Maybe he can! Of course he can! Why not? Thank you Universe!" When the woman asked my son if there was anything he wanted to tell me, he said "F-r-e-n-c-h... f-r-i-e-s." I definitely recognized those words as his greatest love. I stopped the whole thing and threw him in the car. We went to MacDonald's. I bought several containers of fries and babbled on and on with him about how much this would change his life if only he was willing to practice with me. What a different experience this communication specialist had blessed us with from the one wherein the guiding professional said he wasn't going to tell me how to "do it" because he didn't want me to try "it" at home! This woman, whose name I immediately forgot, was largely responsible for all the new possibilities fluttering in my heart. My son had a future, simply because someone had shared a concept. I was more than happy to take over from that point on. I got a napkin and wrote two words: yes and no. I steadied his arm and asked if he was ready to go.

I was completely stoked about communicating with my son. I couldn't get enough. And though each sentence was arrived at in a painstaking manner, we talked at length. I was mesmerized as he composed remarkable poetry and answered questions that shared insightful thoughts on life, love, and the dynamics of our family. Eventually my hyper-focused fascination on Dar's person-assisted, finger-pointing tongue had to end. I needed to make room for the rest of the children. I organized a scheduled time for our "talks" and created laminated alphabet boards for every room in the house. We moved into phase two: assimilation. It was his siblings' turn to support his arm and get some answers. Our lives were changed and—though the method turned out to be very problematic and was ultimately discarded—the beliefs it created about Dar from within our family were forever more bonded, respectful (one day he even brought up the shoulder squeezing memories and explained to me that he "c-a-n g-e-t f-o-r-k… s-o-m-e-t-i-m-e-s") and fully inclusive. I will lifelong remember the good works of that face-and-name-forgotten Nightingale of Speech. Since she merely passed the torch of communication to me and then moved on to teach others, she affected many. It is this model of reaching far and wide that I copied when I designed my career approach to working with and enlightening families.

Dar was selective about who could facilitate him. Initially he chose only me. However, more and more he would answer one and two word questions from family members and school helpers. This selectivity and need for support created enough of a disparity in how Dar appeared to function that the validity of his communication was at all times suspect: He told us what he wanted but always, always, always he needed support on his arm. More often than not, what he wanted seemed to reflect the desires of his arm steadying helper. In an attempt to help him gain more autonomous language, I went to a prosthetics place and had them build me a metal support that could vise grip onto any desk or table and would put resistance on Dar's arm as he tried to type. The new device was awkward and didn't have enough range of motion. You had to move it from station to station, Dar didn't seem to like the way it felt against his arm, and he still needed someone with him as an ATTA-BOY cheerleader because the task was so extremely difficult that he just wanted to quit. In addition, part of the technique in facilitated communication is to pull the arm back towards the body between each letter in order to place it back into a neutral position. This is done in order to help the "speller" reorient his/her hand/eye and also to diminish the odds against spastic movements and twitches causing accidental letter touches. The prosthetic did none of this. Thus, it didn't really work, though we certainly gave it "the old college try."

During this time period all kinds of autistic people were being introduced to the idea of facilitated communication. Shortly after facilitation was introduced to me, I was introduced to the history of using it with populations of non-verbal physically and emotionally challenged folks. It had begun in Australia in 1977, and I learned of it when I saw a dramatized biography about a young wheelchair-bound woman named Annie with cerebral palsy. She was extremely small (despite being an adult, Annie was only as big as a very young child), considered retarded, and living in an institution. Annie had little physical control over her body and was completely dependent on others for self-care and sustenance. (The fact that she lived in an institution was part of the reason she and many others were so small. The place was too under-staffed for anybody to feed her at a pace slow enough for her system to handle.) The movie begins on the day that Rosemary Crossley, a new nurse, comes to work on her ward.

Rosemary brought with her an observer's eye and the ability to follow up on clues in order to generate solutions. As a direct result of these skills and an openness to believe in the unseen possibilities they pointed to, Rosemary came to believe that Annie and about a dozen of the other residents were of normal intelligence. Their bodies just belied their ability. Initially she had Annie use her tongue to point at letters on a Ouija board. (Apparently, we all think of the same thing when it comes to communicating via invisible guidance of an unknown soul. You can see a similar technique in the movie *Awakenings*.) Rosemary created classroom-like programs for the residents and designed an answering system whereby she supported their arms. It actually looks more like a wrestling match as she tries to help them stretch their very spastic (tightly contracted muscles that can also twitch and spasm) arms. She used this facilitated communication technique to help them answer questions about the books like *War and Peace* that they read using a music-stand type of book holder with a mouth-driven page turner. Everything about this story is awe-inspiring. For me, several amazing points were brought up that have shaped my thinking ever since. For example, there is a scene wherein Rosemary is explaining why her "supposedly intelligent" CP ridden students, especially Annie, won't cooperate during rudimentary testing. She explains that they are insulted and also threatened by the whole testing procedure. I remember suddenly understanding the saying "a light bulb went on in my head." It never previously occurred to me that a person who lives in a state of constant misunderstanding might not have my burning desire to be understood. And in that moment, I realized that that burning desire was exactly that, my burning desire, not theirs. Given that autistic individuals are known for not being testable in any reliable manner, I felt as if I was being shown a clue. Maybe my children harbored a kind of love/hate relationship with the limitations that both their disorder and their social environment placed upon them. Maybe they were afraid to trust that we might see them any differently, afraid to pass and afraid to fail, in case they inadvertently confirmed what we already assumed to be true. Maybe they rejected testing out of self-defense as a way of gaining control in an uncontrollable situation. I had gained a new (possible) understanding of my sons and some of their behaviors. Annie's story brought up another heretofore concept I hadn't thought of before: when your outside separates your inside from the world you live in, you are forced to live in the inside which separates your life experiences from the life experiences of the people around you and—according to the outside world's definition of it— makes you crazy. How this concept was relevant in the movie was that Annie's constant defiance came from a place of not being motivated by the same rewards as her contemporaries. "You can't apply the way we think about things to the way Annie might think about things. Our way of looking at stuff is foreign to her," Rosemary explained. I imagined trying to motivate someone like Annie into learning to walk. She may accept my logic, but after years of riding in a chair she has likely built up her own set of beliefs about the plethora of advantages in having wheels. So, though she may think she wants to walk simply because I am convincing in my arguments and tell her she should, her life experience may say otherwise. Thus, she may not want it as badly as the person lifting her in and out of her chair wishes she would. I was blessed when Rosemary explained that any person living a life so locked up and dependent, so removed from the lives we live in and develop from, would lead to different experiences that then lead to different conclusions. Our conclusions are strongly influenced by the varying degrees of ability we each have in our physiological makeup with regard to thinking about such broad concepts in the first place—effectively leaving us in a world of thought that may not even remotely resemble the world within which we live. I was blessed, because these ideas of living separate from the culture around one, helped me to understand my sons' "unusualness" and maybe even a little bit more, my own.

My second to last life-changing understanding wasn't so much explained as modeled by the judge in the court case for Annie's coming out. According to the story someone in the hospital tried to smother Annie. Rosemary wanted to save her from the dangers of the hospital. She loved the spark of thought in this undersized young woman and wanted Annie to live with her. So, in 1979, Annie, who was by then an adult, brought an action of Habeas Corpus in the Supreme Court of Victoria. She won. Annie and Rosemary then wrote the book that became the movie that strongly impacted my children, the world of special education, and me.

In this memorable courtroom scene Rosemary was facilitating Annie. She was trying to help Annie prove that her grasp on reality and cognitive comprehension were great enough for her to be allowed to make her own choices and decisions. Before the judge could accept Annie's testimony, the technique of using facilitation itself had to be verified and Annie's testimony corroborated. The institution was refusing to accept the possibilities of the residents' abilities and denying all allegations of abuse and neglect. Rosemary was counting on her colleague, another nurse, to verify some of her own already shared testimony. The movie employs the usual devices for mounting tension as the clock ticks and the music throbs.

The nurse arrives. She testifies on Rosemary and Annie's behalf. Possibly because of this testimony, when the judge questions the young cerebral palsied woman, he does so with an unusual measure of patience and respect. Still, he needs proof that it is Annie and not Rosemary answering the questions. The judge tries to test the method, but instead of answering his questions Annie goes on long rampages—possibly for the benefit of the court audience—about the morality of the process and the inherent insult in testing her ability to think. This wonderful judge clears the courtroom of everyone but Annie. He lights up a smoke and talks to the CP woman about choosing her own fate and the fate of the nurse who loves her. He models the technique that I now successfully use with autism worldwide: He speaks to her like an equal and leaves the decision in her hands. Finished smoking the Judge gives Annie two secret words to spell and calls everyone into the court. She facilitates the correct words and wins the case.

But it was the scene on the court steps that helped me to understand a more perplexing type of human behavior than any of the ones already described: the aggravation of my neighbors. When the other nurse responded to Rosemary's gratitude her words cleared it all up for me. She said something to the effect of, "You make me so mad. I hate people like you. You come along and make everything different. The rest of us can barely make it through the day. We are just trying to do our jobs but you, you come along and see all these possibilities and follow up on all your ideas. If you are so capable, what does that make us? Just a pile of shit sitting in the sun." Her description fit me. I was the single mother of eight: six adopted, five special needs, four on the spectrum of autism, happy gung-ho anything is possible mom. What a relief! I had previously been frustrated wondering why everyone paid so much attention to what I was doing. And though I didn't like the answer, at least I understood: Some people figure themselves out through comparison. And I was a thorn in the side of many of the tired, worn-out, two-normal-children-only parents living on my street. Being me created a kind of jealous notoriety and was sort of like being Angelina Jolie… only without the Pitt… or the money… and OK, maybe I was just a little less beautiful… (tee hee!) The concept reminded me of the many jobs I'd had as a teenager when the other employees would resent me and in an attempt to defame my character call me "an eager beaver." As a teenager the name-calling worked to upset me because it meant I was too hard working and not very cool (of course it also meant I got the most tips so, cool or not, working hard was hard to give up). Now, as an adult, understanding the concept made the situation optional but my choice stayed the same. Personally, I see it as better to be busy with eagerness than overwhelmed by meagerness, so I maintain the pace. Besides, most of the time I didn't really mind being ostracized. Like I said, I was busy with eight children. Not having neighbors come over for coffee was kind of a relief. (wink)

Meanwhile the media was just beginning to help facilitate the facilitation movement when some unfortunate things began to happen. One of them was that all kinds of allegations of abuse, especially of a sexual nature, began to come forward. Even before facilitation, the number of nonverbal children that were believed to have been sexually molested was (and still is) staggering. On the other hand, these children were nonverbal so the figures weren't verifiable. Facilitation began to change all that. Complicating the picture though was the fact that, by nature, humans are very sensationalistic and quite often take their minds to tawdry thoughts of behaviors committed by others, possibly to feel superior by comparison. Thus, given that historically we tend to carry ourselves away into fabrication and assumption once we began to hunt witches, the facilitation movement was a scary one. The wheels of founded and unfounded gossip were greatly greased by the clucking tongues that spread the news. Limelight seekers took position looking to be heroes and hoping to facilitate the child who would make such a report. And suddenly all the parents and professionals working so hard to give these children language were at risk of being incarcerated by the very freedom they were trying to bestow.

Understanding the signs of sexual abuse is problematic at the best of times. It is especially so when dealing with disorders like autism that most often carry within them a sensory malfunction. Sensory disorders manifest as weird behaviors responding to, or not responding to, the stimulation of any or all of our five and possibly six senses. This translates into a lot of children walking around naked or playing with their feces or tasting, touching, and smelling everyone and everything that catches their attention. As a result many autistic children are kept from circulating with the population because of their parents' fears that the child's desire to self stimulate his or her groin on various inanimate objects might be misinterpreted (Cases in point: One of my sons liked to inappropriately embrace the shoes on the Ronald MacDonald statue while another chose nylon ski jackets as his sensory fixation.) Given that this sensory input seeking behavior is often a symptom of sexual abuse in neuro-typical kids but merely a symptom of the sensory aspects of their disorder in autistic children, assessing the likelihood of an incident using the same parameters and behavioral responses that are based on how a normal child would react is a set up for disaster. Such an approach to fact-finding is a scary response by the uninformed as regards the special needs population; it can get all kinds of people into unfounded trouble. And it did. After a while there were so many reports of abuse that the pendulum of belief in facilitation swung from amazement and support all the way over to suspicion and ridicule. And inside this evolution of either/or thinking, eventually the use of facilitated communication with autistic individuals began to die out. My family was caught up in the milieu from every single angle.

After I began facilitating with Dar I found myself thinking about his birth mother on a pretty regular basis. Ironically, right about then her lawyer located us and forwarded a letter from her. In the letter she updated Dar on his six siblings, her new marriage, and requested that he see her. Dar responded through facilitation: I supported his arm as he typed, "Don't write me. I don't want to see you. Did you think I only wanted to stay in bed and drink white stuff?" I sent the letter to a social worker representing the family, explained that the response was dubious given my involvement, and left the decision about what should be done next up to her.

For the next few weeks the memory of the condition Dar was in when he came home from visiting his mother on that empty-shell-of-a-boy-who-then-beats-his-face-with-a-toy-carpenter's-bench day kept crossing my mind. The social climate around facilitation was, on an almost daily basis, pointing out the fact that it only takes a suspicion told as a story to kill a reputation. (In fact, sometimes it only takes raising the subject matter to create the suspicion that leads to the damage.) And where Dar and his biological mom were concerned, the truth is I had no idea what equaled what. It was all rather confusing: By this time I knew that Dar could simply have been stoned, an opium affect his leaky gut caused his brain to experience in reaction to the casein, in the bottle upon bottle of milk she gave him. By this time I knew Dar may have been the one refusing to eat other foods because they were hard to digest and/or because in the same way that an alcoholic doesn't want to eat a meal so as not to dissipate the high he is getting, neither might Dar have wanted to dissipate the high his milk was giving him. And despite all that new—grounded in personal experience and emerging scientific data—awareness, I still thought of Dar's other mom primarily as having locked him away and left him to starve. In fact, I sometimes still tell the story as if it is a fact. Even though my suspicion is that, it was just a suspicion shared with me by one of the social workers.

The entire subject is reminiscent of a political race or hard-ball courtroom scene in a made-for-TV movie. It's like when rivals are racing to the finish line, and in an attempt to get ahead, use the method of mudslinging on their political opponents, or when a lawyer says something out of bounds and then immediately follows with a "Sorry Your Honor, withdrawn." Even if we disapprove of the methods we have the information—we may hate it but it works. And once the question is in the minds of the people it takes root and grows inter-mingling the founded with the completely unfounded "truths that we tell." And that was the confusing world I was living in on the day it got worse. I returned from a low-paying gig singing on a cruise ship after what is best referred to as a two-week working vacation. As usual there were lots of "Your kids are crazy!" problems to solve and the educa-tor/babysitter I'd hired ran out the door as quickly as I stepped in. I listened to my children's cacophony of tattle telling, defensive postur-ing and sound effects, hugged, kissed, and sent everybody to bed. The following day Dar and Rye (my oldest and youngest autistic children) went to parent-relief camp. When it was time for them to come home, Dar started to scream and jump up and down (something he did at various intervals for most of his life). The camp perceived this as a fear of going home. They sat him down,, pulled out the facilitation board and asked him "Why don't you want to go home?" (I believe they call this approach "leading the witness.")

A couple of hours later two social workers were sitting in my living room explaining to my oldest daughter and me that Dar's response had been, some misspelled word approximations that looked like, "Mom and sister make me sit on her vagination." I broke into spontaneous spasms of laughter until they told me "It's not funny. We've put the kids in foster care." (They took Rye as well as Dar but left the rest of the kids alone. It didn't make sense to me, but it certainly took the smile from my face. I was furious, scared, indignant, and certain that such a poorly thought-out action would put my son into another regression. "Why couldn't they have just stayed at the camp until we straighten things out? At least that's a familiar place!" (Autistic people are general-ly more able to cope in familiar surroundings.) My logic escaped them.

Forty-eight hours later the staff of the emergency foster place-ment home insisted Dar be removed. He'd been screaming and hitting his head and moaning "Mom! Mom! Mom!" They decided that meant he wanted me because—since nobody was willing to have him—it was easier than thinking their previous thoughts: that he was afraid of me. No longer wishing to fix anything but their housing crisis, they gave the boys back saying "This child (Dar) won't stop hurting himself without you!" I hugged Rye who ran into my arms babbling "Roger Rabbit Roger Rabbit Roger Rabbit" over and over at hyper speed and placed my hand on screaming Dar's back. They both instantly calmed.

First I checked in with Rye, who seemed to think he'd been on a campout with people who cook badly: no real trauma there. I gave it a few hours before talking to Dar. I asked him if he was "OK?" He pointed with my assistance "Y-E-S!" Then I asked, "What were you really saying?" He facilitated some gibberish first and then "M-o-m m-a-k-e-s a b-a-b-y-s-i-t-t-e-r w-h-e-n g-o-e-s o-n v-a-g-a-t-i-o-n." Unfortunately I had no witnesses and my facilitating Dar was no more free of influence than theirs had been. The best I could do was assume the communication was valid and help my son feel comfortable with the situation. I wanted him to continue to facilitate with people. I wanted him to feel safe and keep communicating. I told him I was proud of him and that it's OK if other people misunderstand as it always works out in the end. I don't know if he believed me. I do know it didn't really work. At first Dar stopped communicating with anyone but me. Later he communicated with others, but if they got the letters wrong he often hit them. And so we had a brand new problem.

And of course—as was always the case—during that time I was stepping through the daily issues and swirling in the panoply of a million other child-filled happenings. Some of that panoply was less than magnificent. For example at one point the Director of Special Education for my younger children's school took me aside and said, "Off the record, you should move. Dar is having a rough time and we can't fire his teaching assistant because of union rules. Trust me... it's better for him if... well, you should move." So we moved.

I got a new house in a new neighborhood with a new school near by. After several months of searching we found a teaching assistant. I asked the school to run a background check and then he was hired. This guy was great! He was clear and strong in his approach to my son. Dar listened to him. Best of all Dar stopped hitting and/or kicking the other kids. Dar had been working with this assistant about five months when he (the assistant) started behaving in ways that I can only describe as "divide and conquer." At first, since each incident was small, I let it go. But then, as one thing piled upon another and the control techniques began to mount I started to wonder, why? He did things like tell my children I shouldn't feed them so much soup or tell the teachers that I was a bad housekeeper because I had cobwebs on the eaves trough. He said I was cruel to animals because Rye, in a sensory overload *Of Mice And Men* moment, had squeezed another rabbit so hard it died. I assumed that he believed, like many did, that the blame for what my child did fell on me. That's a heavy load to bear without breaking and making a mess. Fortunately, I was pretty strong at this point in my life.

I built four little bedrooms side by side. I was proud of the dorm look and also of the handiwork in my design: I had taken advantage of the lowered ceiling part of the half basement and tucked their cute little beds into the alcove. He and several others reported me for that, saying the bedrooms were too small for habitation. But they weren't meant for habitation. They were bedrooms. I remember having to show them to Children's Aid who simply said, "Obviously none of these teachers have ever been out of the country: in China they use drawers." All that orchestrated "out to get you" attention by my children's teaching assistant was beginning to give me an uncomfortable prickly sensation on the back of my neck.

Then Dar began to act in unusual ways, even for Dar. I was sitting on his bed singing him to sleep one night when, while staring at the ceiling, he peed all over himself. It was very weird and not something he would normally do, so I was surprised and concerned. He did that several nights in a row. Then he added leaving his poop on the toilet seat every time he went. A few weeks later he began to hold his poop and refuse to go. (This turned into an enormous problem that took ten years to rectify.) Dar started to sweat and pace and laugh hysterically whenever the worker came to take him to the pool. He facilitated that he felt bad whenever *&^% put his bathing suit on. And since everything Dar was doing was different from anything he had ever done before, after a while I couldn't help but see a pattern emerging.

I was in a bind because I wanted to keep my son safe and respond to these new weird behaviors in a correct way, but everything about Dar was weird. How could I tell the forest from the trees? All this could be happening because he was maturing and fantasizing about his assistant in a sexual way. A few days later Dar was facilitating with me. We did that for at least an hour every day. He said for the second time that he didn't like it when &*%% helped him change his clothes at the pool. Now remember how this works. I hold his hand and put enough resistance on it to help him steady his aim and use his gross motor system instead of his fine motor system. I try not to influence what he is typing. But I'm always getting guesses and ideas just before he spells what I expect him to spell. Did I know my son very well, or was I subconsciously directing his hand? Working with him was always a bit of a challenge in this way, especially since he misspelled things the same way I did, which made me wonder even more the degree to which I was the author of his creations. (However, no matter how much I wondered, what I actually believed was that all of the possibilities were true, different ones at different times: Sometimes he spelled, sometimes I spelled, or sometimes we both spelled and slowly. If things had gone smoothly enough, he may eventually have ended up spelling alone. All can be true).

So, with all this uncertainty, when he told me in very explicit language that his assistant was sexually violating him, I felt the wall slam hard against my back. I desperately wanted to find a way out. After all, I'd been on the other side of this scenario and had this kind of attention erroneously thrown at me. I knew that Dar's sensory system was so confused that this report of discomfort and even the explicit language he used within the telling could be based on a lack of understanding about what he was experiencing. Still I wanted to support my son and give credence to his method of communication. Because the problem was, I believed him. So even though the accusations made against me had been false, I didn't think these ones were. I had to take some kind of action. I didn't want to do the same thing to someone else that had been done to me, but at the same time I'd seen other symptoms in my son that were congruent with signs of sexual abuse and I couldn't ignore it any more than anyone else could. More than anything I wanted my son safe.

I made a printout of what he'd facilitated and showed it to a social worker. The social worker insisted we share it with the school principal. I believe, in the moment of sharing, each one of us felt heavy with dread. I suggested we just not have that assistant work in the school system anymore, let it go at that. Of course, such a choice wasn't possible: the principal's legal responsibility was to report any and all allegations of abuse. The long and the short of the story is that it was an extremely challenging situation. I just wanted that man away from my children. The principal seemed to just want me to stop insisting he do this or that for my kids and to not cause him any more problems or discomforts. He said, "Do you realize what you have caused, what I have to do? No one will ever work privately with your children now." I really wanted him to ask me how Dar was.

Instead of removing that assistant from the school, they suspended Dar and then assigned the assistant to my other son Rye. He actually brought Rye home the next day intent on picking up bathing trunks so they could go to the pool. I was so fucking mad I could barely dial the phone. Of course, the story doesn't end there. The school was upset with me and I was upset with the school. The feuding grew until I found myself on camera holding a microphone and yelling at the teachers about their lack of understanding. It didn't take much editing to make me look like a shrew in the documentary inspired by that moment in my breakdown. I felt lost and weak and unable to understand the motivations of the people around me. I was keeping Dar home from school and at real risk of crumbling into oblivion. That's about the time I saw the movie about Annie, the girl with cerebral palsy. I started to understand some things that I hadn't heretofore understood. And then I remembered that when raising children the most important thing isn't to prove what might or might not be, but instead to safeguard what already is.

I considered ending the story by moving again, but then I realized it wouldn't work. The story was going to follow me because we were already engaged in a legal battle. The police had laid charges on Dar's assistant. Dealing with the police officer handling the case was the polar opposite experience of dealing with the principal handling my son. The officer was a wonderful man who really seemed to want to "protect and serve" the needs of my child. In order to prevent me from actually touching Dar while at the same time allowing me to facilitate his answers, the officer made a wooden carpet-covered paddle for me to place between my son's arm and my hand. In this way I could facilitate him without touching him. The officer interviewed Dar. I tried to remain neutral so as not to taint the results of his answers. Dar responded clearly via this method and the charges were laid. We had a preliminary hearing coming up.

The whole court experience had that weird déjà vu feeling to it—Possibly because it was so like the courtroom scene in the movie I told you about. Or possibly because that déjà vu feeling can be created by the excessive low wave activity bathing the right temporal lobe when a person is experiencing extreme fear and stress. Dar couldn't communicate independently and the judge was doing his best to be fair. I was expected to facilitate Dar's answers on a large poster-sized letter board that was taped to the wall for all to see. The judge told Dar to approach the bench and look at a picture that he was holding in such a way as to keep me from seeing it. He then instructed Dar to facilitate a description of what he had seen. Interestingly when Dar looked at the picture, I immediately knew the word "lady", and so I resisted as Dar tried to point to the letters leading to that word. I resisted because I was afraid the word was my idea and maybe just a little because I didn't want to be responsible for the ending of this man's career only to find out years later that I'd subconsciously orchestrated the whole thing. I thwarted Dar's communication and turned the word into bicycle. Shaking his head "no" the judge showed me the picture of a lady.

And so now instead of subconsciously orchestrating the demise of the teaching assistant's career, I may have subconsciously orchestrated the demise of Dar's opportunity for respect and the ensuing protection such a light of truth would shed upon all future children in the teaching assistant's career. OUCH! The case was dismissed.

I still don't know what's true here, not even now. Despite the fact that Dar can finally speak—he is hard to understand, seldom forthcoming, and talks on a limited number of subjects—regardless of how subtly we bring the incident up he doesn't have much to say about it. Fortunately, in so far as the unfolding of our lives goes, the truth isn't important anymore. Dar is fully grown, hanging out at home, and helping around the house. He is no longer in any danger. Not even from the effects of his past. Dar's neurofeedback therapy has included a plethora of sessions aimed at calming down his amygdala (think of it as the brain's fear filing and response system). This low frequency neurofeedback training aimed at the amygdala is a good way of easing the effects of PTSD (Post Traumatic Stress Disorder). Given that autistic kids often have problems with over-firing of the amygdala and discombobulated sensory systems that act as if they are being attacked when anything around them moves too quickly, and given that Dar's history included many opportunities for a trauma reaction, when I learned neurofeedback, relaxing the PTSD hold of the amygdala on Dar's brain was one of the first things I tried. The amygdala is of prime importance in the creation of emotional memory. It was (and is) my hope that Dar's has been calmed down enough to effectively intercept, redirect, and reduce the number of connections to fear that exist in his brain, thus making a psychotic break that forces him to relive these events unlikely.

Fortunately I have lived long enough to realize that the saying "Every cloud has a silver lining" is true. Surprisingly enough in some ways we owe gratitude to &%%^$ because it was due to the possible truth of that unsavory incident that my commitment to helping Dar speak independently was reaffirmed. So I kept looking until I found something that could help him talk. Several days after the court case was dismissed, I took the spelling board away. I explained, "You are completely dependent on another human being to help you when you facilitate—and we can't tell what's true and what isn't—so from this point on we are setting aside facilitation, except for a yes and no board, and we are working on talking." I stuck to that decision. But no matter how hard I tried or how motivating I tried to make it, I couldn't teach him to form words in any reliably consistent fashion.

It was another thirteen years before neurofeedback loosened his tongue. Had I still been using the spelling board, I may have been satisfied with just teaching Dar to point. Of course, even that journey could have led to neurofeedback since that's what it took to repair Dar's fine motor skills enough for him to purposely form his hand into an unassisted index-finger-extended pointing position. I suppose, if it was meant to be, my journey might still have led there, but of course that is something I could never know. Ironically, in the end, after all that time-consuming teaching, it was this "no effort required" brain-repair therapy that stimulated Dar's desire to communicate enough to help him to help himself. This enormous change in his functioning should bring many exponentially beneficial returns. Because where Dar is concerned, his wanting to self-teach is a big deal. Previously he had appeared to be sorely lacking self-motivation in arenas that lead to learning things that lead to independence. As I seem to find myself noticing time and again, neurofeedback led to healing both of us. My healing was a pleasant change for the whole family since, where I was concerned, "effortless improvement" had been undesirable. My desire had been to earn a ticket to heaven by having life be difficult and, like many of the professionals reacting to neurofeedback today, my beliefs blinded me from finding value in the possibility of easy or at least easier.

Before neurofeedback, speaking and spelling required Herculean efforts of mind and body for Dar to achieve any measure of success. I believe that closing off his ability to speak through facilitation was the only way to redirect all that effort towards having him use his voice. Still, even though the efforts were directed, the results were not forthcoming. Despite the dust settling upon its face, over the years of speech seeking, the spelling board continued to have an influence on me because it was the memory of Dar communicating that kept me believing throughout all those moments of uncertainty that his understanding was intact and he wanted to speak. Retiring the spelling board was, in many ways, a harsh decision that rather paid off though not necessarily well. This is because, even though Dar now has language, getting good information is not only difficult but continues to be a mine field of dangerous possibilities. Dar prefers to answer "yes" rather than "no". For Dar "yes" is easier to say. It's also more agreeable to the people in his world. He seems to like the fact that his nephews like it cause Dar will take the blame for anything if you ask the question right. This is still a somewhat precarious situation that could easily be abused.

Of course, not every parent gave up on facilitation and, of the ones who did and of the ones who didn't, rest assured there are many more than my stories to tell. Some of those earlier children even managed to grow into independently typing adults and some of them have had an impact.

For example, Sue Rubin, who is considered a functionally non-verbal published autistic author, wrote the Oscar-nominated documentary "Autism Is A World." And though she is often referred to as "using the controversial technique of facilitated communication" in the scenes, I watched how her attention merely had to be brought to the portable keyboard. She did the typing herself.

Sue is not alone in the world of functionally non-verbal autistic authors. As evidenced by the fact that she, along with Lucy Blackman, Tito Mukhopadhay, artist Larry Bissonette, Alberto Frugone, Jamie Burke, and award winning writer Richard Attfield contributed in a published collection edited by Douglas Biklen entitled *Autism and the Myth of the Person Alone.*

As of this writing one of the most talked about non-verbal autistic authors is Amanda Bragg, YouTube phenomenon of 2008. In her amazing video we see Amanda independently typing at lightening speed. We also see her acting in ways our society views as "repetitive nonsensical behavior." She moves from foot to foot wiggling her fingers and humming. Over this visual we hear a computer voice representing Amanda explain that this sensory dance of activity is her way of communicating with the environment. If it weren't for the clip of her typing, the connotations in her overall presentation would lead us to believe her apparent intelligence a hoax. This is the way it is with autistic individuals: they look different than they are. Another similarly problematic disability comes to mind when in the follow-up video Amanda holds a communication device on her lap. The device speaks for her spewing intelligent commentary on life as an autistic while she merely sits. The clip is reminiscent of a Stephen Hawking lecture on life in the universe as he knows it.

The world of special Education is riddled with stories of snake pits and fire hoses, punishment, rejection, restraints, electric shock, pinching, paddling, and learning—or not learning—due to all the heavy-handed techniques intent on creating change. Important to note is that creating change about how we create change requires change. And since the attitudes in our environment, both within the home and without, strongly impact the availability and success of any and all therapies, kindness and curiosity must be taught if they are to be learned and learned if they are to be taught. Only recently have we been curious enough about the easy facilitation of change through the use of neurofeedback to learn enough to teach it. Only recently has neuroanatomy-guided neurofeedback been put into a small number of colleges and universities as a course of its own. It has taken this long even though it's been in existence healing disorders since the early seventies. That's a fact I often contemplate because it's been healing disorders since long before I adopted Dar and began to squeeze his shoulder.

What if Dar had had it then? Personally, based on his age and present rate of change with the therapy, I think he'd be independent.

CHAPTER SIX

OK! OK! Neurofeedback is Great!

But Really, How Does It Work?

Well we don't throw chicken-milk in your faces. We throw beeps. Really!

It turns out brains don't need food rewards in order to be encouraged to change. This is mainly because brains are able to organize themselves and learn based on pattern recognition. In this way they are much like a computer. For example, your computer is capable of everything it's capable of simply because of its ability to recognize coded patterns made from ones and zeros. These ones and zeros are at the beginning of it all. They are called the binary code. I find it amazing to realize that all our complicated computer functionality, all the languages, all the software, everything, originates from a series of combinations using only ones and zeros to represent yes and no. Then, as long as long as the computer hardware is unflawed and as long as we give our computers the right information in the form of this very basic code, we get what we want from them. In this way we are in control. It's the same for the brain because the original "machine" language of the brain is a similar kind of yes/no, go/stop, excitatory/inhibitory binary code.

You teach with it all the time: Like when your baby reaches to topple the ashtray and is at risk of getting burnt so you say NO! He stops and then pulls his hand away. At this point you smile and coddle and praise, he hears "YES!" This is a perfect example of a parentally executed binary code for the brain. However, if while saying "NO," mom or dad grabbed the ashtray away from the child effectively teaching baby that "no" means not you, the pattern has been made more complex by the layering on of an extra message. At this point we may end up getting behavior created by what we taught the child instead of what we meant to teach. (And if we were still talking about computers, this is how we create what is commonly referred to as a glitch in the system. Sorry, I just could not resist such a ripe opportunity for a little commentary on inadvertent lessons. Be careful by being intentional.)

Children learn and generally speaking, if we are consistent in our use of "no" and "yes" eventually our baby learns "not to" and "to." Thus by giving a consistent response to behavior, we supply the pattern and teach our children via their brains' remarkable ability to engage in pattern recognition. This is the how of teaching and learning, but it is not the why. You choose to teach and your child chooses to learn because the brain has a built-in desire for control. So as long as your child prefers it and sees his life as improved in some way by moving toward an action when you say "yes" and moving away from an action when you say "no," he or she will acquire at least some of the knowledge you seek to impart. Know though that nothing is that simple. For example some children—especially if their ability to stay focused is compromised because they have something like ADHD—prefer the energy with which their parents say "NO!" to the energy with which they say yes. If your child is like that, switch the energy and give "YES!" a bigger presence or this type of child will learn to do precisely what you wish them not to do. Fortunately though, for the most part, if all is operating correctly within his/her brain, he/she will just naturally seek the tones and expressions parents tend to pair with the word "yes" to the ones parents pair with the word "no." This preference in the brain is preset, again by the desire to be in control, because in general one feels more in control when receiving approval and agreement than disapproval or disagreement.

To restate: the ability and desire to comprehend and control patterns is hardwired into the brain. Initially the basic teaching pattern is a simple two-signal code of yes and no. Very quickly, however, the pattern is made complex by the consequential layering of the varying responses from the multitude of conflicting signals in the internal and external systems within and around them. However, in its beginnings, just like in the computer, in human beings the root pattern for social learning is nothing more than a binary code of yes for ones and no for zeros.

Many adults think that what is hardwired into children is a preference for the yes response rather than a preference for the tone of approval and/or any other reward that the yes response assures. This is erroneous, as is the concept that learning happens because the consequences of no teach a child what not to do and so the child will then discover a correct course of action as a natural result of trial and error. Though this is sometimes the result when handing out no's without yeses, the actual drive to learning one's way through the conundrum is created from the need for control, thus the driver is the reason for learning. And the drive to learn is linked with the desire for a reward.

So what rewards children or even adults for that matter? Certainly the ability to control the tones or voices in their environment is universally desired and therefore motivating. The existential angst of wanting to know how and why are also presets that guide us to seek directions, especially in childhood. Often we get our directions by acquiring attention. Children, for example, want at least enough attention to see themselves in relation to others. This helps them know where they stand so that they can gain a measure of control and figure out what they want to do next. If the only attention a child gets comes from disapproval, then disapproval becomes rewarding, regardless of the tone or method of delivery. This is the problem with no's unaccompanied by yeses. Teaching is riddled with challenges. For example, our society often passes out consequences based on the motivations of the masses rather than the motivations of the individual making a "'no" more rewarding than a "yes" for the exceptional child standing on the fringe just away from their peers. For example, the child who hates school is punished by being expelled, which is in actual fact a reward. This leaves the parents in the position of trying to make the expulsion more distasteful than the school experience is. Given the often overly busy lives of parents, this role can then lead to having the drama of punishment be the singular experience of attention getting for the child. And Voila! Expulsion is doubly rewarding. Even if the parent is careful to avoid this dynamic, some children will still prefer to hear no depending upon their own personal idea of what is fun and not fun.

The above points are especially relevant if the child is autistic and thinks opening and closing doors is a blast. Since the participants in our society so often teach to the no and then leave the child floundering assuming that the child will be skilled enough to find the path that leads to yes, autistic children are destined to become antisocial. This will only work if our yes is rewarding enough to hold the child's attention and shine bright enough to guide him/her safely home like a lighthouse leading the way. Thus we need a method that rewards the brain by bypassing individual taste and talking to the neurons themselves. Enter neurofeedback. Neurofeedback is especially necessary if one wishes to heal extremely complicated disorders. Since teaching to behavior requires a certain degree of agreement or interest from the student and a definite preference for the yes being taught in comparison to the no being levied, obviously the reward accompanying yes must be even more powerful than the consequences of no in order to pass on the lesson. Thus it is the reward more than the punishment that motivates the student to learn, and this choosing to learn effectively invokes within them the illusion of control. The illusion of control is important because without it one doesn't generalize or own the skill they just learned. Since understanding what does or doesn't motivate an autistic child is difficult for most people, surprisingly it is easier to teach by availing oneself of the neuronal presets. Once again, enter neurofeedback!

Since it is the neuron's ability to recognize patterns (combined with its desire for control) that creates the ability to learn in the first place, the benefits of using a therapy that speaks to the neuron itself makes sense. Better to speak to the actual brain cells rather than wait for those cells to gather together and create desires which create behaviors that explode a person into unacceptable actions and then try to teach to that. This preemptive teaching choice seems like a no-brainer (pardon the pun) to me. Because, unlike with most things in life—in this case—we know what comes first, the chicken or the desire—to make an egg. It is of course the desire—to make a chicken—who can desire—to make an egg—that isn't rotten. (wink.)

Most people resist being told that they have conflicting beliefs causing inner turmoil and unpleasant acting out—especially if the examples of their behavior are specific. Thus having the ability to get around a person's defensive nature when doing things, like confronting behavior, is important for therapeutic success. Neurofeedback enables us to do just that. Thus it is a powerful tool in the treatment of any brain disorder. With neurofeedback we can remain impersonal because people are not all that attached to the nature of their brain-wave behavior. Hence neurofeedback professionals can avoid the usual resistance to change. In addition, neurofeedback works with the brain's natural inclinations by using preexisting neuronal conditions as tools. In this case it is the neuron's desire for control that responds to the neurofeedback's beeping sounds and then changes itself, effectively rearranging the maladaptive firing patterns that have been causing maladaptive behaviors: Much easier than twenty years on a couch. Let me explain, through reiteration: The brain and all its individual neurons have a built-in need to control everything. It is not a futile need; it is a motivator and it is married with the ability to actually succeed—gain control via the inherent skill of pattern recognition. Neurons (hence the brain) are also preset to be in motion, moving towards or away from firing, thus creating a need for change in the form of an action. The command of when to fire or not to fire is passed via chemical changes in the brain itself.

The choosing of whether to move towards or away from (anything) is facilitated by a desire that is shared by all life forms: the desire for balance. You have most likely heard this need referred to as the "Balance of Nature." To summarize: It is my supposition that the desire for balance combined with a neuronal need for control and the ability to recognize patterns is the fundamental reason why neurofeedback is such a powerful therapy.

So how does it work? We throw beeps and we throw them fast. The client has brain wave sensors pasted to his head and his EEG is sent to a therapist computer. The therapist computer then "talks to" another computer upon whose screen one can observe a computer game in progress. Whenever the brain wave combinations that the client generates moves towards a greater state of balance (determined by the therapist) the game beeps. Since the client is alive (one would hope) and is already generating brain waves, all the therapist does is set the parameters of her computer in such a way that the brain can't help but get a goodly number of "lucky" beeps. Once the brain understands what it needs to do in order to keep the beeps beeping, it tries to go to that combination of brain waves more often. Thus it changes itself in an attempt to get more. (Understand that brain waves are related to neuronal firing, which is related to neuro-chemical release). At this point the therapist can—like any good coach or personal trainer—up the bar and ask the brain to move even more toward a brain-wave representation of neuro-typical firing and/or ask it to maintain this balanced firing for longer and longer periods of time. The brain starts to do the dance of "chasing" after control; and the changes created, once it learns the steps required for it to lead in the dance, can be quite profound. So we teach the brain by rewarding it with beeps in the same way that parents teach the brain with a reward system that uses "yes." The reasons for the success of this therapeutic approach is no more magical than the reasons for the success of your parental one. But neurofeedback does have two advantages over normal teaching methods: speed of delivery (the information—or beep—is generated in a few milliseconds of the neuron firing) and that level of precision I referred to that bypasses the resistance of human behavior and goes straight to the neurons themselves. So like I said we throw beeps and we throw them fast.

THE APPEARANCE OF A MIRACLE: Ali, can control her seizures.

Ali is another sweet little pixie of a RETTS girl. She wrings her hands incessantly. She is seven. Her mom handed me a file folder of all her previous tests, QEEG, SPECT, MRI, etc. Each one ended with the same basic conclusion "very aberrant brain wave activity"... "extreme seizure disorder"... "severely abnormal activity," etc. I concur. She certainly had the most seizure activity I'd ever seen in one little brain. She was having a seizure when I met her. At that point Ali spent most of her hours in an oversized playpen wearing a helmet to prevent injury when falling to the ground and hitting her head on the rails. I was told that normally she fell to the ground several times a day. Mom had tried the usual medications and even attempted healing Ali with the ketagenic diet to no avail. Each attempt helped for a few weeks and then created new more intense cycles of seizure activity: Ali cycled through seizures that brought her to the floor for ten days a month leaving her in a recovery state of constipation and sleeplessness for another ten days. She would then have five days of reasonable health wherein one could get a glimpse of the girl beneath the seizures. The final five days she slept through as her sweet little explosive firestorm of a head readied itself for the seizure part of her cycle again. During my initial outreach, Ali was in the middle of part one of this portion of her cycle. Ali was, according to all her family members, friends of family and special education teachers and therapists, unable to speak. With my guidance and some neurofeedback, Ali learned how to move through her seizures. She stopped falling. We removed the helmet. She began to talk. In fact, Ali became relatively assertive about having people hear her ask for help. The first word she (and many of the kids I work with) learned was "ride." She demanded one on a regular basis. She would also stand on the peripheries of our group as I taught everyone how to help her. Whenever someone echoed his or her doubt in her ability to express or comprehend she would sing "Ride" in a confident voice. Mouths fell open as the room vacillated between laughter and tears. But Ali didn't stop there; she indicated the depth of her receptive skills by adding new words like up and down, etc, to this large group conversation whenever their meaning fit the subject we were discussing. Everyone in the room was stunned into listening: A brand new experience for this precious little girl and her family.

THE AFTER FACTS: aka everybody has a life, and life gets in the way, especially when its about death. I left their country for mine shortly after instructing Ali's mom how to continue on without me. A mere six days later she was diagnosed with cervical cancer. She fell into a deep depression at the thought that she might be about to leave her daughter without a parent. Unfortunately people are poor problem solvers when depressed because depression slows the activity in the frontal lobes and the frontal lobes are our problem solving area of the brain. This mom knew she had a tool that could eradicate her depression: She could use the neurofeedback. She could have but she didn't because at the time she couldn't think her way into making the choice of helping herself. During these most vulnerable times, Ali's mom was reaching out to her spiritual healers. One of them apparently said that Ali was in danger and would die in two months if Ali's mom continued with the neurofeedback. The woman's words stopped the progress. It was a very tough two months in that home. Everyone in the extended circle of spiritual supporters focused on the cancer and the neurofeedback units collected dust. Ali's seizures increased and the helmet went back on. Two days before the two months was up, mom reached out for my help. I told mom not to treat her daughter just yet but to treat herself instead. She did. Her logic returned and her outlook grew positive again. She made it through the cancer scare and even treated her own chemo brain. Meanwhile she returned to doing sessions on Ali. I explained that when she had become depressed, every occupant in the house had also become heavy with sadness. (I use the term "heavy with sadness" because sadness increases low frequency brain wave activity. The lower the frequency the slower the wave, so since low frequencies move messages in the brain more slowly than faster frequency waves do, the motor and sensory systems within the brain becomes bogged down and begins to report things more slower. Human beings interpret slow reacting despite a desire to be quick as the sensation of heaviness.) The big problem in such an environmental shift is that excessive low frequency brain wave activity tips the scale of balance in the brain and exacerbates seizures. So Ali got worse. I read mom's reports and instructed her over email on how to proceed with the neurofeedback. Fortunately for the families I work with, with the right support and a willingness to follow directions, people don't have to completely understand what they are doing in order to help their children. In this case mom knew how to run the machines and what to report to me. Thus I knew what to tell her to change insofar as the therapy itself was concerned. We moved forward as a team. Then to make the approach fully effective we included Ali. I explained that she and Ali could work together to interrupt a seizure. Presently, when Ali feels a seizure coming, she can very often stop it by causing sensory information to blast into her brain. In order to do this, Ali chooses to clap her hands: smart little girl. The focal point to Ali's seizures is in a (brain) location that correlates with her right hand. For Ali clapping stops the seizure.

> **THE ACTUAL MIRACLE:** Of course Ali still has RETTS and she also still has seizures. But now you have to be looking at her EEG to definitively know that. At the very least her cycle has grown mild enough for her to no longer be considered as suffering from drop seizures because now, in her worst moments she just looks like a sweet little dreamy eyed happy clapping doll trying not to loose consciousness. I am thrilled to report that even during her cycle she retains her new verbal and gross motor skills. Ali also sleeps normally now. But none of that is the actual miracle. Those changes are merely a good response to a sound therapy. The *actual miracle* is Ali's mom: She has done more than survive her cancer. She has outgrown her fear of it. As a result Ali's mom is not only alive but also aware. Ali's mom sees the miracle in her house, which means that in Ali's house, the people create miracles, daily.

Not only does neurofeedback cut down on the brain's resistance to change by using the simplicity of a beeping binary code—it cuts down on the very normal behavioral resistance that therapists encounter when trying to help clients change how they feel and function in the world. Resistance is understandable. Most people who come for therapy do so after years of dealing with a problem that eventually grew too big for them to handle. During the period leading up to coming in for therapy they have justified, excused, and tried to understand themselves. As a result they have grown fond of and learned to lean on different aspects of the very problem they have come to eradicate. Thus they are resistant to some of the healing they seek. This sort of behavior is reminiscent of a teenage girl who strings her boyfriend along because—even though she no longer likes him—she enjoys getting a lift to school. Seeing the whole picture and making sound decisions intent on "lifting" you out of your "just to get a lift" behavior which colors and creates your present situation is easier when you feel clear and in balance. This is because the brain is an association network, which means it is designed to prove your point. It gathers up memories, ideas, and thoughts that match what you are already remembering, considering, and thinking. Thus, if you feel depressed it agrees and then adds to the story. The power of neurofeedback becomes evident to the client when, once they have completed a session and are feeling clear, comfortable, and ready to change things, they find their brain agreeing and adding to that story instead of the one they came in with. Reminds me of a female forty-year-old client I once found standing in her pajamas facing a wall. She'd gotten herself as far as the office-building hallway and then stopped. She'd been standing in that position for ten to fifteen minutes before I stumbled upon her on my way to the washroom. I guided her into the session room, attached the sensors, and watched her cry. It took fifteen minutes of beeping to change her demeanor and dry up her tears. It took another fifteen to send her home smiling.

In the break between the two fifteen minutes we were able to talk about things. This is one of the ways in which the fact that neurofeedback reduces resistance and helps in a person's healing. With no cloud of emotional angst, it is easier to think and to not feel defensive while examining one's choices. For example, I have a client that had been in intensive talk therapy for twenty-five years before coming to neurofeedback. He did five sessions of beeping and suddenly found himself able to hear, understand, and take action upon some of the "new" ideas I presented him with, the same "new" ideas that I'm sure his previous therapist had suggested many times before. True, I could have just been the lucky number-seven teacher sharing a new oft repeated idea (wink), but in his case I feel certain that it was the neurofeedback which allowed him to actually hear what I had to say. In fact, more likely it was both. The truth is no matter how many times a lesson is taught, it's just plain easier to hear and to learn without defensive posturing. So since my client felt no responsibility for his neuronal firing because no moral imperatives had ever been directed toward them, he didn't resist or hide from information on how they were affecting his state and was thus able to claim responsibility and learn what to do in order to make things better. It was my similar advice he followed instead of his previous therapist's even though our advice was the same. This is because he wasn't taking it personally so he was relaxed enough to take on some cognitive reframes (impressive science term for "take on a change of perspective"). His life improved dramatically.

Of course everything that exists in one form exists somewhere else as its total opposite. And so there are the folks who resist, just to resist. (Remember the Semmelweis reflex?) People like this generally see the act of always resisting as a feature of strength: an important component in their personality. They generally meet neurofeedback with suspicion even though they've chosen to try it. People like this usually wear a tough veneer to hide the fact that they are approaching the therapy from a place of fear. I believe this is mainly because they think that if anything as easy as watching a video game beep (the video portion is less important than the beeps and mainly there to keep things interesting enough to get folks to do the therapy long enough to notice the change) could help them feel better for more than just a moment, that means they were previously making their lives unnecessarily hard. Of course by meeting everything with suspicion, they were making their lives unnecessarily hard, but they are just not OK with being to blame for their pain. Ironically, understanding the physiological reality of your brain and why it is natural to resist actually reduces blame, but people like this can't usually listen to this sort of logic until the session is done. Thus, when I say that the idea is to get the computer to make more beeps, they often triy to make it not beep. Admittedly this is always a little fun for me because it requires a touch more therapist skill; but even if I didn't realize what was happening for the clients, their very resistance creates an unbalanced change in the brain wave pattern and so, by resisting, in a sense it is resistance that gets worked on first. This makes the clients less resistant. And since resistance is their primary problem, they are helped even when they are trying not to be. Now that's my idea of a cool therapy.

This therapeutic help happens because of the brain's very nature and because at some level people want it, or otherwise they wouldn't be in my chair. Fortunately for them, even if they are trying to thwart the process and choose to make fewer beeps, the very desire to thwart creates an interest in the sound which is the tool being used to help them change. The minute any beeps beep the neurons—through pattern recognition—begin to notice how these beeps are aligned with their own firing and move toward controlling the sound. As awareness that these moments of alignment mesh with moving toward greater internal balance grows, the brain begins to prefer feeling good to feeling resistant. Thus, since all life is fundamentally predisposed to try to balance itself, once it knows the way, it follows the path to feeling better. In other words, always assuming I've made good therapeutic choices and am leading the clients toward a more comfortable state, when the clients feel better the neurons will follow the beeps. This happens despite the confusing messages of resistance clients may be giving the neurons via the frontal lobes of their thinking. (An interesting fact of trying to fool this therapy is that if you could control your brain waves enough to control the beeps into silence, you would have to have such great mental agility that you would already be able to balance yourself and not be looking to sabotage things in the first place.)

Regardless of the person's cooperativeness (or lack of it) there are many elements outside the control of the client's brain waves that contribute to the rhythm of the beeps. This list includes, but is not limited to, cortical location of the sensor, degree of difficulty that the game has been set at, the parameters of change being asked for, and how often the therapist resets those goals. Let's look at location. If I place the sensor on a part of the brain that should be firing a predominance of mid-range frequency waves and see a lack of this activity, I may choose to ask for more by setting it so that the game only beeps when that area of the brain fires more waves in the frequency range I perceive as lacking. However, I may instead first let the game beep whenever that area of the brain fires the maximum amount of that frequency range that it is already firing and then, once the brain is enjoying the success and seeking control, ask for more. The difference in the two approaches equates to a difference in the number of beeps. The beauty of this truth is that in both cases the brain would have improved, just as long as beeps were heard.

In my experience one of the hardest things for people to wrap their mind around is the question of, "Why would it work if I don't care about beeps?" Since most autistic kids appear uninterested in much of what is presented to them, many parents and professionals laugh at the idea that young "Johnny might sit still and allow a stranger to attach wires and sensors to his head so that he can watch a game and listen to beeps." This doubting of the possibility that an autistic child with no interest in computer screens might respond favorably to neurofeedback is why I have spent so much time trying to answer the question of, "What makes the beeps matter?" The answer is "they don't have to matter to the child" because they matter to his brain. Which is fortunate because a lot of what needs to be worked on in the autistic brain are areas unrelated to cognitive thought. In fact, often I begin by working on the sensory motor strip at a location that is between the two hemispheres. It is believed that this location helps us read brain-wave activity from the deepest regions, possibly even netting some information from the thalamus itself. This is important because, among other things, the thalamus is strongly influential in a person's regulation of state and ability to focus. For example, when readying oneself for sleep, the thalamus aids the process by going into an "idling mode." The purpose of this idling mode is to prevent the processing of environmental sensory information and to bring the focus inward. It is a kind of beneficial "spacing out" to calm the brain, shield the brain from sensory stimuli, and provide a transition from being awake to being fully asleep. However, some people's brains are stuck in this idling mode even when they are fully awake and trying to focus, listen, or think. They then require the expenditure of endless amounts of energy in order to break through this mode and enter another mode known as the "transmission mode" in which their thalamus sends sensory information faithfully to the rest of the brain so that processing can take place (e.g., listen, think). Again, idling is desirable when trying to sleep, meditate, or recall memories but is not so useful when trying to pay attention and to listen. Point is, in a person with such an "idling mode" affliction, the "spacing out" is not done as a means to escape but runs as the default mechanism whenever their frontal lobes take a break from overriding the issue. As opposed to deciding to daydream, this person must be jolted into deciding not to. Anatomical variation means that our brains are different; the reason for one person is not the reason for another. Thus, in a case like this, telling yourself or your child to stop daydreaming only works for the moments when the daydream is being interrupted by the emergency status given to the command. Some people give a lot of emergency status here and some don't. Again anatomical variation creates a behavioral difference and is not to be judged.

In my observation, as a general rule, we humans are more accepting of people's differences when related to their sleep patterns than we are when related to their awake patterns. We gather in groups and talk about each other with great humor when telling stories of sleepwalkers, sleeptalkers and barely wakeruppers. We share tips and tricks with can't-get-to-sleepers, flip floppy feeters, and feather light zzzzers. But when these same differences happen during our daylight hours we see them as faults, hyper-vigilance, and moral slovenliness.

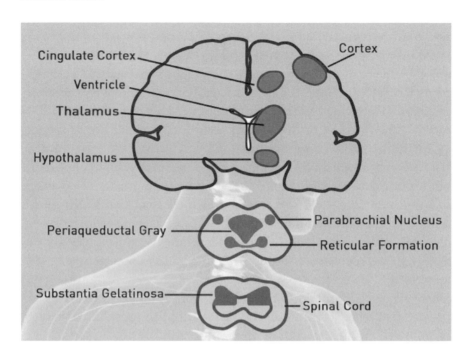

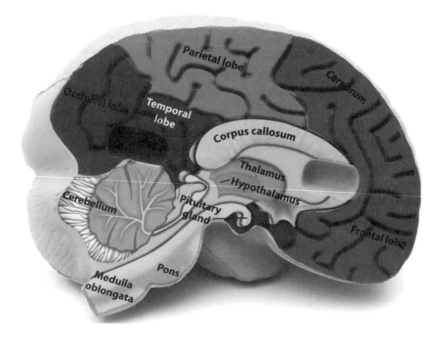

Model Brain © **Karen Roach from Fotolia.com**

Though proper functioning in areas like the reticular formation located in the brainstem (related to levels of arousal) allows the executive functioning of the cognitive regions (frontal lobes) to do their job better, creating permanent change in these areas is not easily achieved via therapies that require the frontal lobes to do all the work. Talk therapy and cognitive therapy both aim at getting the frontal lobes (cognitive) to override the area of difficulty (thalamus for example) in an attempt to achieve balance. Using the frontal lobes so exclusively is a perfect scenario for facilitating extremely hyper-focused behavior because if we focus on the enigma of why we can't focus then we achieve a kind of focus about focus. Such circular thinking is typical of people wrapped up in the "'wrongness of their disorder'" and seeking help through traditional talk therapy, a therapy that is meant to end the very problem it facilitates.

True, there are stories of people healing various regions of their brain that are not involved in conscious cognitive thought through sheer logical decision making and will power. True, some of these stories of hope were achieved through teaching solely to the frontal lobes which very possibly created new pathways to bypass old problems; but normally, approaches like this just lead to coping strategies rather than healing. They also require constant maintenance and are exhausting to employ. This is in part because the message to heal has so far to travel—frontal lobe to thalamus and back to frontal lobe again. (This is of course a very simplified example; the routing system is likely much more complex than that.) With neurofeedback we can leave the conscious deliberation of the frontal lobes out of it and go straight to the area of difficulty. I realize that this is a little bit misleading because neuronal activity of the frontal lobes and its loops with other structures become very much involved as your brain responds to the information of the beeps. However, not requiring conscious awareness is still a quicker more direct route that leads to faster more potent change. We do a system override and go straight to the problem thus repairing it on the spot and relieving the frontal lobes of the need to constantly reroute. Thus, since all life consistently tries to move toward balance, and since a brain uses pattern recognition in order to accomplish its tasks, that means even non-conscious parts of your brain will try to make the machine beep in an evenly spaced rhythm. And its your brain's desire to make the machine beep in synchronicity that will lead it to follow the signal in an attempt to balance, even if it has to change itself to do so. And all of this is regardless of your cognizant feelings on the subject…

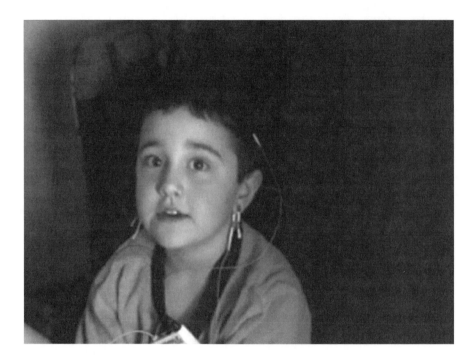

Some parents see their child sitting with wires attached to their head and playing a video game with their brain and fear that it is the Vulcan mind meld or some other mysterious mind-manipulation technology. Other parents minimize the experience, see it as being "beeping hypnotized," but in fact the working of the game is a purely logical response to brain wave patterns, while—for the brain—running it is a lot of work. Since the typical everyday type of feedback happens slowly: (possible simplified example) first neurons fire, then the person whose neurons fired has a behavioral response, and then someone else sees that response making person number two's neurons fire so that she responds to the response of the original person who now sees this response which makes her neurons fire as she tries to analyze the feedback. In the time between the original activity and the feedback, the person's brain has fired millions of combinations unrelated to the original firing. With neurofeedback the "beep" response arrives back to the person's brain around a few milliseconds after her neurons fired. Essentially, by using this technology, we are cutting out the middleman. We cut him out from every pathway. We intercept the message (as in our frontal to thalamus example) of the behavior pathways (in many ways we give the feedback before the firing collects and groups enough to become a visible behavior) and improve efficiency by asking one area to process quicker and another to slow down. A lot of changing is required on the brain's part in order to make this happen. And the feedback beeps request that that change happen at a faster pace than change is ever required by the feedback of everyday life. This speed of feedback response is one of the reasons people often get very tired during the session. Imagine your neurons, which usually have so much time to react, being asked to return the response at the speed of… one of those tennis ball serving machines gone haywire—exhausting to do but invigorating once you catch your breath. And that's how many people feel after a session—invigorated.

The delivery system being faster means that you get there (wherever there might be) quicker. Since neurofeedback is essentially just a behavioral teaching tool for neurons, in my opinion and according to my observations, one session of neurofeedback is equal to a great many sessions of behavioral therapy. This is good news for the parents of autistic children because behavioral therapy is, at best, arduous. It was even better news for me where Dar was concerned because, as I explained earlier, he had really far to go and moving him a long a continuum faster meant he'd get farther. If he wanted to make it into semi-independence, every extra minute mattered. It was also a relief because it meant he had a chance to survive me in life without fear of the abuse so often levied upon the non-verbal. Another marvelous aspect of the therapy is that the effects of neurofeedback continue beyond treatment. Once people get a hint of what clarity feels like, they want more of it. They also behave differently with that in mind. Once a person behaves differently the world responds and begins to give different feedback. Like, "Wow you finished your work quickly today!" or "You were really good at sitting this afternoon." With that information the brain begins to embrace its own changes and heal itself, as the world the person lives in continually redesigns its feedback responding to and reinforcing this evolving brain.

One of the most pleasant side effects of my job is that sometimes a person's brain is cued into a more balanced state simply by the sight of me rolling my equipment up the sidewalk. So I get the credit whenever the sight of me calms a very stressed-out child or mother. However, the credit really goes to the previously felt experience of clarity that the person experienced in the hands of the therapy I have packed into my suitcase. What really happens when they see me is their brain associates me with the beeping neurofeedback directions and jumps to help itself. Thus, it self-changes whenever it is reminded of what it was supposed to be doing in the first place. Some people call this feel-better-when-the-professional-arrives scenario "the curse of the nurse." Your brain expects you to feel better and so you do. I am blessed to be able to have such an effect on so many. And though many parents think their disabled child has no idea they are different and that they won't care about a therapy meant to change their brain function, my experience is that the more disabled the child the greater is the impact of the session; and if I explain what the computers can do for them, even the most profoundly disabled reaches for help and cooperates as I place the sensors on his/her head.

That's how my job begins. I clean and paste their heads with sensors. I watch their EEG (Electroencephalogram) and look for aberrations from the expected norm. I lay what I see on the screen against what I see in their behavior. I ask the parents what they wish to see change and listen to their answers in regard to functioning challenges, sleep, mood, and medicines. After considering all these factors, I set the parameters in the computer and choose the location on the head. It is all just a place to start. The real work comes as we follow the changes. For example, if the child/adult becomes aggravated I make new choices, but if the child/adult becomes calmer and happier I stay with what I am doing. One of the most important skills in working with autism (or any brain disorder) is the skill to follow change while staying focused on the goal and remembering that this is a person who is wonderful to love.

Once I've set the required brainwave parameters into the computer, the game works better when the brain changes how it fires and moves towards the goal of recreating itself according to those parameters. For example, if too many lower frequency waves are firing in the sensory motor strip, one may experience this as a constant feeling of being heavy and tired, especially if the frequency is between 0-4 (called delta waves, aka sleep waves, because that's the only time you are supposed to have them in large amounts). In order to reduce the predominance of this low-wave activity, I set the game to work better when higher (more awake) frequency waves grow in amplitude and lower frequency waves reduce. Since the person is not asleep during this session, the brain learns not to behave—at least for the moment—as if it were. In a sense we are teaching the brain that "no" means "not so much, especially not now."

Learning how to smoothly change one's place on the continuum of arousal is a good thing because having the mental agility to appropriately shift our level of alertness as well as our emotional state is necessary for healthy living with a healthy brain. Imagine trying to stay upright on a surfboard at sea. There is no perfect way to place your weight; there is only the perfect skill of shifting where you place your weight dependent upon the changes coming at you. The ease with which you shift gears determines how likely it is that you will reach the shore intact. Equally, the ease with which you shift focus also determines how appropriately comfortable you are in any given situation. Brain waves wash over you and affect you for reasons you probably already know, like the ability to move between playfulness and sleep. Brainwaves matter because the firing of brain waves is correlated with the firing of neurochemistry. So whether you have an excess of serotonin or a depletion of dopamine, changing how you fire changes what you fire, which changes how you feel and are. This is one of the ways in which I see "teaching" the brain to change its state as superior to medicating the brain to get it there. Teaching changes things in the direction of wellness and freedom while medicating leads to chronic problems and dependency.

For example, a young sixteen-year-old Aspergers boy I work with was given medicine to stimulate his frontal lobes—but since his entire brain was affected his parietal lobes (top portion at the back of the head) became over stimulated. He was focused but aggressive. He was then given another medicine to calm that down but became very nauseous and dizzy. Instead of dealing with all these side effects, I just isolated the regions I wanted to calm from the regions I wanted to stimulate and taught his brain how to do it on its own. This young gentleman's aggression and repetitive conversations were immediately (within six sessions) cut in half. (I should mention here that a session is usually thirty minutes in length). Thirty minutes or more of beeping brain binary codes can have an amazing impact.

So, we use beeeeep to indicate yes or on and an absence of beeeep to indicate no or off—beeps make the patterns—in the auditory form of the binary code. (If likening it to binary code—the original machine language of computers—is too hi tech for your imagination, try thinking of it as Morse code, one of our earlier simply constructed information passing codes that at least has an almost beeping sound to help us communicate). At any rate, contrary to how it looks, I don't put any electricity into the brain, nada, zero, zip, nothing goes in, except information. That's all. Neurofeedback teaches the brain by giving it information—like directions on where to grow. Your brain grows and changes throughout your entire life, so good directions can be invaluable.

And in the case of autism good directions can make the difference between growing more or growing less, exclusively. An exciting thing to note is that recently (as of this writing) it was discovered that several of the genes implicated in autism are not missing, damaged, or mutated in any way; they are just not turned on. Perhaps this is why my experience with neurofeedback is that it's an effective treatment... I can't think of a better way to turn genes on than to tell them, "Hey! You! Turn on!" I know that sounds like one of my *wink wink nudge nudge* jokes but in fact it may not be.

Like I said, my job starts when I put sensors on someone's head. I get the client to sit and play a simple game like Pacman or a more complex game like Space Race. Clients do this without really understanding how they do it. Fortunately, understanding is not required to affect a remarkable difference. Clients play these games without touching the keyboard; they simply power the game by changing their brain wave patterns ("Look Ma; no hands!") The client watches his/her game monitor. I watch mine and I also watch them. I watch for EEG patterns and Paroxysmal (think of it like power surges) events. I watch for over-firing and under-firing, artifact (think of it like static in the radio), and shifts of state. I watch the client, observe their color, expression, physical activity, pupil dilation, and notate any change. Always, always, always I am watching for change because that is my job: to watch for and create change. If I don't notice the shifts in state, I won't know how to follow him/her and ensure that the changes change in the direction of mine and my client's desire. This therapist role is a very out-of-control, controlling position to be in. Out of control because the brain itself chooses what to change. Controlling because it is my choices that choose what choices are available for the brain to choose from. Thus, I do my best to get a clear picture of my client's wishes and stay with that definition of success.

Doing neurofeedback is simple really—for the client. For me, however, sticking sensors on the heads of autistic kids with all their hypersensitivity to new people and new things coming anywhere near their person is a challenge. The challenge dissipates once they've done it a few times because then they come to me. I believe this is because it helps them; they like how neurofeedback teaches them to feel.

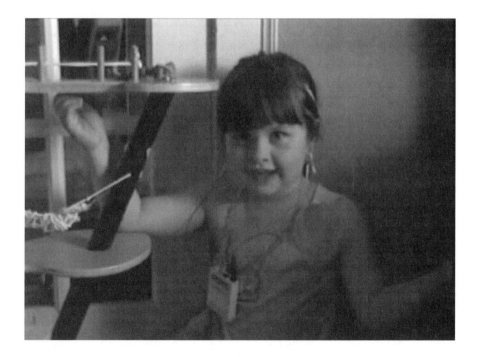

However those first sessions are definitely a challenge. Fortunately I will do aannyyyyything to make it happen.

For example, the first time I found myself working with this little guy who liked to run around saying "fiddle dee dee fiddle dee dee billy bob thorton betty boop bop" I grabbed one laptop and instructed his mom to grab the other. I signaled her to follow me while I followed the cute little "fiddle dee dee fiddle dee dee billy bob thorton betty boop bop" spouting whirling dervish until the moment when I could turn betty boop bop into betty boop "plop" by dropping the sensor onto his head. We continued to run behind him skipping over wires and trying not to disconnect anything. I set the parameters for "CALM DOWN!" and after a few minutes he slowed enough in his pacing for us to set the equipment on the desk. The information delivered via the beeps calmed him because once the sensor was on his head, his brain started to get feedback whether he was intentionally paying attention to the game or not. I have seen this reaction in many children who appear not to care. My suspicion on why is that autistic children live in such a state of cacophonous sensory information that they are driven to control or to block out any sensory information coming their way. Though we all desire control, their need may be even more intense than yours or mine might be. Perhaps hearing beeps in a non-rhythmic broken pattern is just irritating enough to catch their attention despite the appearance otherwise. Despite the fact that some autistic people may not care if they get points or make the game work in the same way that a neuro-typical person might, they do seem to attend quite well to whether or not the sound of the beeps is continuous and smooth. Hence with or without a cognitive buy-in on winning the game, the need to control the beeps is the only desire necessary in order to make the reward powerful enough for neurofeedback to treat the brain.

Fortunately, the game will work even if the child is zooming around or just daydreaming while I run the machine. And fortunately, the working of the game will affect change because, contrary to popular opinion, this therapy doesn't care if the child is paying attention with the part of the brain that pays attention because there's so much more to the brain than that. To recap: Since the brain has an innate ability to recognize patterns and a desire to change itself accordingly, when the sensors send his brain wave activity into my computer, my computer reads that information and tells the game computer—the one they are looking at and trying to play (or running around and trying to ignore)—my computer tells the game computer, "Hey, when he makes less energy in those problem frequencies go ahead, beep; when he doesn't, don't." And as I mentioned before, we are talking to the brain, just like when you teach your child's brain with do's and don'ts – only in this case it's a beeping code doing the talking.

To help you imagine the games I'll describe a simple one called

Mazes. It has a little Pacman head moving through a maze and eating dots. Whenever Pacman eats a dot the game "beeps" and, as you now know, when it beeps the connected brain hears "oh yes brain oh do that good brain good." Now when Pacman doesn't eat, Pacman doesn't beep, and when he doesn't beep the brain hears "oh no no no no now brain listen up, you too neurons we're saying don't fire." It's kind of like Pacman is spanking the synapse and saying, "Don't fire don't fire don't fire so many of those sleepy time waves right now—he's trying to be awake".

So with neurofeedback your neurons "listen" to me tell them how to fire and your synapses respond. Hence as I explained previously we affect neurochemistry.

Now, unless my count is extremely off, I've only mentioned the below points six times thus far so I'll sum it all up once more in order to hit that lucky remembering number, number seven, so we can move on, fully informed. Your brain is always growing and changing, basically restructuring itself. In the early years of life the neurons in your left hemisphere are still migrating into position. Your frontal lobes— the part we think we think with—are under construction throughout your entire childhood. Since parts of the neuron go and grow where the signals of your life tell them to, the neurofeedback beeps are kind of like a tracking device that beeps faster and faster the closer you get to the right position. Another good analogy is to imagine that your therapist is like the guy with the flashlights directing the plane into position: "Keep coming, over here, keep coming – Whoa! Stop!" It is a good analogy; the difference is instead of flashlights we use beeps—to direct those migrating and growing neurons into position. The beeps truly are like those flashlights because they don't have any more power over the brain than the lights do over the plane. Still, even though he doesn't have to, the pilot follows the beams, just as your neurons follow the beeps.

So even though humans are resistant to change because our brains are set up to want control, fortunately, like the pilot who accepts the rules of his vocation, our neurons' vocation is to gain control through pattern recognition and a desire for balance. Neurofeedback uses that reality and benefits from it in order to stimulate change by giving the brain some patterns to look for and try to control. So, next time you are tempted to call someone a control freak, think again. You would only be stating the obvious. Since resistance is a function of neuronal behavior and hence also of human behavior, we all do it. We do it individually and we do it in groups, as medical professionals, politicians, and families. My family was no exception. We were like many families with autism—making our way through—managing to change and learn—the hard way.

Once I started using neurofeedback on the whole family everyone got better. My youngest, Rye, stopped thinking he was the terminator and punching holes in the walls. I stopped eating caffeine pills to make it through the day. Chance stopped having night terrors. Cash started processing quicker and keeping up with the conversations his newfound friends were having. Both Cash and Rye—who were afflicted with fetal alcohol syndrome—moved off the continuum of retardation. These are only some of the reasons why I think biofeedback for the brain should be available to everyone. I also think it because neurofeedback stops those self-perpetuating crazy thoughts. It clears your head, brightens your mood, rather like Starbucks. (wink) I know I winked but actually, maybe that part is not a joke; maybe that part is a good idea. Neurofeedback *should* be available on every street corner just like Starbucks (wink again). Nah, that is not a good idea, neurofeedback should be made affordable, unlike Starbucks (final wink for now). Besides Starbucks is downsizing and neurofeedback should grow. (see? no wink)

This touch of lightheartedness—stolen in bits from the comedy portion of my live show on the subject—is meant to keep the information interesting. But comedic or not, I really do wish it were readily available because I think easy access to neurofeedback would be great for things like stopping inner-city violence. Think about it. Since all you need to do is dial in the necessary mood effect, if there was one on every corner and you see some guy walking through Central Park wielding an angry expression and a pair of clenched fists, all you have to do is guide him to the corner. Then his therapist could sit him down and beep his brain into calmness, almost like giving morphine, only better, because morphine makes you dependent whereas neurofeedback makes you independent. Of course no good therapist would purposefully cause a morphine effect. She could. But she shouldn't. Something less overwhelming is preferred. Trust me, I know from personal experience how detrimental it is to live the morphine effect. In fact, the first time I had neurofeedback the clinician took one listen to my constant patter (actually I still like to talk—yap yap yap yap, neurofeedback neurofeedback neurofeedback, incessant chatter really...)—anyway, that therapist listened to me tell her about Dar and said, "Girl, you need a little calming down; you are way too revved up."

I understand why she thought that, but the fact is she was wrong. What I really needed was revving up so I could calm down. I know it sounds weird, but I probably had an undiagnosed case of ADHD and needed help to relax and focus. The concept was the same for me as it is for those kids using stimulants like Ritalin or Adderall because without it their brain is so tired they have to run around just to stay awake. When you wake their brains up you take the burden off their bodies and voila! They can relax. Without help undiagnosed kids like this self medicate through the use of behaviors like hyperactivity and extreme sports. In fact, a young fellow I work with says he likes the rush of wake boarding because it relaxes him. At the time when I was first introduced to neurofeedback I was kind of like him—only without the wakeboard—I needed a little rush in order to relax. So, before neurofeedback I used Starbucks. (Now you know where the jokes came from: my life.) Where others might drown their sorrows at a bar, I drank coffee. This was especially true if I was depressed about a divorce. [Which left me needing the excitement of a new husband just to fall asleep. If no new husbands were available about five cups of coffee would do just as well. (wink)] The point is it took lots of stimulation to calm my body down enough to relax. So, because it's hard to tell the difference between hyperactivity caused by low brain-wave activity and hyperactivity caused by high brain-wave activity, the clinician guessed wrong and was approaching my brain totally backwards. With the best of intentions she placed the sensors on my head and pushed a few buttons that beeped my tired brain into the state of even more tired. This is what I call the morphine effect and that, by the way, is not such a good idea.

She didn't know my brain well enough yet though, so she dialed in the coordinates that she thought would change my mood into a calm Zen-like place. And it did. It really did! When the session was over, even though I felt a little weird, a bit "zoned," I was definitely calmer. I headed for home not really saying much to the clinician. Now the effect of a neurofeedback session becomes greater after it's over—in fact, what appears like a subtle change in focus when you first leave the office can incrementally magnify itself for anywhere from fifteen minutes to two days after you've stopped playing the "brain game." It was about forty-five minutes into my hour-long drive home when I noticed that I was starting to feel like I was on morphine.

Now do not imagine I know what morphine feels like because I was a drug user. I never did drugs, illegally. [Unless you count two months of pot smoking when I was fifteen. Well? Do you? Actually don't bother answering; I can't hear you anyway. (wink)] The truth is the reason I know what morphine feels like is I had lung surgery, which in case you were wondering hurts a lot. Anyway, they gave me one of those self-administering morphine machines where you just push the button every time you want to fly away from the pain.

Now being on morphine for pain while you recuperate is OK cause all you are driving is an IV pole. However, astral projecting because your neurofeedback session put you in a morphine-like state while your body drives a speeding-down-the-highway-at-seventy-miles-an-hour CAR!!!! That's not so good! Because it's a CAR!!! I remember watching the world zipping by and taking on a kind of glowing amber slow-motion underwater effect. I tried to shake it off and wake up but I was beepin' stoned. My brain was slowed down to the speed of molasses. It took me forever to think the orders out, "Pullllll ovvvverrrr! Stttoppp! Ggettt ouuuttt!" I was definitely out all right, spaced out! It took at least ten minutes to realize that I had to put my hand in my pocket in order to get the money out for the coffee that I hoped would be the antidote for my slow-motion state.

This story is why I said I know how detrimental to being alive a morphine effect can be. The power of that first neurofeedback session was incredible, and dangerous while driving. The truth is, my state was more altered and much longer lasting than anything I ever got from morphine. I was stoned for days. So maybe neurofeedback shouldn't be on every street corner dispensed by baristas without proper training (wink). It definitely shouldn't be dispensed at a drive-through (wink wink double blink). All teasing aside, neurofeedback is safe. In fact, it is actually both the strongest and the safest brain-altering therapy there is, really, because the effects of neurofeedback are reversible. Which was lucky for me or I'd be on some beach right now saying "Whoa! This grain of sand is Cool Man!" while some vacationing doctor diagnosed me as high-functioning autistic. Fortunately, it only took two additional brain biofeedback (alternate way of saying neurofeedback) sessions to make me function like myself again, which as you may recall wasn't that much better: instead of driving while drugged, typically I was driving while daydreaming!

Fortunately, after four sessions of neurofeedback I wasn't myself, or rather, I was more myself than I'd ever been. I was clear, bright, and able to focus all the way home. I felt like a brand new version of me. Now that was a trip! I felt like I was on a—better than downing all the coffee in Cuba—bright-headed buzz. It was so exciting! However, that wasn't the best part. The best part came when I learned that even though, at the time of the morphine-like effect, it didn't feel as if that slow-motion session was helping me get brighter, it turned out it was. Apparently every session was working toward healing my brain because all that agile flipping back and forth from one focus state to another exercised it and made it flexible. And, like I said, according to the literature, a flexible brain that is able to switch focus and shift states easily but not frenetically is a healthy brain. What that meant to me was that biofeedback for the brain is a fairly safe therapy to apply—especially on yourself (always assuming you have learned enough about the therapy and the brain to do so) because even the mistakes can become a blessing. Thus, even if you used the neurofeedback computers to self medicate—which I wouldn't advise—your brain would get healthier as you just naturally follow your own changes, tweaking and shifting the protocols in search of homeostasis. In fact, seeking balance is what all junkies are doing, especially once they find themselves avoiding the crash and reaching for more. Only as I already mentioned, with neurofeedback we don't create dependency like drugs do; we create independency and work towards healing many different disorders.

So it is great right? After all, it is legal! Think of it: you can get a buzz without getting busted! (OK, OK, enough joking) But it is great because instead of losing touch with reality, with neurofeedback, your buzz is one of clarity and comfort. For me achieving clarity of thought was like finding the pot at the end of the rainbow. It was such a life-changing heretofore-elusive windfall of health that I became convinced everyone would benefit. Because of that conviction I often joke that I could make a fortune by hiding in the back alleys as the woman in the trench coat full of drugs to sell. Except that my drugs are computers and instead of hurting I help. I like the image because it is a funny thought with some actual issues imbedded within: Drugs and therapies when kept expensive and secretive become "underground" elitist. Sometimes what works to improve the quality of life is not what is readily available to the masses.

By (possibly the pharmaceutical industry) keeping things rare, the price is driven up, which means people like me get to work less and make more. And that's a problem. (Don't misunderstand me; I like making a goodly amount of money per hour and I adore being paid to sit on an airplane and watch movies whenever I work Internationally. But even though I work hard, make a difference, and like to buy nice things as much as the next gal, I don't like knowing that there are a lot of parents who just can't afford my kind of help. And since the main cost of home training is buying the units themselves, I can't do all that much about the expense.) So it's a problem because, even though I am well paid for my time, the fees are prohibitive to many clients and my dream is affordability for all. In a way I got this idea of making a lot of money by making things cheaper from a friend. For years I was blessed with the company of this very rich very good mentor friend. He was extremely generous and included many people in his projects. His answer to the question of dilution of income was always the same. "It's better to have a small piece of a big pie than a big piece of a small pie." Whenever he said that I would imagine how much more I would gain from a small piece of Wal-mart than a big piece of an upscale boutique. I think it is partly because of his influence that I have come to believe we all gain when the prices go down. So I believe we would all benefit by seeing this therapy go mainstream. In the final analysis I am just selfish enough to want more: more happiness, more health, and more financial security for everyone.

I want a happier healthier society wherein we all fight less and succeed more. If neurofeedback can help create that, then I want to spread the word. This long-range grandiose goal is why I write with humor. I believe if we laugh a little while we learn a lot we gel into one united force. We become the "big pie" and exert a greater influence. Thus, I will reach more people. Of course I realize that autism, science, and humor are unusual bedfellows and that being light about textbook information can be construed as disrespectful to the serious nature of the subject matter. I realize that this could be hazardous to my career, but I'm OK with that. Because I enjoy laughing more than I enjoy worrying about being misunderstood—which in my experience—is inevitable at any rate. Cautions like "Joking about autism and brain science is unprofessional" simply tell me that my approach is needed. Because learning enough brain science to help your autistic child at home inevitably requires a PhD in parenting, and nobody survives that career choice without a sense of humor. It's the *messy-haired meet-the-teachers night; spewed-on jogging pants you also slept in; here, wear my wedding dress to prom; I'll watch the recital as soon as your brother stops screaming in the car, immediate-responding techniques that presuppose a need to jerry rig the solutions until you get to the end that never comes, part of raising an autistic child before you have the means or ability to do so,* that makes laughing a basic need and changes your life for the better.

So perhaps there is a reason why most professionals in the field of mental health don't reveal the history of their own challenges when sharing the jewels of what they know, but that doesn't mean it's a good reason, at least not for me. I think not sharing is a missed opportunity to lead and connect. I think it's the "used to be" in the crazy, from within myself and my own family, that gives me the credibility to teach. If I were in that back alley hawking my wares to all the people who found me repulsive, I'm sure I'd be saying, " Come back here! Dontcha get it? I'm better now! You could be like me—healthier—stronger than I was before I got all blissed out! Heck, I'm not even stupid anymore."

That's because intelligence is basically a function of processing speed, and I found a way to increase mine with neurofeedback. As I said before, it gives your brain directions on how to help itself, and part of that help leads to getting your brain to process at a more desirable pace. Personally, I've done a lot of sessions. So nowadays I comprehend at a pretty good clip. In fact, I've turned into a kind of a speedy thinking brainiac, well, according to me. [What can I say? It's a comparative thing (wink).] But seriously, (because after all, I did promise to stop joking) I have noticed a lot of differences in my functioning. For example, my couldn't-focus-enough-to-make-it-through-high-school IQ was so turned on that I could learn neuroanatomy. This was unlike my previous college experience of taking mainframe computer languages that required an insane level of hyper-focusing and a maniacal attention to detail. (Trust me; no one would want to live with me then. I even flow charted my salt and pepper shakers.) Neurofeedback made neuroanatomy a fairly easy course. Interestingly, though, this teaching the brain how-to-learn process meant that I became a very different person than I had previously been. Remarkably, no matter how much I changed, I always managed to stay the same me. I believe that this is because the "who of who I am" is made up more by my motivations than my brain capacity. For example, though my mental acuity for brain biology and electronic processing improved a lot, other aspects of me improved but only a little. At present, I'm still challenged in the things that don't interest me, things like politics and math. However the new me—unlike the old me—is challenged in these areas not because she's not smart enough or able to stay focused, but rather because she is smart enough to be otherwise focused into something tangibly valuable. [Of course tangibly valuable and smarter are both just my personal assessments; you know, comparative things (wink).] Getting smarter itself was motivating for me. As it turned out, to make the journey I had to learn a lot about my brain, which made my brain better at learning a lot. I felt so much better I had to share it. That's when I started using neurofeedback to fix other folks—who also got smarter—enough for me to teach them how to fix other folks who also got smarter and then other folks who also got smarter and so on.

Spreading the healing is what therapists do, because they have to, in order to spread it to themselves. When I first began to take classes in biofeedback for the brain, I discovered that all those MD's and PhD's in the class were either there for continuing education points and not very interested in actually doing the therapy or had come to the class as a result of their own search for mental health (either in their own lives or the life of a family member). Not to belabor the point, but since all life is seeking balance, it is not too surprising that most people are attracted to the field within which they believe they will find balance. Thus the financially challenged seek to gain money and the emotionally disturbed seek to gain comfort. "Physician Heal Thyself" is a revealing mantra because, as it turns out, most health professionals I meet are trying to do exactly that. I see this as a good thing—as long as the professional in question is mostly done healing when he becomes your practitioner—because it is our journey of sameness that helps us to help each other. I believe that a willingness to share one's own foibles with honesty leads by example and helps others do the same—effectively shortening the time it takes to unravel the pain and heal the brain.

THE WAY WE WOULD NORMALLY DESCRIBE THIS MIRACLE: She was a beautiful elderly Psychiatrist with Parkinson's. When we met she was either in a wheel chair or holding a cane and leaning on walls. She had been a pioneer and singular force as a woman in the field of mental health back in the sixties. Forty years later she closed down her practice and sunk into a depression. After thirty-five sessions of neurofeedback, she was a medium-paced cane-only walker reopening her office and wearing "happy socks" with Santas on them.

THE FACTS BEHIND THE REST OF THE MIRACLE: Even after reopening her office, she was still having difficulty talking and her balance was often unpredictable. She was faking it with her clients and letting them do all the talking. She decided to include neuro-feedback in her practice and took a certification class. I tutored her through as she tired easy and her cognition was still fairly affected. She began treating herself first in order to gain more experience and then told her story to a couple of long-standing patients. She offered to use this new therapy on them for free as a case study. One of the patients agreed to try it.

THE PASSING OF A MIRACLE: Dr. M. discovered this treatment because she needed it, and because she was helped she passed the treatment to her patient, and because she was willing to share her story her patient agreed to try it. This lucky patient, whom Dr. M. had treated for years, this lucky patient whom Dr. M had been unable to lift from his depression in all that time, this lucky patient stopped needing his meds. He then spent a Christmas with his family for the first time since his wife passed away ten years earlier. It was a beginning.

I have chosen to try to work with whole families rather than individuals because families—like clusters of neurons—reflect and reinforce each other's position when trying to create balance in the group. So, again, because of this homeostatic urge it appears to me that if I want to heal individuals, I must also heal their group. (This thought expands and expands outward into cultures, nations, and global communities. Another reason for wanting to bring this therapy into the mainstream is because healing my group actually requires also healing yours, since at some level we are all part of the same family). I tell you about my family (composed of myself and my children) in order to help you learn about yours. In my family we all changed together and maybe that, almost as much as neurofeedback itself, is why Dar no longer regresses, though his progress is slow.

I began to understand autism and this therapy by learning on myself, and my variety pack of a family. Fortunately for me, I had a plethora of heads and disorders to practice on. Since they were my children, I was able to bypass the need to proceed according to the norm. In my experience many clinic decisions in regards to treatment are driven by the fear of future litigation created by unrealistic expectations on the parts of the patients. Thus with thoughts of possible court dates in mind, many clinicians proceed with prudence based on protocols already known to have a particular effect, albeit for somebody else. This approach meant to maximize safety minimizes experimentation, slows down the rate of learning, dilutes the therapy, and prevents creative thinking. It also prevents strongly individualized programs that are only loosely based on what is known about others. I didn't have to worry about any of this.

I proceeded with excitement and curiosity, wearing that familiar old *Sherlock Holmes of the Mind* hat. Everything I learned became part of my toolbox, so mixing and matching according to the evidence presented became my style. Because the brains I began with belonged to my children and me, I just followed the clues in their behavioral, emotional, and cognitive responses. They blossomed before my eyes. I was fueled by the information I gained as I learned neuroanatomy, brainstormed on neurofeedback, read about autism, and saw every single one of my children as capable. I designed a can-do approach for whole families to follow. Nowadays, I walk into a home and three days later when I walk out everyone is happier, more comfortable in his/her own skin, and also in the skin of their family. Rather than leave them to deteriorate in my absence, I leave them with tools. I leave them with neurofeedback, reams of knowledge, and a life-long commitment to ongoing support. I leave them equipped for the future so that they can continue to benefit at a lesser cost than would be possible ii they had to go to a clinic for their treatments. (Autistic children need hundreds of sessions. Add to that the forty or more required by each other family member and even my math skills can see the benefits of home training as compared to paying approximately a hundred dollars a session in a clinician's office.).

Having learned from following the changes in my own children, my overall approach is based on following evidence of neuronal change by being observant to changes in behavioral responses. I am lucky. I get to observe a lot of change like the exciting emergence of both expected and unexpected skills in all the children I work with. I am lucky. I know so many culturally diverse, wonderful parents who learn about their children from me as I learn about their children from them. Together we work to heal larger and larger groups as we make new protocol choices according to the differences we see and the similarities we seek. And so we learn, together, how to follow the shifting of the mind in order to recreate health. And in following each other follow the evidence I have learned this: that every family is beautiful and that the best-case scenario for healing brain disorders like autism is with neurofeedback, a united front, and positive reinforcement, by the whole family, of man, as one.

And that's why I called this chapter OK! OK! Neurofeedback Is Great!

CHAPTER SEVEN

Neuroanatomy as My Guide

I daydreamed a lot as a child and my understanding with regard to where my body landed in space was a little challenged. So I spent a lot of time bumping into things. On an almost weekly basis I drove my head into the cubby door that was generally left hanging open above our stairwell. However, even though it being open was a common occurrence, I still bounced whenever I trounced down the stairs, always forgetting that the darn thing was laying in wait. So on the hip in my hop I'd pile drive into it damaging the top of my skull and dropping into dizzy again and again and one more again. The irony in something like this is the more times you hit your head, the less likely it is that your memory skills will be intact enough to help you remember to not hit your head. To complicate the picture my mother was known to fly into rages of hurricane force. So I was shaken, punched, thrown down the stairs, and brain bashed with blunt objects every weekend and at least once during the week. For me being slapped from side to side was an almost daily occurrence, and as a teenager my nose was broken straight up and into my sinuses. On top of all that were the innocent accidents that befall every child in the hood. For example, at about six years of age my babysitter turned out the lights and we all played ghost tag. It was fun but I couldn't see, so I fell into the coffee table and damaged my skull just above the right eye.

At the age of thirteen I began to attempt suicide and over-dosed on every household cold medicine and painkiller my mom ever bought. I had aspirin-induced tinnitus (ringing in the ears) for six months after one of these episodes. For two months after another my vision was blurred in a swirling pattern and it seemed as if I was trying to look through a rainbow-colored gasoline slick that slid and shifted with the tilt of my head. Between the ages of two and eight I had Synesthesia (saw sound as color), smelled rubbing alcohol all the time, and my vision was pixilated (saw people in pieces and couldn't recognize them in different environments). The edges of things wiggled until well into my thirties. Due to this mosaic mess I have no idea if any parts of my brain functioned normally. I do know I definitely had *marry-men-like-you-are-following-the-directions-on-a-shampoo-bottle* brain damage. No, I do not think that is an actual diagnosis, (wink) but it is possible that the injury I sustained while playing boo in the dark may have damaged my right frontal lobe and compromised its ability to inhibit romantic impulses. I do know I was different.

As I have already mentioned, neurofeedback helped me to focus and changed my life dramatically. Initially I simply worked on lifting my spirits and replacing all that coffee with faster happier brain waves. I pretty much concentrated on strengthening the left hemisphere (more of a detail-work and logic-oriented hemisphere) even though all my mentors and teachers said I should be working on healing my right hemisphere (more of a big-picture-concept-oriented hemisphere that knows how to get married but not so much how to stay that way). The problem was every time I tried teaching my right hemisphere to calm down and stop monopolizing my state I ended up feeling stoned and nauseous. Contrarily, whenever I exercised the left hemisphere I felt bright and happy.

Brainwaves come in frequencies measuring anywhere from 0 to 60 or 70 hertz, depending upon which professional you believe. When reinforcing brain-wave activity, the basic school of thought is to reinforce the activity generated at 13–17 hertz and higher on the left hemisphere and around 12–15 hertz and lower on the right. The effects of these are similar to what one might expect. Training higher frequencies to increase generally causes a brighter feeling while increasing lower frequencies creates a more calming effect. However, this is just a general statement and depending upon the original state of the brain being trained, opposite effects to what you might expect are often achieved.

As I progressed through the sessions I could literally feel my ability to understand and remember increase. This, as I have said, caused a subsequent rise in my IQ. Thus I often did neurofeedback just before tests in order to increase my scores. (Interesting to note: what worked best for my brain was a fairly high training frequency of 19–22. Much later I was to learn that the benzo bump occurs globally in the brain as an increase in activity in a similar high-range-frequency group. The benzo bump is a curious happening not well understood by science. It appears cortex-wide for a small period of time as a result of taking any of the anti-anxiety medicines known as benzodiazepines such as Valium. I wondered if I hadn't stumbled on the same "feel good" I would have gotten from the drug without the drug actually being necessary; certainly my anxiety had been relieved. I smiled to think that I may have made a discovery even while having no intention of following up and figuring it out with certainty if I had because, finally, I knew how to stay focused on the goal. In this case the goal was helping rather than researching Fortunately, with neurofeedback, it's OK not to be able to connect all the dots because the brain does that for us.)

Regardless of why I needed this frequency, since this type of training made me "feel good" I followed the effect and encouraged my brain to make more activity in the 19–22 hertz range. Since this felt good while nothing else did, I ignored all the advice I was getting from others and followed myself. In my opinion "following a person's state change" while keeping an eye on the long-term goal—whatever that might be (for the purpose of clarity, let's say, "better behavioral control")—is a skill that should be taught to anyone wishing to make a beneficial difference in the mental health of another (or in the mental health of him/herself for that matter).

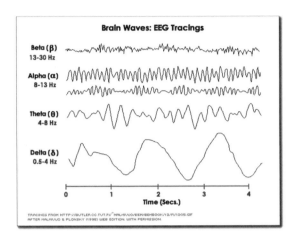

Brain Waves: EEG Tracings

Beta (β) 13-30 Hz

Alpha (α) 8-13 Hz

Theta (θ) 4-8 Hz

Delta (δ) 0.5-4 Hz

Time (Secs.)

TRACINGS FROM HTTP://BUTLER.CC.TUT.FI/~MALMIVUO/BEM/BEMBOOK/13/FI/1305.GIF
AFTER MALMIVUO & PLONSKY (1995) WEB EDITION. WITH PERMISSION.

In order to help you follow the manner of influence neurofeed-back has over the brain I will share some basic knowledge, bit by bit, as we move along in this journey of stories. To begin with, as I just mentioned, brain waves range in frequency from 1 to 60 or 70. They are then divided into groups of low frequencies, sort of low frequencies, medium low frequencies, sort of high frequencies, high frequencies, and jeez, I think these ones have something to do with the collective consciousness frequencies. That's too much to say so in order to talk about them we give the different groups of brain-wave frequencies names. At first they were called delta, theta, alpha, beta, and gamma. Then in the middle of this group was added (an overlapped frequency name) SMR, which stands for Sensory Motor Rhythm, and was the allocated grouping of activity (when on the sensory motor strip) first discovered to be trainable in the original "cat" experiment. Each of these frequencies is represented in the brain at all times and dependent upon the location, anatomical variation, and the activity the person is engaged in, the weight or "balance" of which group is firing as the dominant frequency shifts and adjusts in order for the brain to do its job well. Flexibility requires a healthy brain.

Some people have difficulty shifting gears. They get "stuck" in mania or depression or just "wigged out" by transitions. These people may have a physiologically inflexible brain that is trying to stay in control by staying put. Neurofeedback works beautifully to teach the brain a new "be ahead of the curve" "duck and weave" "shift and sidestep" method of control. I use these sayings because they are cute and easy to relate to, but they are also only partly true: too far ahead of the curve means too anticipatory of an action and/or too impulsive. As any touch-everything person with ADHD or any parent of a young child with her still-undeveloped left frontal lobe asking the lady at the checkout stand why she is so fat and ugly can attest, being too impulsive leads to a pot full of problems. So perhaps a more desirable epigrammatic phrase describing a healthy brain would be "on the curve" and "ready for action."

It appears that once again we are talking about balance because, like for the surfer on the crest of the wave, "perfect balance is an ever-shifting state" and comfort comes from the ability to maintain that fluidity. My brain was not fluid. In my brain I found an extreme predominance of delta everywhere. Since delta is the term used to describe low-frequency brain waves sometimes referred to as sleep waves—because as previously mentioned, that's the only time you're supposed to have them in large amounts—it's not too surprising I was caffeine dependent. And that's why I felt best when I used the neuro-feedback equipment to ask my brain to give me more of those bright high-frequency waves and fewer of those dreamy low-frequency waves: nothing like a good strong dose of caffeinated beeps.

Many things improved. My twenty-year bout with diarrhea cleared up (I often track alterations in bowel behavior and shifts in a person's sleep patterns in order to judge the direction the neurofeedback changes are taking us), my mood lifted, and my caffeine intake dropped in half. Even more important, I began to finish things. Always before, I would hyper focus—learn the skill and then quit—just before completing the project. Now all of a sudden I went until it (whatever that might be) was done. My math skills were still embarrassing but I figured, "What the heck; they have calculators for that." The truth is I kind of enjoyed my numbers' deficit. As a child math answers had come easy, but the steps I took to get those answers was unknown to me. The teachers considered this a problem and marked all right answers with a zero unless accompanied by the appropriate steps. I felt invalidated and confused. I couldn't share what I didn't know, and I didn't know the steps since I hadn't actually taken any in the first place. I did know the answers, but since that was met with suspicion by others it was met with suspicion by me. I stopped knowing even the part I did know, and remained unable to grasp the part I didn't. According to everyone around me, the problem was I didn't try. They may have been right. After years of avoiding math I was suddenly lost and barely capable of simple arithmetic. Fortunately, most of my children were too disabled to need help with algebra.

As I write this I realize I am not representing things in an accurate manner: I could add and subtract (especially when aided by an adding machine) and at sixteen even got a job as bookkeeper for an affiliate of Singer Sewing Machines. However, in order to attend to the details of step-by-step processing I had to block out all sensory input, and the effort required was exhausting. This type of steel-trap focusing hampered my more spontaneous side. It just wasn't fun, and quite frankly I didn't want to do it so I quit the job, just as I had always quit whenever math was required. I tried to find ways around the problem and learned to enjoy other people's need to caretake the situation. Eventually I noticed I was doing this. It happened while playing Scrabble with my best friend who totally rocks at math. As usual I was letting her keep score, but then I noticed that she always won—hmmmm? Now, now, settle down. According to the rules of science "correlation does not always prove causation" so I ignored her successes because that was easier than checking on her scoring. I chose to love laughing at the jibes made about my lack of mental math prowess. I chose to love laughing more than learning how to make the jibes no longer true because—in this arena—avoidance was my preferred activity. We bonded over laughter, her at my math, me at her serious more competitive nature, and us at our crazy words. So, for me the problem had become fun, except when it wasn't.

I avoided math so well and for so long that I even lost my ability to keep the books for my own company. Unfortunately, though my friend was happy to keep score at Scrabble, she wasn't willing to take over my bookkeeping. In fact nobody was stepping up to the plate and offering to help me with that. Though generally happy with my life, I lived on an undercurrent of nervousness about money. Sure, my checking account stayed healthy, but even when my check book balance sheet said I was doing OK, I just didn't trust my own answers. I wasn't bouncing checks or missing payments—just always a little uncertain of my own skill. To be safe I would add buffers to the amounts. There was no real downside to my solution. In fact, it led to a little extra money from time to time, but the feeling of uncertainty undermined my comfort and kept me from really going after success in business. This fear of figures played out in many ways. For example I never negotiated payment terms or read the financial forms from my investment company. I often paid too much in interest, never checked my credit-card statements, and stressed every year over my taxes, even though I paid someone else to do them. I preferred all of this discomfort to trying to understand the world of finance because I believed myself incapable. I excused myself with the term artsy because my fear of failing at being businesslike was overwhelming.

By the time I noticed this addiction to math avoidance via my friends Scrabble scoring good-natured jibes I had already managed to fix some of my problems simply by using neurofeedback to increase my ability to focus. I've always been good at pattern recognition, and so I leaned heavily on this skill as I became comfortable with reading EEG's and gaining a relationship with the mathematical equations buried within the therapy I was using to heal my family. The need to know had created a need to heal and I was partially there. Partial healing created a craving for complete healing. I was quickly reaching a place in my life where I wanted to "walk my own talk," and as my Scrabble games were easily pointing out there was more to be done. I worried that I couldn't really encourage others to heal themselves if I kept avoiding healing this part of me. I knew I really needed to do therapy on the top part of the back of my head (parietal lobe), especially on the right side. But I was afraid.

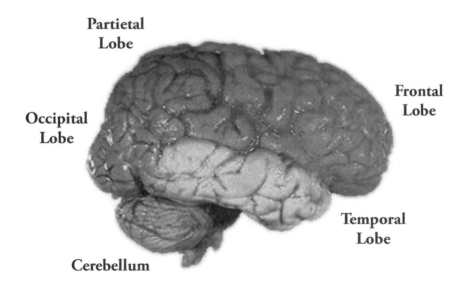

My last experiment in this area had left me ill and disoriented for a week, and I just couldn't stomach the thought of trying again. On top of that my original mentor in the field of neurofeedback had said I would never be able to treat this area as it wasn't "right for me." She said something to the effect of "treating the back brings you into the back and that's not good for you." Even though I knew her explanation was void of neuroanatomy and a little too non-specific for me to be certain of its validity, I remained nervous. Still, I was tempted. I'd learned some things since my last attempt and thought that the new information could change the result. When I had tried previously I had done the session at my normal reinforce-the-faster-wave-frequency choice of 19–22 because I hadn't yet learned that different areas needed a different predominance of different brain-wave groupings.

In fact, at the time of that experimental effort I hadn't learned a lot of things. For example, some autistic and sensory-disordered people have the desired brain-wave balance of activity between the front and the back parts of the brain reversed: They fire too much beta (higher waves) in the back and too much alpha or theta (lower waves) in the front. What they then need is to have the slower waves reinforced in the back and the faster waves reinforced in the front. Given my autistic-like history of sensory challenges, I figured I'd gotten half of it right (I was treating for a deficit in low beta—aka sort of high frequencies—on the left prefrontal and frontal lobes). I had definitely helped myself with the frontal training, but my parietal experiment had probably just reinforced my own problem—not because I couldn't treat this area as I'd been told but because I shouldn't treat it at a high frequency—thus I had been right to fear beeping that area with feedback, at least until I learned more. Once I learned that my response to this area had been my own error and that the parietal lobe and the frontal lobe work in association with each other to facilitate focus and since focus had been a life-long problem, I continued to wonder if maybe I shouldn't give it another try. I don't think I would have though. My life was improving and I was happier and since I was now more focused than any of my friends, I just couldn't imagine it getting any better than it already was. So, except for the nagging feeling that I should have more subjective knowledge about everything I taught, I just wasn't all that motivated to experiment. Until…

Three things changed: I got tinnitus, I got vertigo, and I entered a Scrabble tournament.

For every big change one simply needs the right motivator (remember this statement because it is true of autistic people as well). The first thing that happened was (shortly after smashing my temple into a speaker while practicing a comedic stop-drop-and-roll move for my new show) my right ear began to ring incessantly. Remembering the old overdose-of-aspirin days I cut out all my allergy meds and hoped for the best. Result: Nothing but an increase in volume. I researched and theorized and tried many things. I even decided to attempt right hemisphere low frequency training, which sent me back to a kind of old-news lethargy that I had to treat my way out of, and over and over I kept remembering a picture I'd seen of an auditory tumor (benign) in a patient's right parietal lobe. Now, my head had sustained many injuries by this time so I wasn't really giving that enough weight as a possible cause because, after all, I was used to them. Whereas, since my dad, my mom, and my niece had all dealt with brain tumors of varying types and I had not, suspecting something of this nature seemed quite logical. I also had dizziness and headaches to confirm the possibility and could well have gone for an MRI and followed the path of (who knows?) believing it into being a tumor (?), but I decided to look at the evidence differently.

I considered the fact that I had already followed the logical first steps of investigating my Eustachian tubes, allergies and nightly teeth clenching to see if they were at the roots of my tinnitus. I bought a mouth guard, had my ears checked, and underwent a cat scan of my sinuses. Wherever there was a problem I had it treated and still the ringing rang on. I checked my vitamin B levels, adjusted my hormones, and added zinc and ginko biloba to my supplement regimen, all while listening to my ears whistle a high-pitched wail. I continued to consider the possibility that the problem could be treated with neurofeedback. I wondered if an imbalance in my sensory system was causing the tinnitus and treated my sensory motor strip. Since that didn't work I went nearer the auditory pathways and treated my right temporal lobes again. At the same time I was doing a parasite flush to get rid of the little critters I'd picked up while drinking cow's blood in that Masai ritual in Kenya. (When in Rome? Ok! Ok! So I shouldn't have done that!)

These nasty little devils create cysts and tumors in the lung, liver, and brain; and according to all the tests I'd done, my lungs and my liver were loaded with benign blebs and cysts that could be encasing dead bits of parasite. OOPS! So it was only logical that while being serenaded by imaginary dog whistles I began to wonder if the parasites had gotten into my brain. Again my thoughts turned to more dire possibilities. This time, instead of refusing to look, I researched brain cysts and tumors. Though the parasite was a good theory, it wasn't an easy one to treat; and I wanted something I could get my hands on. I researched the benign auditory tumors whose first symptom is often "ringing in the ears." I found pictures of them located in both temporal and parietal locations and read the various treatment options. The general reaction is either surgery or—if the tumor is small and the symptoms are mild—a wait-and-see approach. This helped to ease any sense of urgency I was creating and allowed me to think once again in terms of neurofeedback. Since the tumors seemed to show up in the temporal lobe (which by now I had treated extensively) and the parietal lobe (which I was still avoiding), it occurred to me that the auditory pathway near the angular gyrus (located in the parietal lobe and seen as the intersection of various sensory systems) could be compromised.

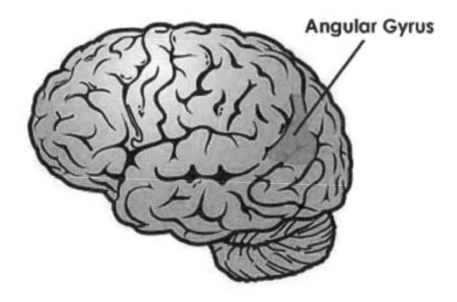

Angular Gyrus

I thought about one of my clients: Bob had had bad tinnitus but I had been treating him for focus. Coincidentally, as his focus improved so did his tinnitus. I looked up his protocols and saw that I had done a lot of work on the right parietal lobe near a location we label p6. (Locations are allocated by using a letter to illustrate the desired lobe or area. In this case 'P' stands for Parietal. We then add to that letter a number that is based on a 10/20 system, which denotes distance from 0. Zero allocations run from nose to neck in the middle of the head between the two hemispheres. Which side of the head one is treating is indicated through the use of evens and odds. Even numbers indicate right hemisphere training; odds indicate left. Think of the skull like a globe and the mapping system as lines of longitude and latitude and the concept becomes clearer and easier to understand.) The Parietal zone I'd done on Bob was the only area in his treatment plan that I hadn't successfully done on myself. So I was tempted to try it. However, I didn't want a repeat of the last time I'd treated myself there. My clients and family just couldn't afford to have me out of action for a week. And even though it had worked for Bob, that didn't mean it would work for me.

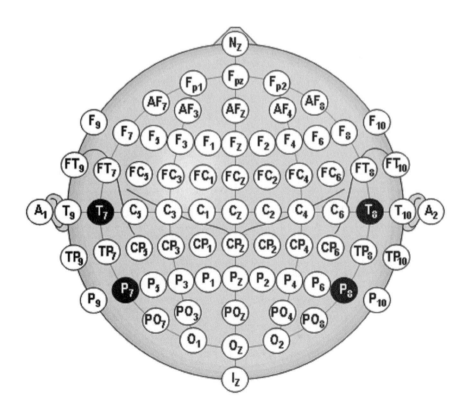

One of the things I've learned from helping so many different brain disorders is that very often the part of the brain that needs the most help resists it with the greatest intensity. This kickback can cause some very uncomfortable temporary side effects. On the other hand, since that's the area needing help, giving it feedback could also cause some marvelous healing to ensue. So a little creative insistence with an eye to the goal of total health is always a good idea. I have an edge over many neurofeedback clients because I am self training. Thus I am able to listen to my own reactions and adjust accordingly. I knew that if I gave feedback to my Parietal lobe for just a few minutes, the subjective info of how I was feeling should help me know when to stop, even if that was immediately. I also knew that since I was already struggling with a rolling dizziness, any increase in that direction would be made quickly obvious to me. Best of all, if it did happen, I knew how to fix it: I could immediately right myself by returning to the left front and reinforcing it at my usual 19—22 hertz.

Thus it was that I was considering treating myself in the right parietal when I entered my first Scrabble tournament. The tournament was an interesting experience. My friend won second place for our division; I was way down at fourth or fifth; and though playing had been fun, scoring under the pressure of a timer had been stressful. The laughing and coffee club conversation was kept to a minimum by the tournament director whose main job was to say "Shhhhh!" approximately every three seconds. In order to enjoy the experience and stop getting shushed, I tried to take the competition seriously. I immediately panicked over my fear of simple math. It was quickly made obvious that adding my score took me much longer than creating words out of a mish mash of letters, and my pounding heart and slow addition was costing me oodles of points. So I just stopped. I ignored my score pad and let my opponent do the math on hers. Surprisingly, I lost using this approach [That was sarcasm (wink)]. But I did feel better, at least until I thought about it. My friend loves this game and wants to do more tournaments. I love my friend so I want to join her. But for me social time (and work for that matter) must be fun. I realized that to play in more tournaments and have fun, my math skills more than my spelling skills would have to improve. I went home and hooked up my right parietal lobe. Why? Because some math solving brain issues are located here.

I had finally been motivated enough to fix this area of my processing. I went slow and easy, training only a few minutes at a time. Within the first two sessions the dizziness and nausea stopped. After another five sessions the ringing began to diminish in volume… eleven sessions later it was so quiet I had to force myself to hear it… two sessions more and it was gone (hopefully for good). As for my math skills, well, I guess at some point I'll enter another tournament, put the timer on, and find out; but by that point in my story I had forgotten the whole math issue and was just happy to enjoy the quiet. It lasted for a year and a half until…

I was doing an outreach with a new family in Florida. I'd had an awesome and productive first day and I went to bed happily tired. I fell asleep around 10 PM. Then, at 4:12 AM I heard a loud SNAP! BOING! inside my head just above the right ear. Surprised awake, I opened my eyes and the room began to spin. Let me interrupt myself here to say that I had heard of and even treated vertigo before, but until that moment I had completely underestimated how totally debilitating the experience actually is. It isn't at all like in the movies or even in my overly graphic imagination. It isn't an experience of "seeing" the room spin; it's an experience of the room actually spinning. The room spins despite the fact that the parts of your body in touch with the floor or bed or tub or toilet are telling you it's not. The experience is like being split into two distinct halves: The back half stays pressed to the floor while the front half spins and swirls and tries to separate, arguing with the brain that such a thing is possible. It makes for an unacceptable sensory experience that forces the system to vomit up, all over oneself. Thus, while parts of my body did not seem to spin other parts did as I tumbled and fell and swirled into an *Alice in Wonderland* vortex that unhinged me from my planet of self. I awoke to find myself sweating and puking. I tried closing my eyes but my body separated and spun even more intensely, so I dropped from the bed to the floor. I dragged and rolled and belly crawled from the floor to the tub to the toilet, but I was too sick to lift my head to the rim. I tried spotting the wall like a ballerina, but still I couldn't get a hold of myself for the motion. My internal dialogue was simple and focused. I kept telling myself that "this is just vertigo— get a hold of yourself—you have to work in the morning—get to your units—get to your units—get to your units." Even while lost in this experience I found myself grateful to have the knowledge to not be terrified.

It took me four hours, but eventually I made it to my neurofeed-back computers by sliding down the stairs or rather pouring myself like a cartoon figure made flat against the carpet. I got to my units and plugged myself in.

Knowing neuroanatomy I realized that some minute little calcium deposit or protein particle could simply have come loose in my inner ear and set my world reeling. I approximated the location, placed the sensor on my head (at c4) and started to beep. It worked: The session helped and the spinning slowed to a mild undulation accompanied by low-grade nausea. I went to work. As long as I steadied my eyes and sucked on a piece of gingerroot to calm my stomach, I was able to do my job and move effectively in the playroom. I made my way through the day and even succeeded in teaching that little guy to talk a bit.

I will go quickly through the process of healing but understand that I "coped with and kept the vertigo at bay" for months. I did neuro-feedback daily—sometimes twice daily—always in the same location: at c4. Every time I treated the vertigo my world steadied but left me with that mildly undulating walls and ceiling effect. Sucking on gingerroot became a constant pastime.… until the day I realized that the problem was similar to the one I had had with the original tinnitus. Unbe-lievable! Again I was following the rules instead of my own evidence. After all, the treatment was working to brighten and steady me but it wasn't making me bright enough. Always I had been negatively affected by training at lower frequencies, but according to the teachings when training at c4 (over right inner ear) one is training on the right side of the head. And according to my training, when training on the right one must reward at frequencies of 12–15 or lower. But… I…don't…do… well…at…these…frequencies! Feeling like I was about to blow up my brain I took a shot and rewarded 17–20. The vertigo, the undulation, the low-grade nausea, all immediately went away. Eureka! Whenever the vertigo threatened to return I did it again. I performed this rule-breaking treatment on myself seven times over the next several months. Each time the spinning disappeared and each time, it was less intense when it did return, until eventually the problem was gone altogether. The last time I even experienced a hint of wooziness was a year ago. Yippee! Yahoo! Look what I can do! I brightened up my brain, by trust-ing myself again. Yay! Yay! Yahoo! Look what I can do! Pay attention to me and become vertigo free! (wink)

The truth is the tinnitus and the vertigo could have been caused by the same problem. And it's possible that I hadn't actually cured the tinnitus but rather that it had just grown quiet for a time until another particle broke off my cochlear and banged about inside my inner ear. It is probable, in fact, that I have Meniere's disease and that I was just in tinnitus remission before the big one hit. But given that medicine has no cure for most forms of tinnitus and none for Meniere's (nothing but coping techniques) and that the prognosis is a lifelong chronic disorder that can vary from total debilitation to chronic low-grade annoyance (with the odd unexpected fall thrown in for good measure), I can't help but feel that having the vertigo stop every time I treated it meant something more than coincidence. Perhaps by skipping the known science I may have stumbled upon a cure... called "follow the patient."

THE APPEARANCE OF A MIRACLE: He was four and autistic. He had very little language, bumped into things all the time, and was unable to keep food down. While playing with him I noticed that his eyes moved rapidly back and forth in a saccadic movement. It occurred to me that it may be nystagmus which could result in vertigo. So I treated him for Meniere's just in case. He stopped falling, kept his food down, and started to play with his brother.

THE FACTS: I had no idea if I was right about the vertigo I just knew it was possible and that even if he didn't have vertigo the protocol was a good one for him since it also helps sensory with integration, anxiety, and much more. Besides, I can reverse anything I do with neurofeedback; so if the protocol didn't make him feel good, if necessary, I could put things back the way they were. And if it did make him feel good enough to keep his food down I'd effectively save his life, autistic or not.

THE ACTUAL MIRACLE: It worked.

That's the reason I'm telling this story, to illustrate the art of following the clues. Nothing I had personally read about the application of neurofeedback for tinnitus or vertigo would have suggested treating at c4 or p6. And yet there I was using it. In addition, though, there was no real reason other than heredity and symptomology to think that my problems may be due to an auditory tumor and no real reason to believe that even if I did have one neurofeedback could impact its growth in any way, I saw no reason not to preventatively try it. I'd had no MRI's or CAT scans serving up solid evidence of brain parasites or cysts. It was only my history, my childhood visual and auditory sensory confusion, that pointed to the angular gyrus, that pointed to the sensory strip over the cochlea, that pointed to the higher frequencies, that pointed to the possibilities. So it was when I "used but wasn't dictated to" by science's preexisting thoughts on the subject that my knowledge of neuroanatomy began to inform me about my symptoms and a path was illuminated that was personally designed for me. Thus it was that I knew where and how to treat the problems. And it worked.

Neurofeedback is often like that, full of miracles by trial and error. Because the brain is designed to "fill in the blanks" with guesses based on associative thinking in order that it may know what it does not know. If aided by just enough information, given its desire to find balance, it is indeed equipped with the recipe for self-healing. Since the referred to brain is contained within the person, this fact is universally true of human beings as a whole: we can heal and we can hurt, ourselves. Neurofeedback takes advantage of this reality. It is a special therapy that combines the precision-oriented data-driven science parts of what we understand about neuroanatomy with our inherent ability to "make a story" thus allowing us to use a little knowledge to get a lot of result. And because neurofeedback relies on the brain's ability to heal, or more accurately, create itself, a therapist can use a more generalized "guesswork" styled approach than a surgeon or architect would dare to try. Thus the most important part of creating change with this therapy (in my opinion) is the therapist's ability to keep her eye on the desired goal.

NEUROFEEDBACK ROCKS! Because it works… with who we already are… and is the most effective non-intrusive therapy I know.

I think in our world we get so busy manipulating inanimate objects that we forget just how uniquely different life is from machines: You can't fix a plane with the same "atta boy, you can do it" approach you can use to fix a brain because the plane won't build itself. Given the right directions, ascertained by just a little observation, respect, knowledge, and guesswork, if the brain has the parts to do it with, then the brain will heal itself. I'm sure my pointing this out will infuriate many neurofeedback professionals who would prefer you believe that armloads of training is necessary to effect any consistent results and to ensure the safety of the client. These same therapists would prefer you not use home training to help your child and your family. These therapists and I will have to agree to disagree. I train and teach families what they need to know when they need to know it, and because they have units in their homes they are able to help their child handle the moments as the moments come up. This is invaluable for a population that is historically very hard to help.

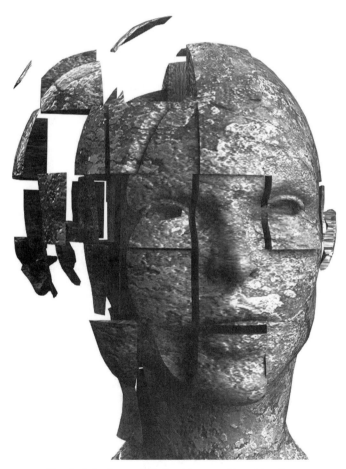

Esprit de la femme © Julien Tromeur from Fotolia.com

If I had limited myself to the tried and true locations and frequencies other people were using to treat my tinnitus, my vertigo, or my ADHD, I might still be dizzy with ringing ears and a morphine mentality. I say might, because with the brain, as with many things, lots of different approaches lead to the same end. The fact is, even if I never treated the parietal area of my brain that area might still have healed simply as a result of the work I had done elsewhere. It's because of the passing of information that travels from lobe to lobe and its domino affect of changing balance as one section heals and then leans on another that we are sometimes able to create waves that recreate the ocean of our brains and pave out new roads to the same end. After all, if everything is moving toward homeostasis, then nothing can happen in a vacuum and one change must denote another. Thus I am presenting you with powerful possibilities.

That very power might have intimidated me out of using neurofeedback if its effects weren't reversible. However, since they are, since I am able to undo any mistakes I make along the way, I am able to relax and use what I learn to make a story about it, solve the problem, and try the solution. With enough information, experience, and this ability to follow change, much can be discovered that was not already known. This is the kind of thinking that carried me to answer after answer as I tried to solve the challenges contained within my various sons' autism.

My son Rye for example: The day his autism was the most heart wrenching for me to observe was when at six years of age he was kicked out of Special Olympics for being too special. He was a boy in perpetual motion and too exhausting for the Special Olympic coaches to bear. Rye was more than disappointed. He was hurt. He'd been ostracized by the group that was supposed to accept you if you'd been ostracized, as he had, by group after group after group. He punched his head, scratched his face, and screamed, "I need a new Brain! I need a new brain! PREEEEESE BUY ME A NEW BRAIN!" My tearstained little peanut of a guy was undesirably lucid on the subject of not being liked. Thirteen years of shopping and countless temper tantrums later, I finally found and bought him neurofeedback. I did my best to give him that new brain.

Again all the literature of the time pointed to right-hemispheric treatment and again the therapist looked at a member of my family and thought "calm down." She told me Rye needed to be "made warmer" in his approach to life. So she "calmed down" his brain—which left Rye in a "cold" "actively angry" state of hysteria. On the way home Rye lost control when I drove past our exit. He called me a "fucking stupid bitch" and then, in order to help himself feel better through release, he punched the windshield, which cracked into the shape of a star. He had created his own kind of art therapy! This was unusual—not the star shape but the unexpected outburst. Generally Rye built towards anger. Almost always he needed a more dramatic reason than overshooting exits to destroy my property. The fact that Rye's anger threshold had been affected seemed to me not a bad thing but rather evidence pointing to the power of neurofeedback. If this therapy could turn Rye's anger button up, then maybe it could also turn it down. I wanted Rye's mental anguish reduced enough so that he could have access to himself and learn how to solve problems, not flail against them (and not just a little so that I could keep my windows intact). Maybe this new therapy could do that for him. I considered blaming the therapist for Rye's reaction but quickly decided that she was just in the process of discovery and needed to reverse her thinking where Rye was concerned. Peering through the sparkly new comet's tail-like crack in my windshield that ran across my line of sight, I pulled a u-turn and headed back to the clinic for an undoing session.

My introduction to neurofeedback, as you can see, was anything but trouble-free. There was much to learn and many experiments to be done before I, and my children, could experience the miracle of cognitive healing. However, from minute one of my own therapy, I knew neurofeedback—more than any other touted cure I'd used thus far—had the power to teach us how to affect our moods and unstick our thinking. I knew this because the impact on my level of comfort, my problem solving skills, and my reaction time was immediate. Once we figured out the right protocols for each of us, our lives were permanently impacted to the positive. As a family it changed how we felt and hence how we behaved together. I learned how to do the neurofeedback at home as it changed us for the better. Because that was the goal upon which I had my eye.

I am often struck by the irony intrinsic to the fact that many families like mine are searching for alleviation, and yet, though they search for alleviation they do not believe in it. It appears as though human beings are often more convinced of the "truth" of a thing when the so-called "truth" is a negative response. I understand this conundrum. In our society the story is never really over until the hammer falls. Happily ever after just means there's an "ever after" to live out—an "ever after" within which the story could change. And in our society "innocent" often just means "innocent for now." I doubt that the media will ever stop asking Brad and Angelina how their marriage is doing until their marriage is over, and to many people OJ remains to be found guilty even though he already was found not guilty. For the most part we accept a no as more definitive than a yes because a yes leaves the door open to more questions which means more and more opportunities to find a no. Thus, as a society we are often more convinced by (and desirous of) the relief that we feel when we find out that the story has ended, even if the only way to get an ending is through the death of a dream because at least then we can let go of the story and move on.

When we see acne in our mirror we know we are ugly, and when our skin clears up we know we are tricking the world into thinking that we are pretty but that we are actually ugly because our acne is in the air just waiting to settle back upon our faces. We humans are, as a race, often just that silly. For example if I say "I love you" to a new partner, he/she may actually be afraid to feel good in case later feeling good leads to feeling bad and so (as I am here to attest) this new partner chooses bad now instead of bad later by doubting the validity of my statement. Contrarily if I say "I can't stand you!"—unless this hypothetical person is suffering from delusions of grandeur—he/she will generally believe in my expression of state.

So "I can't help you" is easier to buy into than "I can." And families like this are more easily convinced of the power of neurofeedback from the problems it creates than from the ones it alleviates. Perhaps I was no exception to this societal proclivity. It seemed to me that if the therapy could affect us so negatively as too make me drive like I was under the influence of morphine and Rye to rage without warning, it might also have the power to affect us just as much in a more positive direction. (Neurofeedback has no "side effects" in the truest sense of the term, but it can have "incorrect effects"—at least until the clinician knows the client well enough to pinpoint what he/she needs.) Perhaps if we had just felt good, I'd have chalked it up to coincidence. But regardless of what might have happened what did happen was that once the correct frequencies and locations were figured out we experienced only improvement, alleviating symptom after symptom day upon day upon day. (One of the mom's I work with calls neurofeedback the "gift that keeps on giving." Probably because even once you stop the therapy the improvements continue to grow.) So, the original motivator for my becoming a professional in the field was that once I became convinced of its effectiveness, considering the number of people I had to treat in the house, I quickly came to understand that though this was a therapy for the whole family, I couldn't afford to treat us all. Given the cost and my income at the time I would have to pick which among my children I could afford to help.

I've never been very good at the *Sophie's Choice* moment of prioritizing with my children, so I refused to go that route. I knew I understood my children and their behaviors better than anyone else so I figured I was probably their best expert and decided to become their therapist. The more I thought about it the better the idea seemed. I was already trained in play and counseling techniques so why not learn neuroanatomy and neurofeedback too? I was especially excited at the thought of having the equipment close at hand. Being able to help my child in the moment of an upset (if you've ever dealt with an autistic temper tantrum you know what an understatement the word "upset" is) was preferable to having to schedule an appointment for after the "upset" was over. It was also preferable to trying to represent my child in a believable manner by going on office visits wherein I pointed to this calm teenager and explained that he'd been the Furniture Eating Tasmanian Devil for the past week unable to calm himself until just moments before walking in the clinician's door. It was logical to me then, as it is now, that teaching the brain to fire in a more comfortable manner for the person in the very moment that it's firing in an uncomfortable one is more likely to make a quicker, and hence bigger, difference over the long haul. Also it would be a lot easier for me, the parent, to be able to help my child in a proactive manner in the moment of a tantrum rather than dodging breaking glass and waiting for some clinic to open as the weekend came to a close.

As it turns out, exchanging the helpless feeling of "WHAT NOW!!?" for one of "Here Honey, let me help you feel better" empowerment, knowing that there was finally something I could do to ease my child's discomfort was the best part of all about finding Neurofeedback.

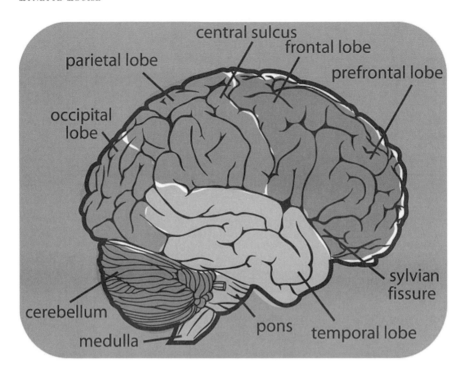

So I got my own therapy computers, took some classes, and began. The first thing I did was to follow Rye's behavior and conclude that—like me—he would benefit from high-frequency training in the pre-motor strip. This decision was based on the fact that he was a pretty depressed guy who seemed to use anger to brighten his sensory system. I'd learned that faster waves firing in this prefrontal area could help one feel happier and lighter in their body. A clue supporting this theory came from the fact that Rye had seemed more successful for the short period within which I had given him Ritalin. Thus stimulating his neuronal firing made sense. Much to Rye's teachers' chagrin I stopped the Ritalin at his request because, according to Rye, it made him feel lonely. It also kept him calmer during the day but unable to sleep at night. I decided if the neurofeedback had this affect, I could just train him to be calm at night and then train him again for awake, happy, and functioning in the day. This did not turn out to be necessary, though, as having his brain learn to stay stimulated rather than be stimulated by medicines actually improved his sleep. In addition to Rye's mood and focus problems he had a very low IQ (probably as a result of the fetal alcohol syndrome which is the leading cause of retardation in children). Rye was considered educateably retarded. Rye was very easily confused and slow to understand so increasing his processing speed near the area of the portion of the brain that deals with executive functioning seemed like a good way to help him up his ability to focus and think clearly. Another component in the decision was the fact that his speech pattern was still very stilted and his sentence structure poor. He seemed lacking in the necessary skills to do the detail work required in creating expressive language, so I wanted to be somewhat close to the expressive speech center.

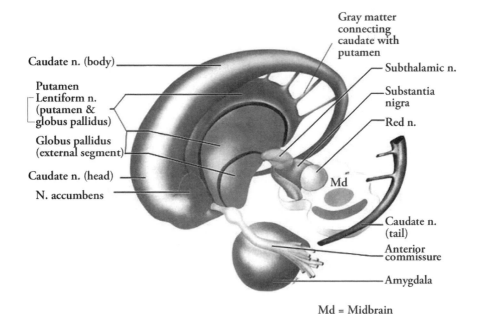

Md = Midbrain

Basal Ganglia – Nuclei: Medical View

Finally, he had a lot of tics and I surmised that they might be due to a difference of processing speed between the pre-motor and the motor strip and also as a result of problems in the basal ganglia and dopaminergic system.

Having learned these various influences in neuroanatomy class, I kept them all in mind and chose to treat my son at a high frequency in the left prefrontal lobe (f3 19–22 Reward 0–11 + 22–38 Inhibit). I observed my son carefully during the session. Fifteen minutes into the therapy Rye's body relaxed and his tics diminished. He spent the day happier but seemed a little tense in his body. I considered that he may have been too stimulated and the next day when I treated him I dropped the frequency a bit (f3 18–21 Reward 0–11 + 21–38 Inhibit). Voila! He began to improve, and the whole family experienced a greater state of comfort from and with him than since he had been adopted at the age of one and a half. And so it went as I used what I knew and guessed at the rest… using my sons' behaviors, neuroanatomy and other people's learnings as my guides.

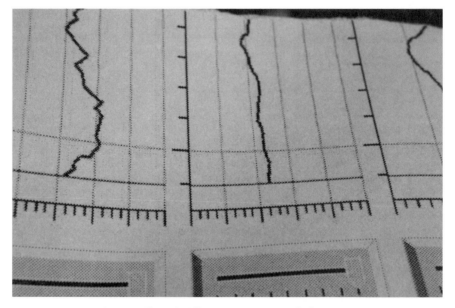

Compare Charts © **Allyson Kits at Bigstockphoto.com**

Four years have passed since Rye began neurofeedback, and though I have occasionally ventured from this protocol, for the most part Rye's best neurofeedback results still come from a repeat of the first thing I ever tried (high frequency training at f3). At present he tics so seldom that no one is aware of them, lives on his own, and runs a small handyman business. His unrealistic perseveration about becoming the world's only car designer and making everyone drive square flat cars by the year 2016 has become a healthier, more realistic desire to put his car designs on You-Tube and try to influence the market that way. Rye is no longer retarded (to reiterate neurofeedback can increase a persons

IQ score up to 15 points), but he is still a not-so-smart normal guy. And we are very proud of him.

The field of neurofeedback has many such success stories. It is truly an amazing world of sudden possibilities. Part of the reason for this is the fact that—since the therapy itself is so effective—the clinician/technician or therapist doesn't need reams of knowledge in order to make a big difference. This statement is underscored by the fact that even though some of my original thinking was made up and strung together loosely, I came to the same treatment choices as many others who followed different logic. Why? The common denominator I believe is that we were all following behavioral changes caused by the brain's response to training… so the brain itself leads us where we need to go. Thus, since we follow what works as we seek to help our clients achieve balance, we follow the brain, which seeks to do the same and we can help without knowing exactly how we are doing it. In some ways we are like the nurse assisting the surgeon—unable to perform the actual operation—yet having knowledge and a vantage point that makes our input invaluable: Of course in this analogy our surgeon boss (the brain) often only talks in behavioral signals that gesture toward what we need to do next, so it is up to us to interpret well enough to follow his/her directions. (I know a few nurses who would say the same about the doctors they work for).

Thus the brain, in the case of this therapy, functions as the expert while we suggest changes in order to assist in its evolution. Regardless of all the studying I've done, thus far, I have found no hard and fast rules about how to proceed. There is no set-in-stone order of operations for how to lead the brain to heal itself from person to person or disorder to disorder. And the best way I have found for choosing the changes I want to suggest is to be willing to make up a story out of the evidence I see. Without this sort of audacity there is no way to collect the info and move on ideas that lead to solutions. So with a little knowledge and a lot of chutzpah many of us march toward the answers we seek even if this marching includes a goodly number of u-turns. The fact is many great scientific discoveries have been based on erroneous thinking that was acted on and then learned from. For example, in 1922 Sir Alexander Fleming discovered an antibiotic that killed bacteria while leaving white blood cells alone (unlike carbolic acid, the most used antiseptic of the time) because he was willing to experiment. Fleming had a cold and was studying the fluid from his nasal passages. He had been trying various chemical substances in order to find something that could kill bacteria but remain harmless to human tissue when a tear from his eye fell into the dish. The next day he found a clear space in the yellow culture. The clear space coincided with the location of where his tear had fallen. He "followed" the clue buried in the behavior of the bacteria to conclude, correctly, that his tear contained a substance that killed bacteria but was harmless to human tissue. In 1928 he was reminded of the incident when a similar thing happened after a bit of mold fell into a dish full of staphylococci. He isolated the mold and discovered penicillin.

One discovery always leads to another. Science changes its story and the world goes from being flat to being round as solid answers liquefy and evaporate when new info comes to light. But it's because people "make up" answers as if they are solid that they are able to uncover new questions and feel brave enough to quest for more answers, especially as others make up different answers to the same questions. Often it is the controversy that causes the quest. And quests lead to trips in search of India or the horizon. It is misinformed journeys like this that lead to a whole new world instead. I'm sure that many things have gone undiscovered when out of apathy or lack of self-confidence we deny our inherent curiosity and name miracles and un-understood happenings as coincidences or oddities instead of problems to be solved and made into solutions. Just as I am sure that many things are wrongly discovered due to calling correlation "proof." But in my opinion it is our and our brains' ability to make patterns out of the milieu, combined with that very arrogance of thinking we know what we are doing, that is the secret to our success (yes I said success—personally I think people are awesome) as a technological race. It is our audacity that makes us human. And since one can't begin to surmise without inventing a plausible story it is OK to guess, though I do believe you will achieve more with an educated guess than an uninformed one. Thus you will avoid the need to reinvent what has already been discovered. But still, even after you've educated yourself on the options, if you want to move forward and don't know the answer you have no choice but to choose anyway, or remain ineffective, because the real trick to action is to act... hopefully after ensuring that what you are about to do is reasonably safe.

And herein lies the beauty of neurofeedback: it is safe because it is reversible. All you have to do is follow.

In order to do that we (clinicians and parents) do need some way of organizing our thinking and making our choices. Some folks study other people's work and use that as a guide; some study psychological constructs and follow the thinking derived from that. I study both. But most often I study neuroanatomy and its influence on behavior. This is a crucial approach for me because the majority of my clients don't talk so I have to watch and interpret as their behaviors talk for them. Thus when I see a child rocking on her forehead it means something different than when I see a child rocking on the back of his head. And that something different comes from a basic understanding of neuroanatomy.

Here's an example of how educated guessing can play out: At one point I learned that many autistic children—especially the ones diagnosed with PDD NOS (Pervasive Developmental Disorder – Not Otherwise Specified … now there's a mouthful)—don't have enough mirror neurons. Mirror neurons begin to migrate into position at a pretty young age. They fire when a person uses his or her face or hands to copy an act. If you have ever watched adults play with babies, then you know we are assisting this migration by becoming copying buffoons for about the first year and a half of a babies life: They make a face, we make a face; they make a sound, we make a sound; they wave, we wave; and back and forth the copy-cat tag game moves throughout those first five hundred or so days of the child's existence. If the child I am working with has a history of shunning this game of imitation at an early age, I assume a mirror neuron migration problem and stimulate the left frontal lobe, but if the child's history shows a sensory overload I assume right temporal lobe dysfunction or sensory motor strip issues and begin there. These assumptions are based on a combination of neuroanatomy and behavioral clues. However, from the moment therapy begins behavioral clues come first and neuroanatomy second, making "following" the most important component of this type of work. This is merely my approach; as I have said there are many, and the beauty is most of us see great results.

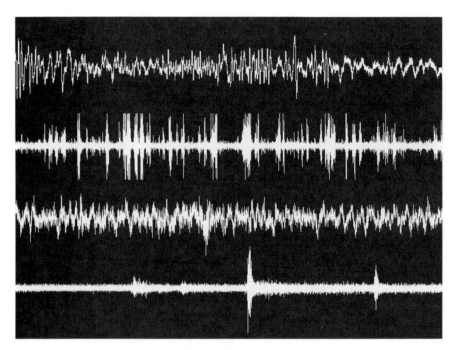

Vector Oscillations © **Stan Tiberiu Fotolia.com**

I believe that getting great results relies on congruence in three areas: definitions, expectations, and limitations. Let's look at each.

<u>Definitions:</u> What is one's definition of "good results?" This is an important point and comes up over and over again in every therapy meant to help a handicapped child. If I define "good results" as "he claps on cue" and you define good results as "he does his chores without being asked," we are clearly not in agreement about when we have achieved "good results." Understanding the definitions and making sure you are working with people who have similar definitions to you is part of building a good team with consistent attitudes and approaches. So it is important to understand with specificity what is meant by "good results;" otherwise you might get there without even knowing it. Or worse you might already be there without your therapist knowing it.

For instance, early in my career of traveling into homes to work with children, I was hired to help a boy who had CP (Cerebral Palsy) caused by a birth accident and oxygen deprivation. He was also diagnosed autistic. I was hired as a play therapist. It was an exciting opportunity for me. Until two weeks before my visit his basic sustenance consisted of a bottled concoction of pabulum and milk. However, just before my visit a great event had taken place: Mom had managed to help him swallow several teaspoons of mashed baby food. Everyone was excited. I felt certain we could find ways to help him grow even more capable.

This twiggy little guy's gross motor skills were quite good, but his fine motor skills and visual processing were so damaged that chewing or following your movement around the room with his eyes required total concentration and some strange posturing in order to make his gross motor system compensate for the failing in his fine-motor execution. Talking was, in the family's mind, out of the question. He was one of those kids that is described as "so ugly he's cute." He had no body fat, big teeth, hollowed-out cheeks and knobby knees on a bum-less body. He drooled constantly, ran around with his head tilted sideways, and reminded me a lot of my son Dar when I first met him. My heart melted immediately. I think I wanted even more to help this little fella because I hadn't known how to help Dar when he first came to be mine.

Whatever the reason I made a lot of assumptions on that trip that taught me a great deal in retrospect. For example, I assumed that since all my clients came from word of mouth about my playroom expertise at getting non-verbal kids to talk and/or violent kids to calm (I had only just begun to include neurofeedback as a tool in my practice and so this special skill had not yet become what people shared about me and my services), and since this nonviolent little fella was non-verbal, I figured speech was what the family (Mom, Dad and one child) wanted from me. So naturally that's where I started. I went into his enormous and very fun playroom and looked for any independent skill he seemed capable of. Bart spent most of his time rocking and pounding his chest against the floor while drooling and burping. This happened immediately after each bottle. He would drool and pound and burp and rock and then, after about an hour of this, he would lay and stare and twitch. Once his energy returned he would reach for a new bottle and begin the process anew. This rocking combined with his sideways glancing and lack of language and his need to pull his body away from contact with people were the main reasons he'd been diagnosed as autistic.

I had other ideas. I believed he was pulling away because he was in pain. He also seemed to be seizing during many of these episodes and so I shared with the parents my observations and suggested I bring my neuro-feedback equipment with me next time. The parents appeared surprised. They then informed me that he did indeed have a seizure disorder and that they mostly controlled it with meds. Up until then they had thought that the meds made it so he only seized at night, all night, every night. I suggested that they might want to try for a more complete solution since it didn't sound as if the meds were controlling very much at all.

The next day I watched as the child and his mother did a beautiful silent gesture dance of unspoken communication from moment to moment throughout his day. She was busy with his needs one hundred percent of the time. She seemed calm in the quietness of her environment. He seemed to be so busy dealing with his body that there was little room for more than being serviced and assisted as he managed his digestive struggles. He burped constantly. My mind flashed on the image of an acquaintance who had had throat surgery and used his air to speak through a hole just below his Adam's apple. Then it occurred to me that this little guy might be able to use the force of his burps to shape language.

Back in the playroom I rolled up my sleeves and began. Whenever he would drink his milk I would pound and pat and rub his back until the pain, twitching, and drooling subsided. Then as his eyes came back into focus, I would rub his feet and compliment him on his manly burps all the while explaining that he could use them to talk… then when I could see by the gurgling in his tummy that a burp was about to erupt I would stop rubbing and request he try to talk. At first I just pretended the burps were words but then I began to ask for more shape to the sound; closer and closer approximations were required in order to get me to keep rubbing. Before long (by my personal assessment of time so it was likely three or four hours later) he was burping out close approximations of the word rub.

Whenever this game began to bore him, in order that I might keep him interested I did gymnastic-like maneuvers about the room in celebration of his newfound language. I hung from edges and ledges, hid in cupboards, slid on slides, and did summersaults and cart-wheels. I was noisy and lively and he seemed to be responding well. On my second visit we picked up where we left off while also adding neurofeedback during his sleeping hours in an attempt to improve his seizures. He was highly drugged with Trasadone to help him sleep. He was also seizing. I began the treatment and after about an hour these on-and-off seizures stopped for the rest of the night. The next day he was more alert and began to run and play with me. By the afternoon he was verbally demanding loud and proud in a very clear burp voice "OPEN! CLOSE!" over and over again at every curtain and cupboard in the house. This had been our game of the day and it was paying off. I was thrilled and expected the same from the parents.

With the outreach nearly over I sat and went through some last-minute details with the mom. We had to speak up over the sounds of the house. The normally quiet dog that I had been playing with during my breaks was a little thrown by the sudden vocalizations of his mini master so he began to bark whenever the little boy said "Open." I thought it was wonderful until the mom in an exasperated tone blurted "Oh My God! You've even got the dog talking!" I looked clearly at this woman who appeared to be about to crumble and finally saw the moment through her overwhelmed eyes.

I took a moment to breathe some awareness into my own under-standing. The job I was expecting this mom to embrace was mammoth. Looking at things realistically this darling boy may be able to potty train and learn some easy-to-copy repetitive language skills from us in the first year. He may even stop seizing and be able to reduce his meds. However, given the damage in his brain and its lack of connectedness with his body, anything even close to independence within his world (their house) would likely take ten or more years of total commitment and family re-creation. It's nice when you get there, but the journey is gargantuan in its need for the implementer to constantly see the evidence while simultaneously shaping that same evidence into the goal they were keeping their eye on. This was a quiet woman with an energy that emoted stillness whose purpose and whose husband seemed to be held in place by her special relationship with this child and his disabil-ity… at the end of the day independence may not even be what she wanted… it was a conceptual surprise for me… so I asked her.

It had never occurred to me before that there might be times when I should not go full force into the doing of what I do. (Remember I like being the *eager-beaver-do-it-all-doll*!) It also had never occurred to me that I might be hired as ammunition. I never imagined that I might be brought into a house to be employed as the one who would agree with her employer. I never saw myself as the professional whose job it was to defend a position of hopelessness. But that's what had happened. Apparently I had been expected to inform spouse and neighbors that nothing could be done to teach the child. Meanwhile I was trying to be the professional proof that indeed something could be. So I had just barreled ahead and created a whole new set of problems for this family. This woman wanted very much to keep things the way they were, but to have her husband become more aware of how overwhelming it all was in order to keep him home more. And it was obvious to me that her desire was no less perfect than mine, no less righteous, no less loving. It was their life to design just as it was their child to help in the way they wished to help him. It was them, not me, who would be living the daily ritual in this dynamic dance of silence.

As it turns out, not everyone prefers the sound of noisy kids! I'd had no idea.

Nowadays I try to be the person that wants for the family what they want for themselves while at the same time still showing them that they can want something else. I suggest that you seek this type of support. Thus, before you give your allegiance to any therapy, clinician, or school system, find a common language wherein you all have the same definitions and concept of the goal.

Expectations: Even though I used the definition of expectations as my example of definitions, expectations are a subject unto themselves. (You might have to read that sentence twice.) Expectations and definitions are quite different. Definitions can be as simple as what you mean by lunch? Anything eaten midday or a balanced grouping of foods set out around noon? Whereas expectations are more of a long-term/short-term belief system that play out in the choices made by the people working with your child. In other words, if no one believes your child will ever be able to speak, then whenever he does make a word approximation it will be seen as gibberish or nonsensical noisemaking; contrarily, if it is believed he will speak then—as little burping Bart proved—any sound can be shaped into language.

I was observing an example of this just a few days ago when my friend's brother and his wife were playing with their rather brilliant one-year-old child. She was consistently saying things like "da" and "hi" and "out there" and "nose," but whenever anyone pointed out that she was talking her parents questioned the likelihood and asked if she had said it unprompted and if so had she done it three times consistently. Ironically they were thrilled to see her say "pup" every time her dog went by, so much so, that she quickly built upon the attention-getting concept and was soon identifying all dogs as "pup." I use this example because this child is quite advanced and will definitely not be stopped from talking by her parent's lack of vocabulary appreciation. This particular little one may be slowed down a bit or, more likely, she may even be encouraged to try harder given that she is quite short-fused about not being understood.

However, with a child who is struggling to make these connections or to even get their mouth and body to behave according to the directions their brain gives, if the assumptions made by the people around them are created by the need for their communication to seem "valid" enough to be believed in, then the child is set up to fail. These assumptions and their subsequent devaluing of unclear attempting come from the expectation (in this case) that the child is too young to talk (possibly in your case that she is too autistic). These assumptions lead to un-rewarded attempts and can be enough to stop many a verbally challenged child from trying.

I teach to this in almost every home I go into because it can make the difference between success and failure. I know because I learned it from setting up to fail.

In the early years my expectations and beliefs about what my children's capabilities were was always higher than the expectations they received from their teachers. The effects of this "expectation disparity" between the two environments became most obvious with Dar. Each summer was spent with only family to reflect him back to himself and—from five years old to age nine—each summer his word approximations became clear enough to bridge the gap between verbal and non. That is, until he would go back to school. And with every day spent in school we could literally watch the words whoosh away until, by the end of September, he would have regressed from greeting us with approximations and eye contact to guttural screams and contact avoidance. As the years wore on, the influence of Dar's school environment won the battle and the disparity gap closed until eventually all this yo-yoing from one style to another left him with fewer skills than he had had to start with. He was without words, attempts at words, or hope for words. Even I began to wane in my belief of his possibilities.

In fact, before I discovered the existence of neurofeedback my expectations had dropped so low for Dar that they had grown a million miles apart from my hopes for him. I *hoped* he could be independent some day. I *expected* he might eventually wipe his bottom well enough to keep from smelling so badly. It is truly interesting to me the complete 180 my expectations took when neurofeedback came into the picture. Previous to that I looked into therapies while experiencing the same trepidation I felt when I fell for a handsome man and then became afraid he might notice me falling. [Hmm… there is a strange theme to my analogies—(wink)] Fear of believing and a need to believe coexisted within me as I tried to help my sons. I trembled with that mixture of fear and hope each time I reached for something new. Sometimes this flirtation with the belief in my children and their ability to grow more capable via the next miracle discovery on the rise led the way and sometimes the fear of not getting what I wanted. So I oscillated from one extreme to the other. Mostly though, I tried to believe in all these new things. Mostly though, I tried to believe that I had found my science-created soul mate solution each time I looked… especially for Dar.

And so, with the heart of the eternally hopeful, I wrote testimonials for everyone whose approach, supplement, or technology had even the slightest positive impact on Dar. I felt so much appreciation for even the tiniest development and so much hope that it might grow into something bigger. I remember one "way out" therapy wherein I would phone and talk to an anonymous man called Dr. C whenever twenty-two-year-old Dar would throw himself naked on the floor and hit his head on the ground. It was weird (not tantrumming Dar that had become "normal" for us) phoning a strange man with invisible technology. But weird or not the call did help. Dar would calm. Just not for long. Even so, at that time, I was thrilled to have any tool at all to reach for. That's around when I started neurofeedback. And that's when my idea of success was redefined and my expectations rose.

I became aware of how different my idea of what was possible had become when I found myself cleaning out an old drawer. I came across a file folder full of those testimonials for advances gained but not maintained. I cried… with joy. I was so happy to no longer have to perceive Dar's inches of development as if they were miles of change. Because now he actually was changing inch by inch, foot by foot, yard by yard, day by day.

Interestingly I also realized I'd finally become comfortable with how extremely challenged my son was. At last I was able to see and accept the truth about him because at last I could actually do something tangible to help him. I was experiencing so many internal changes, simply because I was no longer overwhelmed by the impossibility of the job I could never do, simply because that was no longer the case.

Since more can be done and in much less time, obviously I would never write those testimonials now because getting two seconds of eye contact as opposed to one is no longer enough change to get me to put ink to paper. However, even though both those out-of-the-box and in-the-box therapies were nothing but momentary band-aids for Dar and me, they did give relief. They also, however, stole time and were distractions from continuing to search for something greater: like the act of waiting for a husband to make good on his promises of security while he gambles away the mortgage payment. [OK. Enough! I am over it! No more dysfunctional mate analogies. I will do some neurofeedback on my nucleus accumbens and let the post-traumatic stress disorder go? (wink)] It is refusing to see the truth while waiting to see what happens that effectively detours one from her desired future. Since I like to make the most of my life experiences, I am trying to spread the lessons I learned from all my waiting in order to save you time. (And, not incidentally, to validate all the time I wasted.) Thus, though I still write testimonials, I only do so if the therapy changes our lives enough to make a difference in some dramatic way: like moving a child from exclusive to not.

At this point the most I can say about diets and supplements and long-distance healing and speech therapy and occupational therapy and cranial sacral therapy and chiropractics and behavior modification and oxygen and hormones and this and that and this and that is "these were good augmentations to a very all-inclusive program." But none of them were effective enough to stand alone and still create constant change. At present the only thing I give Dar is neurofeedback and acceptance, and so far he's continued to grow. As far as my other boys go—well they've healed—all the way off the spectrum.

So, other than pressure to come home for Christmas—all I give them now is a little long-distance love. One thing my life has made me acutely aware of is that, like with the tinnitus, if all I expected was occasional relief or baby-step movement, then my end point—even if I kept trying until I died—would have come at a very different place. I am too greedy to settle for that. I don't want to be satisfied with a little less hearing loss instead of a clearly heard world of beautiful sounds. I don't want some. I want it all.

It was because of my experience with neurofeedback's power that I expected total relief from my tinnitus. Thus I didn't give up until I got there because I knew that getting there was possible. In my show I have a joke that says I talk about me—not because I'm self-centered—that's just a coincidence! But in fact like all good jokes on some level it's not a joke. I do talk about me and my life and it's not because I'm self-centered; that is just a coincidence. (wink) Actually it's because many people believe you are stuck with what you are given, and since my life proves otherwise, I share my story to combat that belief. Hopefully I can help you to replace your limiting ideas and become infected with expectations of possibilities.

The point is: your point of completion is defined by your expectations.

In summation: Incongruent definitions create confusion and a kind of lazy attempting, but low expectations are worse; they can actually lead to a lifelong thwarting of skill acquisition.

Limitations: Learning about the brain has been liberating and limiting at the same time. I used to think anything was possible but then—as I came to understand our physiological presets—I realized that like gravity preventing me from using my arms to fly, some things are simply limited by nature. Thus even though I found a way to ask the brain to grow differently and at a faster pace than usual, the results were and still are limited both by developmental starting points and speed of processing range. Comparing the changes possible in a child with Asperger's to the changes possible in a PDD-NOS child is not unlike trying to race a small GEO car with a four- cylinder engine against a caddy with a V8—some advantages in small spaces and cheaper tank fill ups, but a definite disadvantage on the straightaway. Understanding this "reality versus opportunity" scenario helps one set up for success by picking a life wherein agility or steadfastness or hyper-focused hard work is more valuable than speed. For example, as previously stated three of my boys were not only on the spectrum of autism, they were also adopted afflicted with fetal-alcohol syndrome. Thus they were considered retarded and learning disabled (kind of redundant I know but diagnoses can be that way). As I helped them reach for more in their lives, I also relocated my family to a township with lower IQ scores in order to surround them with reachable goals: a society within which they could grow to become the norm. Choices like this, made from understanding that everything is a variable, made it so that I could go for everything possible.

A few years ago I heard the words "call it by its name" in some movie in reference to something about mental health. This phrase echoes in my head whenever I teach to specificity. Because knowing what to call a thing helps to liberate us from making up self-perpetuating pain. For example, I remember being liberated in neuroanatomy class when I heard about the diurnal rhythm of cortisol, AKA the stress hormone. Apparently it is released into one's system in the wee hours of the morning to help break down proteins and stimulate the brain into wakefulness. It rises in level and peaks between 5:00 and 7:00 AM. At this point it begins to recede and diminish like an abrasive wave leaving its mark upon the rocks and heading out to sea.

I remember thinking "WOW! Surges of anxiety-creating stress hormone. Guess I should never take myself seriously before 10 AM!" I used 10:00 AM because I was giving myself a little cushion for comfort, you know, just in case. You see, generally, 10:00 AM is just a little longer than the time required for this physiologically necessary, unrelated to the happenings of life, stress to dissipate and complete its rounds as it circulates one's body. So if I don't take myself seriously before then. I won't make decisions based on my body's need to break down proteins. This is good info to spread if you want to prevent early-morning road rage. After all, if you know it's all about you and your hormones, AND that you will feel better sometime between 8:00 and 10:00 in the morning, you may not choose to shoot the guy riding his brakes in front of you on his way to work. Personally, I was never at risk of that sort of behavior, but this information did mean an easier life for my children: I no longer woke up looking to blame someone for the way I was feeling. I would just smile, breath deeply, and wait until it passed.

Liberation and limitations are bedfellows when working to create change. Which one is taking the driver's seat is dependent on the moment of evolution. For example, as I have already mentioned, according to another of my classes it takes seven repetitions for the brain to retain a fact. I struggle with this concept. On the one hand it is liberating because it releases me of a need to understand why even though I may have taught my children something over and over again when they hear it from someone "cooler" than me, they treat it as if they are hearing it for the first time. Suddenly missing out on the "Ta! Da! Moment" isn't frustrating because suddenly I understand that it never would have happened without me, because I was like the supporting cast; responsible for numbers one through six.

However, I do sometimes catch myself thinking "Darn! She got the lucky number seven!" In these moments I like the concept. On the other hand, I rail against any belief that says we know something about individual brain functions with this much certainty. It seems limiting. I question its validity, especially as I work with people whose ability to remember is completely determined by their ability (or disability) to focus and understand. Having such a basic rule seems terribly misleading. I ponder these things often. What if on every twenty-fifth brain it only takes three repetitions to retain a fact? What if I am teaching someone who is the exception to the rule so I repeat myself and bore them until they lose focus, daydream, and miss out on the rest of what I say? Will they then look stupid from grade four through grade seven? Or? … Was that just me? (wink wink nudge nudge say no more) What about that little girl whose parents—aside from the word "pup"—listened to her screams rather than her word approximations. Will she get bored of not being heard and only scream? What if only screams counted? What would you do? Scream? I suspect so.

Sometimes when we don't listen to our children, the thing that becomes limited is our patience. This is especially true when a parent comes to the realization that their autistic child needs more like seven million repetitions in order to retain a fact. I actually don't believe this is due to limited intelligence. What I think is usually happening is that the child has a hard time focusing on and understanding us so he is unaware of most of our repetitions just as we are unaware of most of his/hers. Thus, it's not so much that it takes more repetitions to learn, as that it takes more opportunities to be heard. However, regardless of why, if you were in my neuroanatomy class and came to believe that it would take your child only seven repeats to learn but you have to say it more than that, you may also come to believe that for your child learning isn't possible. You might be sad or you might just scream in frustration, "I told you a million times!" (In fact you might do that with or without neuroanatomy class.) But however it affects you it is unlikely to leave you filled with hope.

I know I certainly felt frustrated and hopeless and said those words. Many times. And I said them as if they mattered. And then one day I realized how often I had to repeat myself was irrelevant. After all, they were my children. I was expecting to be teaching them every moment of the day anyway, whether by example or by direction. So what if what I was teaching remained the same day in and day out. At least then I knew what to do each day. Maybe I was luckier than other parents: I didn't have to search for the next thing to teach. Or maybe all parents are that lucky at least on some level. After all, as I mentioned previously, parents often effectively teach their kids a skill and then, panicked by the unknown next step, regress them just enough to start again. At any rate, whether that's our personal M.O. or not, it's the belief that our child should learn quicker and that we are somehow disadvantaged when they don't that leads to this frustration.

The fact is, when it comes to any kind of focus disorder, hyper-focused child [friend, grocery store clerk, or mate (wink)] you probably will have to make your points a million times. So make them seven or seven hundred, whatever it takes until Eureka! They get it! Just say it, say it, say it, say it without attitude or tone that can be interpreted as "You are making me exhausted!" because your obvious stress is contagious. As such, your stress can multiply the stress your child experiences just enough to increase their low-wave activity and compound the problem. This low-wave-run-amuck response is a brain mechanism designed to separate us from the trauma of the moment. This physiological safety net is likely intended to help us handle extreme danger. Unfortunately given that we live in a high-stress time, wherein we comprehend danger at every turn, such a design probably contributes to the evolution of our population having more and more members with increased difficulty staying focused. Stress increases feelings of separation and decreases focus, just as living with high stress dynamics in the home can increase the problem of attending to details for each of the members within.

Understanding the brain helps one to understand the reason to repeat, and the reason to do it with reason. So read about the brain; it's interesting and it'll give you great ideas.

A couple of quick examples on how knowing the workings of the brain can help one to work with it:

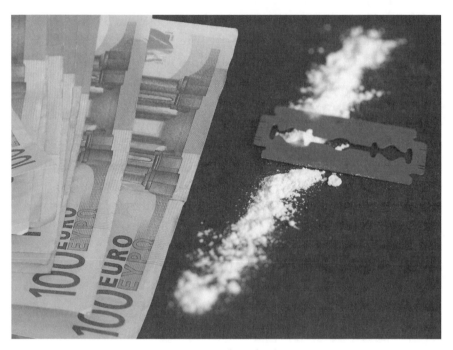

Cocaine Drug © **c from fotolia.com**

1. I was trying to heal a cocaine addict—I researched the effects of coke and decided to use the neurofeedback to ask the brain to up the stimulation in the mesolimbic dopamine pathway because cocaine gives you a dopamine buzz. So I figured if I could help his brain to increase his euphoria by upping the release of dopamine (or any other stimulating neurochemistry), then he would have a lighter crash and hopefully a lesser need for the drug itself. It was just a theory based on a little bit of knowledge but worth trying. He couldn't believe how easy it was to stop the cravings—though admittedly it took several sessions a day to "keep him happy." As the intervention wore on he explained that since he was rich enough to afford his drug he didn't

want to quit using until he had made all his drug fantasies into realities. This, I explained, was his choice. The most an intervention can do is to present a person with an array of possibilities so that when they want to make use of them they know where to go. He wasn't ready but he knew—for the first time—that it didn't have to be so uncomfortable. Last I heard he had gone full circle (fallen off and gotten back on the wagon) and was doing well. There is no way to know what kind of influence or long-term effect the neurofeedback had. Possibly none.

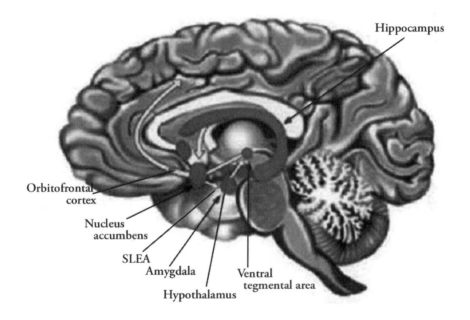

So why tell the story? Because for me, the miracle of being able to act as midwife to emotional comfort, sustained or otherwise, is the gift this therapy can give. I can always aim for recovery but I can't always give it. Degenerative illnesses are great examples of that fact.

2. When I met my first client with Parkinson's, I again found myself researching the issue of dopamine. I was working in a clinic at the time where we were using the usual alpha-frequency-reward approach. We were doing a lot of cognitive exercises together called APT (Attention Process Training) and though he was working hard to regain the twenty

or more IQ points he'd lost, his improvement in so far as memory and speed of processing were concerned was minimal. Overall, although he was more emotionally stable, his ability to think and move on his feet had hardly improved. Since Parkinson's is caused by the substantia niagra loosing its ability to make dopamine, I figured asking the brain for stimulation of any kind that could take the place of the dopamine in the necessary pathways and assist the basal ganglia in controlling his ability to coordinate and balance movements might help.

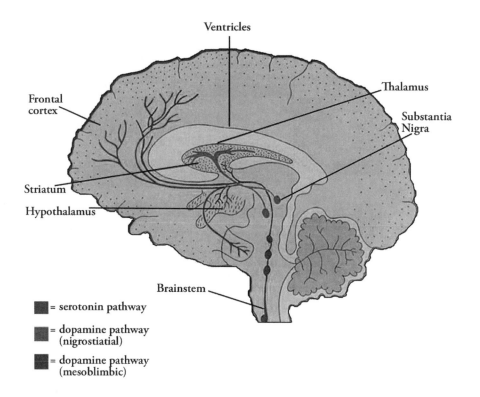

He had first entered the clinic as a foot-shuffling, arm-rolling bundle of depression who would soon need a walker. Following this new thinking, in his treatment I used high-frequency training in the left frontal lobes accompanied by more high-frequency training between the two hemispheres on the sensory motor strip. His symptoms began to recede. He stopped barking at his kids and resumed relations with his wife. I have now used neurofeedback to help several other patients with Parkinson's; and though the thinking is similar, anatomical variation has required slight differences in the approach. So far, it always improves the clients' mood and movements. The question I have no way of answering is—is the therapy healing the brain or just causing it to compensate for the problem. Will we eventually lose the battle as the system degenerates given the nature of the disorder? I have no idea. But to quote a client, "Who cares as long as it helps me now." The truth is that's more than he had before, and maybe while he is feeling better a new more complete healing tool will be discovered.

Some quick examples of various cases and the thinking behind their solution:

1. One of my autistic clients was showing signs of auditory schizophrenia, so given that hearing voices is often accompanied (correlation noted, no causation known) by too much dopamine in the right temporal lobe, I decided to discourage stimulation in this area. I used a low-frequency reward and placed the sensor just above the right ear. After around ten sessions he stopped listening to the sounds of ghosts as his imaginary voices quieted to a whisper and then went away.

2. A young girl I worked with was a chronic liar. I read that lying activates the anterior cingulate, which when under-active is often complicit in ADHD (Attention Deficit Hyperactivity Disorder). Given that many ADHD kids tend toward telling lies (possibly self-medicating through behavior?) and that she had some of the ADHD symptoms, trying to stimulate the anterior cingulate through the use of an fpz placement (front middle of forehead) and encouraging activation with a high-frequency reward made sense. I accompanied this therapy with some "how to get out of the grave you just dug yourself into" approaches like "When you catch yourself lying, make it part of your sense of humor to embellish a story and then admit—' Yeah! That's a lie,' and then laugh." She became known for her unpredictable sense of humor and outrageous stories. So though she still lied she did it with flair and with thoughtful preparation rather than uninhibited desperation. And as a side-benefit her grades improved.

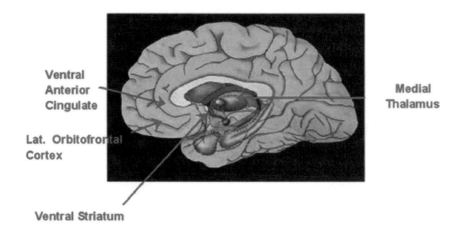

3. A young autistic girl had problems with facial recognition and what everyone referred to as "an irrational fear of spiders." I explained that a fear of spiders and/or snakes is actually built into our brain and that it is filed by the amygdala. If hers was overactive then her fear would be intense but I would certainly not call it irrational. (I remember when my son Rye acquired one of his fears—a fear of toilets. I had just finished voiding my bladder at a public restroom. Since he was known to slide under all the stalls and scare the women, I was holding him on my lap. I pulled myself together with one arm and then dangling Rye from my hip leaned over to flush the toilet. His head was positioned down and almost in the bowl. It was one of those really powerful very loud toilets. It startled him in a big way. For the next year he would scream, spit, scratch, and block the doorway in a fit of panic anytime any one of us tried to enter the domain of an unfamiliar toilet. Each of his therapists, in turn, called Rye's behavior of barricading buddies from bathrooms irrational—even after I told them the story and explained that, to Rye, the toilet was a danger zone. It's because of this memory that I challenge the concept that any fear is irrational. I am sure that, to the person with the fear, there is a rationale.)

Anyway, this young scared-of-spiders girl had a myriad of symptoms that we plucked away one after another. For example, she seemed really incapable of recognizing facial expressions and their messages. In fact, she seemed really challenged to even recognize the faces themselves. I knew these symptoms (and many other aspects of autism) might be related to problems with her amygdala (a common problem spot since with autism the amygdala is often inflamed). I was most concerned with calming her amygdala enough to reduce her panic, while at the same time hoping to affect her ability to know her people when she saw them. She had a lot of sensory issues as well so it was amazing to me that she allowed me to treat her by putting a sensor beside her right eye on the bridge of her nose. There was no question in my mind that it was helping, because no self-respecting autistic person is leaving wires next to their eyes for half an hour just because I ask them to. I treated her several times at a very low-reward frequency of 2–5. She soon (several months later) began to "know" her people and calmly call for help whenever she saw a spider. (Understand that treating autism is highly complex and requires hundreds of sessions aimed at different processes; I am telling you what and why while also simplifying in order to explain some of the neuroanatomy connection to neurofeedback protocol choosing.)

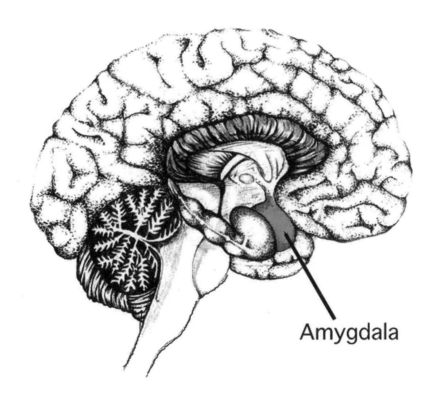

Amygdala

4. I worked with a young man who loved music so much he would get stuck in it. Whenever this happened I would brighten his left frontal lobe to diminish the hold his right temporal lobe had over him... after a few sessions he would get too into numbers and become too manically happy so we would treat the right temporal lobe to calm down the effect of the left frontal lobe. This seesawing approach went on for months until he reached a point where he was cooperating, answering questions, and showing spontaneous affection. (Interesting to note that his affection wasn't always welcomed because it went through a phase of -lobe-based inappropriate behavior. This was a challenge for the family, and although the problem is common with autism they read his new touches as a dire indication of possible past indiscretions. They began to look for culprits. It was a responsible reaction but it did waylay them from continuing his therapy for a time while they dug at family skeletons. Fortunately they found their way back. We treated his right temporal lobe and completed the job of getting to their goal: integration.

5. Since I read that focus is controlled by the left frontal area as well as the right parietal, I began using a combination with many extremely focus-challenged kids, doing half the session in the back right and the other half in the left front. This has become one of my favorite protocols for many children with autism—one boy even looked at me midway through this low-frequency calming of the right parietal lobe and said, "'I'm getting that happy Ritalin feeling." But even though he said that, when I treated him only on the right parietal lobe he became depressed. It was the combo that really worked to help him be social and happy.

6. A nine-year-old girl I work with was very into genital stimulation. This obsession was causing some very uncomfortable moments for her family. There were several possible causes for her fixation, like the right temporal lobe or the sensory motor strip. I began by treating the sensory motor strip, but much to her family's dismay this only increased her behavior. I had some decisions to make. I could try the same thing at a lower frequency or move to a different area altogether. Then, since in autism there is often a lot of inflammation in the right temporal lobe (as well as various other places) and since she had this behavior whether she was being bothered by other sensory input or not, I decided to go in a new direction and reward at a low frequency

in the right temporal lobe. This slowed the interest in her genitals but also made her more exclusive and "daydreamy." Then I realized that she acted as if she couldn't feel much of her body. She never really reacted to my touch or noticed if I was moving her body until her eyes saw evidence of motion. So I moved the sensor away from the cluster of neurons that was creating the sensation in her genitals. I adjusted just a little to the left on the sensory motor strip; this brightened her whole system enough so that she could feel other areas of her body, not just her genitals. Then just to be sure I rewarded the more calming frequencies on the right temporal lobe for a few minutes at the end of the session. This thinking worked.

Note: Remember how this works. It's not me doing the "brightening" or the "calming" as we move to achieve balance; it's her brain responding to the feedback I tell the computer to give.

Sensory homunculus

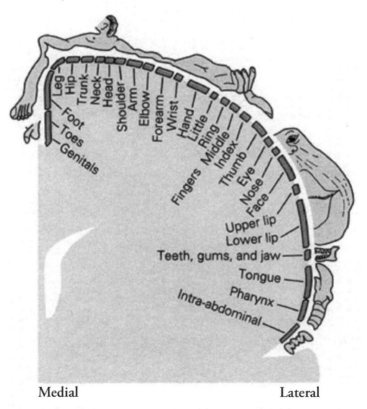

Medial   Lateral

Understand that you don't have to understand what I'm saying to benefit from the information. The point of these detective-like maneuvers is that learning about neuroanatomy can guide you to some great ideas. Even had I not been using neurofeedback to help her help herself, this thinking would still have led me to assist her sensory system as I created games that kept her body moving enough to bring sensory information into her limbs. Or I may have simply tried pressure on her joints (much like the squeeze chamber Temple Grandin designed) or rubbing on her skin. In my experience the ideas that help the most come from knowing that this disorder begins in the physiology and is more than just a person who doesn't want affection or interaction.

For example, I see a young bilingual autistic teenager with very few social skills and an intense sensory disorder. When we began he would repeatedly hit his face and head. By watching this behavior I was able to ascertain that they came from different sources. It appeared that his face was numb, especially around his mouth and the front gums (common problem area in speech disorder autistic kids, unusual with someone so gifted in the area of speech); it seemed as if he would hit these areas until they had feeling but that once they had feeling the sensory stimulation would grow too great in his brain and then he would develop a headache. In the initial stages he refused to let me try neurofeedback so I used this thinking: Whenever he began to push on his lips I added to his sensory input by squeezing his shoulders. This helped him relax and then he let me massage his face with lotion. Once I gained his trust he let me add neurofeedback. But even without the neurofeedback I was already helping him. So I used the same thinking again. It was important to locate the sensory area related to his face and then stimulate it. This was then followed with an overall calming of the cortex to prevent the stimulation from causing a headache. At present he is no longer self-injurious though we do still have a lot of exclusivity to deal with. The point I am trying (repeatedly) to make is: *being right matters less (especially given that neurofeedback effects are mostly reversible) than being proactive in your observations and solutions, because taking a "wrong" action can help point you to the right one.*

Motor Homunculus

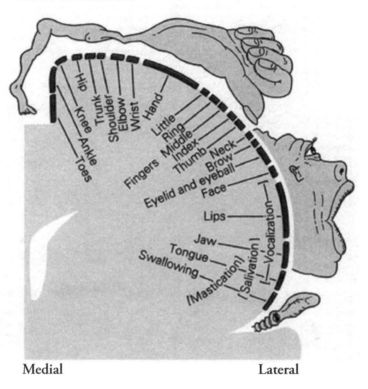

Medial   Lateral

Note: The homunculus that diagrams the clusters of motor neurons executing directions for movement in various parts of the body is slightly different than the homunculus that diagrams the clusters of sensory neurons creating sensations in various corresponding parts of the body. This is an important difference to note when creating protocols for your family or client. Be clear that the problem is sensory as opposed to motor when you choose the placements. For example, I have a client with Parkinson's who can feel everything in his right hand but not control its movement. Treating the corresponding sensory part meant I wasn't covering enough area as it is smaller than the motor representation. This did very little to alleviate his rigidity and tremors. But by giving feedback that encouraged more stimulation in the rather larger motor strip location, he was able to overcome—at least for now—the rigidity in this location.

As you have seen, I don't talk just about autism in this book about autism. I talk about other brain disorders as well, partly because they are buried within the whole brain issues of autism itself, but also because I treat the whole family, not just the autistic individual within. Why? Because it is common to find the entire grab bag of brain dysfunctions embedded within a group of relatives. And because people that help themselves function better are better equipped to help their people function better as well. That is why I teach people to teach themselves about the brain. Many bits and pieces of neuroanatomy information can be found by doing a quick search on the internet, buying a text book on neuroanatomy, or getting a magazine subscription to autism brain facts. It's really not hard to find out what's being found out. The challenge comes in knowing what to do with that knowledge you gain once you look. It is my hope that by the end of this book you will be fueled with enough proactive detective concepts to get some of your own individualized answers, based on the behavior of you, your family, and your child. It is my even greater hope that you will be self-trusting enough to act on them.

This is easier to do if you remember to trust the person you are trying to help over and above everyone else. At the end of the day I trust my client's answers because they know how they feel; they have the subjective knowledge I can only guess at. So when Barry sings that he can't stop singing I believe him and sing too. And when I make a neurofeedback choice and train the frontal area, but autistic Andy asks for a center placement, I listen and change the spot. A deep understanding of this subjective superiority can only be gained by self-training and exploration. Thus moms who use neurofeedback to train their own brains and heal their own focus or emotional issues can grow to become the most amazing therapists for their children.

Choices can come from the subtlest bit of information, especially when working with such a safe and immediately effective therapy. A word of caution here: Though I continually point out the safety of this therapy, it is only safe when used with an eye towards change and an understanding of how to follow. Nothing that can have such a profound effect could also at the same time be benign in its ability to do harm. However, as long as the person—parent or therapist—follows the changes and keeps an eye on the goal, while wrapping in a desire to see the client feel better and happier with each session, then this therapy is safe. This is another reason parents make great technicians:

they want their kids happy and easier to help. However, sometimes parents need to be taught what that looks like. Once informed, they follow the clues to that end helping the child grow towards self-confidence and independence. Regardless of the therapy being employed, if people doesn't use their observational skills to follow up on changes with new ideas, and instead believes that proper learning must follow an order of operations approach, they will often ignore the anatomical variation of the individual and thwart the learning process altogether. This happens when the person needs the child to say "pup" before she says "outside." Such a blind eye can make any safe therapy no longer effective, and somewhat unsafe.

Care must be taken to at all times do what appears to be needed in order to move towards balance. Our brains seek balance; life seeks balance. If we value one skill over another and seek an imbalance for our client or children, something happens to tip the boat. An example of a way in which this can play out follows: I had a client for whom t4 had a calming effect. The mom loved it so much that when this boy was no longer benefiting in an optimal way from that prescription she just did more on the same spot, and when that didn't look good she did even more and more and more. More is not necessarily better. He was so slowed down by this refusal to switch protocols that he ended up returning back from whence he came—into total exclusivity. At this point the mom had a choice to make—come clean with me so that I could guide her better or quit neurofeedback and call it ineffective. Fortunately she came clean.

When I arrived to reintroduce myself to the child, he seemed very distant. His pupils were dilated and his face was pale. I chose to be an unavoidable force in his world for five days. It was a crazy outreach because I added all kinds of noisy, gregarious play to his high-frequency training aimed at stimulating, stimulating, stimulating the brain. Five days later he was back!

I miss this beautiful boy. I spent a lot of time with him that year. His family had some very ambitious plans. Despite the fact that this was a boy about whom the previous therapist had said, "He's the most autistic child I've ever met," the parents chose to believe that it was possible—with the help of neurofeedback—to move him from extreme exclusivity to school-ready in less than a year. However, after the experience of miscommunication and over-training on t4 they were leery of doing the work themselves. They wanted me to do the job. I was hired for eleven weeks that year.

We made great progress during that time. So much so that this awesome group of people spread the therapy to extended family members and had me take a look at their cousin: She'd been injured several years before when a bank of school lockers came loose from the wall and fell on her. One arm was deformed, paralyzed, and overly sensitive to touch—so much so that she jumped at the thought of contact. She contorted her body with the arm turned inward, possibly to protect against such an assault. She had become frozen in this position. I found a cortex-wide anomaly in her brainwave activity and inhibited it. We did several sessions and by the end of the first day she could allow touch. She could also move her thumb. It was a summer full of miracles and love.

Unfortunately, spending this much time together with me in the role of expert meant that this family was at risk of becoming dependant upon me—which put me at risk of being resented, and/or worrying about being resented. Meanwhile, even if we managed to escape the trap of co-dependency, we were all at risk of becoming overexposed to each other. It's called the saturation point and happens in all walks of life. A common example is when an actor crosses the line between exposure meant to increase public awareness and "Oops! I see him everywhere!" If he has too many well-advertised movies wherein he is the star being released simultaneously, we are overexposed and his popularity wanes. It is a natural function of the brain to filter out and stop noticing (or appreciating) anything (or anyone) that is too evident in our lives.

Despite these possible potholes we reached their goal and the child was introduced to school where, according to all reports, he has continued to grow. However, the family has moved on so I don't get many reports and am no longer an authority on the subject of this child. It wasn't until a year after last seeing them that I got an email saying he was doing well and handling school, but that in retrospect, the family wasn't sure neurofeedback had had anything to do with his progress. This family's reaction, like the reaction of many practitioners who choose to use phrases such as "misdiagnosis" whenever a child comes off the spectrum of autism, is to be expected. After all, the brain does all the perceiving, even about the past. Thus professionals who work in the field of mental health run the risk of being obliterated from the story by their clients and/or colleagues whenever they accomplish their goals. This is especially true if, like me, they suck at organization and record keeping. Sorry! That's way too much like math! (Wah! Wah! Wah! OK. I'm whining a bit!) Truth is I'm not really complaining. I think the concept liberates us from caring about being credited and instead releases us into the joy of helping others because it helps us to help.

It turns out that when the brain assimilates the changes enough for us to hear echoes from our clients stating that perhaps the neuro-feedback had nothing to do with their new state of balance, we can be encouraged to note that said clients may be nearing the point of completion to their therapy. In other words, a lack of credit can be a positive sign for the clinician. Since this therapy is not meant to be done forever, in most cases having the clients take responsibility for their life and how they function within it while no longer needing or wanting us is a good thing. In my experience when a parent resists—just as when my teenagers resist—it can mean help a little more—hand out a few more tools and then let them go. It's time for the new feed-back that the world is about to give them to complete the job and give them the credit. As well it should.

When working in the field of brain health, this rewriting us out of the story happens at least to some degree every time a client is fully helped. It is a reality one must become comfortable with, even if s/he is the parent.

So, to be clear, neurofeedback works via feedback loops to the brain. This feedback teaches the brain to change itself. The brain then takes ownership of the changes made. At this point the only way for changes to become an integral part of the person is if they are assimilated. So the brain assimilates even the memories. This is really cool, especially if you'd like to change the story of your life. It turns out you can, and do. The reason this hasn't happened to me is twofold.

- One: It actually has. But I am constantly being re-impressed by neurofeedback because I am always at the beginning of this story watching the magic unfold with a new client or family of autism.

- Two: My son Dar. He was twenty-three and not talking. He wasn't going to change on his own or via any of the other therapies I tried and he wasn't misdiagnosed. I know this because he was just plain too old. That's why when I catch myself wondering if I'm wrong about my other came-off-the-spectrum-kids and grandkids, I think of Dar and hold fast to what I know: Brains heal!

And neurofeedback changed my story.

I do admit I miss being more a part of not only that family but of the other families who have fallen away. This revolving-door reality is why I never wanted to be a teacher, though the job has been offered to me many times. It is why I adopted instead of fostering because I wanted to stay involved. But I finally get that that's not the point. This lesson that being able to be truly loving meant having a willingness to give the gift of freedom took a long time to learn. But I learned it—just in time—to enjoy the fact that my children grew up and got almost as independent and almost as busy as me. It turns out that there's always some child to mother, to teach, to help. And the more kids that get better the more kids that get better. So now I enjoy the present while looking forward to the future of letting go. In fact, I set up my practice to that end. I aim for therapeutic independence. It is because of that choice that my way of working and teaching parents how to do without me evolved.

So what do I teach? How do I know what to do? Where do the ideas come from? *They come from us, applying knowledge to a problem.*

An example of how subtle a life-changing, soon-to-be-assimilated idea can be happened when my neurofeedback instructor was talking about autism and the cerebellum. He said two things that led me to make some very unique therapy choices. One was to describe what is called an intention tremor. He mentioned that people with autism have seriously compromised cerebellums and that one of the issues created can be that the client has no tremor unless they reach to touch something; then at the closing in on the desired-item point, a tremor emerges possibly moving the hand away from the item the person is aiming at. This makes success extremely difficult to attain. I immediately thought of Dar and all his difficulty when trying to type or pick up requested items. I remembered taking him to a speech therapist and having her line up ten items. She asked him repeatedly to pick up one of the items; instead he picked up all nine of the unasked for ones. He did this three times and she declared him too retarded to learn to speak. I suggested (with a little desperate annoyance at her calling my son a lost cause) that she was overlooking the obvious. It seemed to me that his getting the wrong thing every single time was against the odds of coincidence. Obviously he knew what she was asking for. She refused not only to entertain my logic but also to take him as a client. Then there I was many years later in neuroanatomy class coming to understand what had been going on all along. I thought of Dar trying to get a fork and—more often than not—getting the item next to it. I realized he had a tremor that was moving him away from whatever he aimed at. I felt a little guilt over not having known sooner, but then the instructor said something very cool.

He said, while pointing to the back of his head near the neck, that the cerebellum is tucked way down here and nobody really does neurofeedback on it. Then, as if he was talking to himself, he muttered something like, "I guess you could." He went on to explain that most clinicians just work other areas of the brain that hopefully create new pathways that will lead the brain to heal in this area as well. He kept talking but I kept thinking, "I guess you could." And I wondered if I hadn't just learned a secret. So I went home, placed the sensor in a spot no one else was using, fussed with it repeatedly to get rid of the heartbeat artifact (interference) created by the veins there, and started training Dar's cerebellum at a low frequency. I watched his hands relax and his tremor settle. And slowly, ever so slowly, session after session his intention tremor faded in intensity. He began to play short games of Scrabble and type a word or two unassisted. Oh happy day!

Knowing neuroanatomy helped me stick with things even when they didn't look good while at the same time making sure that they did. For example, Dar couldn't speak and the things that helped him speak best were placements on the left near the speech center and the sensory motor strip at a mid range of frequency reward— unfortunately this also made him hit himself and sweat and pace and he seemed in general very uncomfortable. The healing needed to happen, but it hurt him too much for me to work in that area. Periodically over two years I would try this type of protocol and each time he reacted in this way, though with less and less intensity.

(Understand that I knew how to immediately reverse the effect and make him comfortable again so trying wasn't cruel, just necessary in the cause of information gathering.) By the second year Dar could do half a thirty-minute session at this location. But the sessions themselves had to be spaced out. At present he can do the whole session about three times in a row, then on the fourth we need to settle his system down. His speech is better and, in fact, it improves even as he is doing the sessions. Some of the improvement stays while the rest recedes. So we train again.

This slow-moving miracle is one that requires patience and persistence. But the improvement is clear. My intuitive understanding that I should keep checking to see when Dar could handle being treated on the part of the brain that is responsible for expressive speech was rewarded. This gentle persistence is another reason I believe in home training, because Dar had done about four hundred sessions before he could handle this area At the normal office rates I never would have been able to get him talking, even clumsily.

I can't stress the art of following change enough… I have three clients whose protocols were the usual t4 low frequency placements. Three of these kids became very calm but also very exclusive and unmotivated; one of the two first cried and then fell into a deep depression. Doing a protocol just because that's what everyone else does for autism is limited thinking. Of course we are back to definitions and expectations again because if the definition of "good results" is "no longer hyper," and the expectation is that this therapy can make them calmer and easier to deal with, then those are examples of a "job well done." However, as one mom put it, "I used to think I just wanted him to stop hitting himself; now I wish he cared enough about anything to hit." So we got him interested in the world again and, for the most part, he doesn't hit.

So much more is available through retraining of the brain than calmness. Expect it all! Appreciate what you get. And define "a good job" as closer to the goal today than yesterday.

One of the things that I've learned from looking at the brains of autistic people and their families is that lots of eccentric brains like mine seem to have an excess of delta waves otherwise known as sleep waves because, as previously mentioned, that's the only time you are supposed to have them in large amounts. I found myself wondering why I was finding such enormous amplitudes of delta waves in relation to autism at around the same time that I got a possible answer. I was studying these waves and researching the lack of pruning in autistic brains. (Just as your skin sloughs off its dead cells, so should your brain prune away the neurons that didn't migrate or grow properly—in autism the neurons often just keep coming but the pruning gardener is not at work. This leads to children with oversized, over-crowded heads under pressure and a well-known fact about neurons is they don't like to be squeezed.) I was engaged in a brainstorming session on the excess inflammation in the autistic brain and found myself wondering if these things went together. "Maybe," I surmised, "the excess delta is caused by broken ion pumps which are caused by the damage created by the inflammation which was a response to the pressure of overcrowding." Now there is no way on earth in a normal field of science one would be comfortable making such a leap; after all, correlation never proves causation. It's always just a clue of coincidence until you prove it to be more, but holding back on building stories that create cohesive thoughts based on the flimsy evidence at hand is why Dar was considered too retarded to speak. To my way of thinking sometimes correlation points to possible causation, and if the quickest way to get an answer is to assume that as truth and proceed accordingly, then as long as the assumption and pursuant course of action doesn't put any one at risk but does create possibilities for healing, well then, I'm happy to spin a story that puts cause and effect together to give it a try.

THE NEUROANATOMY CLASS MIRACLE: Seven-year-old autistic Joe showed no interest in food. I remembered a neuroanatomy class on a similar problem with mice who had lesions in the ascending dopaminergic pathways. Thus I rewarded low beta activity and inhibited delta in the left prefrontal area just above the temple. Joe began to eat.

THE FACTS: Joe's parents had, at the suggestion of other professionals and well-meaning relatives, tried many times to wait out Joe's disinterest. "Leave him long enough and he'll eat!" they were told. They said that they had gone so far as to stop feeding him

> while leaving the food out for two days. Joe never bothered with it. He showed no inclination toward it at all though he salivated when smelling it cook. And though he never wanted to eat he always allowed himself to be fed.
>
> **THE BEST PART OF THE MIRACLE:** Once we got him eating on his own, he never stopped.

Of course I didn't really need to create a story of "why" in order to know that I was finding too much delta and that asking the brain to make less delta might be a good idea. But the story allowed me to create a pathway to follow in my thinking, and as long as it unfolded by creating positive behavioral change I followed the path. The trick in asking for change is to put all your energy into making it happen while at the same time being open to the possibility of being wrong. In other words, be prepared to wash your hands if it turns out you've been spreading germs. This is easier to do when you stay in touch with the fact that it's just a story you're telling to help you gather your thinking, thus new evidence can mean making a new story with no blaming for having previously written a different plot. Of course this sort of big assuming only makes sense because we are simply teaching to behavior and giving information—albeit to neurons—because even neurons can be taught to change their collective "minds," hence the reversibility of neurofeedback. Such an approach is not OK when using intrusive therapies like medicine or implants or surgery: it's preferable if the surgeon knows what the liver does before he decides to take it out and then realizes that OOPS! You need one of those!

Fortunately neurofeedback doesn't take anything away from you; it merely helps you to restructure what is already there. This is done by teaching the brain which frequencies it should increase in amplitude while simultaneously telling it which frequencies it should decrease. And even though—as we direct the brain on how to do that—there is a lot of "difference" in the field among practitioners for the frequencies we ask the brain to make more of, as a general rule, there is a great deal of "sameness" in the things we ask the brain to make less of. We call the "make less request" inhibits. Since most professionals inhibit the same basic frequencies, perhaps that is where the true power of neurofeedback lies: in its ability to make less of the problem. In fact, the brain itself expends more energy and allocates more neurons for the act of inhibiting neuronal behavior than it does for exciting it. So the mathematical odds favor the likelihood that the majority of cognitive problems lie in the brain's inability to inhibit itself. Perhaps the fact that all neurofeedback professionals are helping the brain to become stronger in this regard is the true power of the therapy and the reason why "there appear to be so many ways up the mountain" because in fact our different paths are an illusion: In our sameness we are the same.

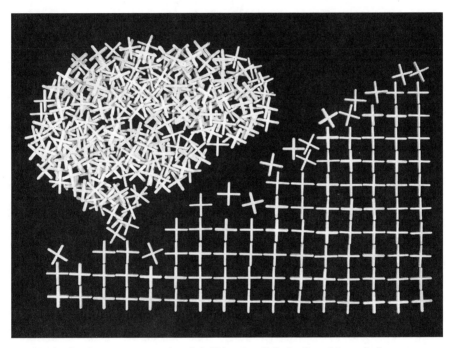

Human brain overcoming an obstacle © **Valentina Shibeko from bigstockphoto.com**

I often use analogies like exercise when trying to explain neurofeedback to clients. I say things like, "You cannot play the game perfectly because I keep making it harder, in the same way that a good coach will start out asking for what you can already do by requesting that you run one block but as soon as you are capable he will up the bar and ask for two. And so it goes, for as long as you are motivated to work toward improvement, he can ask for more and increase the level of difficulty forever because one can never run out of blocks." I do the same for your brain. However, in some ways this is a misleading analogy that just allows me to begin a glimmer of understanding by basing the explanation on something already known to most people. The misleading aspect of the analogy lies in the fact that things like exercise or facials or massages or pedicures (hmmm, I must be wanting a spa day) only benefit you as long as you continue to do them. Whereas neurofeedback begins a process that actually gains momentum rolling up hill: it's kind of like struggling to leave the earth, and then the atmosphere of the earth, and then the gravitational pull forcing you to orbit the earth, until the struggle ends and you do… suddenly find… yourself able… to just go and go and go.

As I have mentioned before the reason for this amazing development is that once you begin to function differently, the world you live in begins to give you different feedback (even more so if the entire family is treating and improving their brain function). As the world begins to tell you how much better you talk, or kinder you are, or faster at tennis you have gotten, you begin to believe it. And what you believe you are, you become. Then as you experience yourself anew, new things come into your horizon and you perceive more as possible. In other words the world you live in becomes your neurofeedback machine.

These points are useful even if you as a family or as a professional don't wish to use neurofeedback, because they underscore the importance of positive thinking and open-minded believing with regard to your child's abilities and possibilities. I work with one family who has some religious convictions that disallow the use of technology and still we have fashioned the child's life around these concepts and made the same (albeit slower) gains as we would if she were using neurofeedback computers. The fact is, intentionally "feeding back" in order to achieve a goal can be done at any speed—high or low.

An example of how a simple little change in one's demeanor can effect everything in a relationship came when I was working with Barry. His mom was afraid of his violent outbursts and so avoided saying "no" while not saying "yes." It was confusing to watch, and her expression at all times when looking at her son seemed worn and tired. I suggested she say "no" when she meant "no" but that she also follow that with an explanation of why before offering a substitution. I also suggested she "sparkle her eyes" so that every time he looked he saw acceptance. I explained that this would help him to feel encouraged to try harder and listen more. It was a simple thing that immediately made a big difference. Because you can't sparkle your eyes and feel sad at the same time her mood lifted and so did his.

I added that she should keep sparkling but with less intensity whenever she said "no." He threw some tantrums but she was OK with it so he eventually stopped. This mom became quickly proficient at following her son's needs; his violence lifted and she changed her ABA therapy to a more child-centered approach. However, true to her instincts as a mom, she kept one of the old behaviorists because that girl knew how to sparkle.

CHAPTER EIGHT

Don't Drink the Poison

I had a brother and sister set of clients whose changes were miraculous enough to take the girl off the spectrum in less than a year. But then I got a panicked phone call from the parents who were terrified that their children had begun to regress. I arranged for a personal visit and arrived to find children who were screaming and fighting at an unnatural level. At first it appeared that indeed the children were regressing but after some careful questioning and some attentive listening, it became obvious that the parents had been fighting a lot over the past few months. They had put their children's needs so far ahead of their own that they were buckling under the pressure and finding fault with each other. This habit of martyrdom is what I call the cup of poison. It is also why the families that prioritize their own therapy help their children the most effectively.

These two little cherubs were simply mirroring their parent's anxiety and behavior. All kids do this but autistic kids mirror you without the filtering component of waiting until you leave the room. They also do it at a high level of skill that is so magnified and caricatured that it becomes unrecognizable to you as something you've modeled. Conversely they may also react by withdrawing from the chaos and becoming more exclusive. This connection between environment and cognitive functioning is why so many people try to blame parents for their children's deficits. This is an unfair conclusion since the deficits were pre-existing but it is at least based in some semblance of truth. And rather than look for whom to blame with this evidence we can look for how to solve. I think this connection is why Cognitive Behavior Therapy is so successful and such an important addition when implementing neurofeedback because a quicker brain is just quicker at learning from its environment. So being cognitive of what you or your child learn can make the difference between happiness and misery.

As I mentioned before when I began this journey of trying to raise children out of autism in 1983, many people still believed that the disorder was caused by a psychologically driven state: a child hiding in a world of his own, a child who was purposely rejecting his family and the society that they represented despite the fact that he/she was fully capable of embracing them all. THIS IS NOT WHAT I MEAN WHEN I REFER TO THE INTERCHANGE BETWEEN BRAIN DEVELOPMENT AND THE CHILD'S ENVIRONMENT. Back then it was believed that autism was something to rise out of, and that belief was the only benefit I got from this time period. Because though children don't really rise out of autism they do heal away from it. Even though this belief about the possibility that my child could emerge from the autism blanket unscathed kept me motivated to reach for change, it also cursed and exhausted me. This is because believing that a good mom could remove the blanket meant that if my child wasn't rising out of autism, then this lack of progress was something for me to be ashamed of—something to be blamed for and something to hide. And that pressure almost defeated me. As it turned out, in order for children to be truly helped, it was the mothers that needed to be lifted from the blanket of autism and found guiltless because righteous mothers are relentless. And that's the kind of energy this takes. Unfortunately at the time that all this "mom blaming" was going on, the people that needed help to "rise up"—parents and their children—were a minority that carried very little weight: Because at the time autism was very, very rare.

Back then professional helper's—intent on doing good—sprayed water in the children's faces and trained them like dogs. Or conversely people like myself held them and gently sang words of love until they passed out—exhausted from screaming—preferring to be left untouched. Trying to love them into choosing to come back to our world only sometimes and even then it only worked if we loved them in a way that they could perceive as loving. This is something most people still don't understand. But back then it was worse. Back then a concept like that was so completely alien to everyone that I would have had just as much likelihood of being understood if I wrote out it in hieroglyphics. Back then autistic children were seen as frightening and mysterious, psychic, magical, and proof that there were aliens living among us. Back then we called them retarded, which has never been seen as frightening and mysterious, psychic, magical, and proof that there were aliens living among us. So in my opinion, back then, we pushed and pulled and spouted our silliness while making no sense at all. In some ways those days aren't really all that different from right now. For example, there is a school in Canton, Massachusetts that still uses backpacks to shock children when they behave inappropriately. It's an aversion technique for "bad" behaviors. (God forbid anyone should flap their hands except when waving.) At present we still have uninformed observers spouting silliness that stings. In fact just a few years ago (when I first began writing this book) Michael Savage—a radio personality—gained notoriety from angrily stating on air that parents were to blame for the behaviors of their autistic child and that all they needed was a good bit of discipline. Celebrity slander is a problem for parents, like within the pages of Dennis Leary's book when he jokes about autism, blaming laziness on the part of the child, for this toe-walking trend of not learning to talk (Yes, I am being sarcastic!). It seems that we are still a little confused. And despite the public outcry these statements drew from us—as mentioned in the discussion on facilitation—once it's said it's in people's heads. And quite frankly it's ridiculous!

In my experience it takes a lot more energy and commitment and time to stop people—brain disordered or not—from learning than it does to teach them what they want to know. The fact is everybody learns, at one speed or another. So let's teach things that lead to everybody getting better; better at being together, with respect. A good place to start would be public opinion (hence, year upon year, I invest more than I earn into my show and the cause of autism awareness), but in these pages we start with parents and professionals because the public is composed of them and they are the people that can make a difference now, in this moment, day upon day.

So how do we put the two approaches of behavioral therapy and neurofeedback together?

EXPLAIN, EXPLAIN, EXPLAIN! FOLLOW, FOLLOW, FOLLOW!

But first determine what the client's long-term goals are. I often loosen people's limited ideas of what's possible with this question: "OK, I'm the Magic Brain Genie and I have the power to give you anything you want from your brain. That means things like speed of understanding, physical reaction time, focus, emotions, better math skills, sensory awareness, IQ, anything. What do you want most?" This question often dislodges a confession of the person's biggest impediment to their daily lives and overall success. At this point I create a plan of attack and explain my thinking to the client. I do this even if the client is a nonverbal child and the Brain Genie question gets rephrased into "Since telling me what you want doesn't seem easy I'm gonna start by helping you talk… that way you'll be able to pick."

Explaining is a way of thinking out loud and helps me to check on my own logic. It also implies that I have enough respect for you to include you in that process. I see no reason to exclude a child just because they are non-verbal from this type of respectful treatment.

Besides, people generally (though not always) give back what they get. For example, I was invited to work with a young lady who was very, very disabled. She bit her hands so much they were kept in protective foam wraps. She also had leg braces and a walker in order to move about. She was an only child in a very rich family. She was beautiful, about eleven years old, and when I first met her she responded quite quickly in that she was affectionate and looked in my eyes right away. Admittedly I had gotten on the floor beside her in order to make looking easier and by my position almost unavoidable. In fact, looking away from me would have taken more effort than looking at me did. (This is a great technique by the way. It's called "be in the way—with a smile. We do it to babies all the time.) For the next few days I followed her around making notes on the various aspects of her life as we moved through her pre-existing schedule going from therapy to therapy.

The first thing I noted was that this child who everyone said would just melt down and burst into self-injurious behavior for no reason at all had very good reasons. For example, at one point she was at physical therapy where she was helped onto a table. A lady put the little girl's leg in a sling, whipped it up really high to the point of pain and the girl cried out "Don't!. She didn't pronounce well though so it came out sounding more like "doe." Nobody believed she could talk so nobody listened, especially not this lady who was busy telling her to behave and stop crying out. Since words didn't work the girl tried hitting. So the lady called her a bad girl and tied her into the device all the while treating me as if I agreed with her techniques. I intercepted at that moment and attached sensors to the child. I translated her words and used the neurofeedback to relax her muscles.

But this was to be a one-time trip for me, and it looked as if I might end up walking away knowing that what this girl was going to learn was that her voice had no power. I feared this was true because in my absence from the room I overheard (through the door) "No matter what you do young lady, this exercise has to happen." It was an interesting challenge. The girl had every moment of her day filled with that kind of activity, and there was a way in which everyone was being wonderful and using the skills they believed would help her. They had good intentions, very good therapies for her, and only when she acted like that did they have voices that were commanding and unforgiving. The rest of the time they smiled and were sweet and they actually loved her very much. They just believed that this was the way to get the job done. I just believe that if I were the child, I'd have bit her too.

The point is when she was given explanations, when her words were given power, and she was allowed to set the limits of how far to take the stretch, she was cooperative. She didn't act out, hit, or bite. In addition, when her therapists were given explanations, when they were shown that her sounds were words and they had a chance to understand the workings of her brain, they didn't act out, pull, or push. Given the right information almost everybody is ready to learn. [That is as long as they aren't afflicted with the Semmelweis reflex. (wink)]

In my experience special children are ravenous to learn and happy to be redirected as long as we are too.

The real challenge is teaching the neuro-typical folks who help them to understand that many special people look as if they are ignoring you or not responding even when they are. Thus when they do speak we assume a lack of communication because their posturing is odd. Consequently their language is perceived as having an accidental similarity with words regardless of their sounds. (We do a similar but different version of this when the child speaks clearly but in peculiar ways.) We assume a lot. Like in the movie about the young Australian CP girl who was one of the first to use facilitated communication: what we appear capable of and what we are capable of are not always the same. I want to share a memory: I was strolling a one-mile circular path with my then (new to neurofeedback) twenty-three-year-old son Dar. I was talking and explaining that we would not even have to turn around to end up back at home by going on this route. I explained that, though it felt as if we were constantly moving forward, we would end up back where we started from having actually gotten nowhere. I likened it to some of his repetitive behaviors saying, "It's the same as when you are doing the same thing over and over again while not learning anything new." He said something I didn't understand. I asked him to try again. He did. And I still didn't understand. His face got red; he kept trying and trying, his forehead dripping with sweat as he attempted over and over again to tell me something that seemed to be very important to him. His panic rose as my lack of understanding grew. He began pulling and pushing and guttural-whisper shouting the same unintelligible sound over and over again. Cars were beginning to slow down as their occupants stared and pointed at this desperate thigh-slapping man they were passing by.

Dar was, at this time, still perceived as retarded by most and very, very, very, very hard to understand. In fact, nobody but me even believed he was talking, though sometimes they pretended they did. (I had always believed Dar was smarter than he appeared; however, in retrospect, I guess I didn't believe him as smart as he was.) So, there I was repeating myself and explaining in terms that grew simpler and simpler because I assumed that I had somehow confused him with my lesson. Finally after half an hour of trying to enunciate I heard him say it—his ever-so-important-to-convey thought—"Like Metaphor!"

WOW!

My kids have often amazed me with their conceptual perceptive-ness, especially since autism is supposed to be a literal disorder: One day I was walking that same stretch of circular road with my young-est (twenty-one at the time) son Rye. He had been fired from his job. I told him he should be careful because he was burning bridges. He asked me what the saying meant and I tried to explain the concept. After several variations on the definition we began to walk in silence. I assumed he had begun to daydream and considered finding yet another way to explain the meaning when he said, "You know what Mom. I think you are a bridge that's hard to burn."

WOW! WOW! WOW! and WOW! AGAIN!

I worked with a young girl who had no language aside from the ability to hum a tune. I explained to her that she could talk and that my computer would make it easier to do so. I stimulated her pre-motor pre-sensory strip by using a high-frequency reward and then gave her rides on my back whenever she made any approximation of the word ride. At every turn I explained the benefits of speaking and pointed out that she was already learning. Several helpers and both her parents also got in on the act. After six weeks of this program, Joanne was able to name many vegetables, sing several songs, and even occasionally answer from another room when her name was called.

It wasn't until after my experiences with Joanne and DW that I began to understand just how much knowledge about autism was stored in my head. Since I had acquired this knowledge over so many years of trial and error, and since my guys had improved one problem at a time, I never really experienced it as anything other than living and learning. Life just isn't like that edited movie version of a miraculous instantaneous windfall of health. And yet three of my kids and two of my grandkids HAD gotten better. The more homes I went into, the more I realized what a really big deal that was. So I decided to share what I know and started to—among other things—put this book together.

As I have previously mentioned, nowadays I go out and teach all kinds of parents all over the world how to work with this combination of play therapy and neurofeedback. I begin by enjoying the child's game while complimenting everything he/she does that resembles typical behavior. I say things like "Wow you are great at pointing," and then increase his ability to cooperate and learn by adding the technology of having the child balance her brain wave activity while playing a video game with his or her brain. I stir in some teaching to family dynamics by showing the parents how to do things like give the quiet (sibling) child the attention that the screaming (autistic) child seeks (all the while explaining to the children that it's quiet I notice most). And then we all recreate together by examining our thinking about the thinking of their autistic child. We open up our minds to stay aware that just because she looks only for the flash of a second from the side of her eyes, that doesn't mean she didn't see, and couldn't have read, the entire paragraph. We learn through observation what might be helping in order to grow the healing even more and notice other things. Like maybe she is listening only when she is chewing her hand, because the act of chewing mixes with the sensory input and stimulates her brain waves enough to keep her focused enough to hear. Rather like a truck driver chewing ice to stay awake and notice the blaring horns whenever he wavers from his lane.

We discover together how to reward properly, always keeping in mind the desired goal, so that if he appears to respond with excitement when we yell then we whisper what we don't want him to do and cheer for what we do. We brainstorm and observe each other, looking for ways to respond that will get us more quickly to our goals. Thus if she screams while we are talking and Mom goes into autopilot and hands her things to hush her up, we laugh: Because laughing clears the air and makes it easier to think. Then we think and search for other ways to handle the situation knowing that if we don't come up with something new we better learn to enjoy the ritual because we are reinforcing its existence by participating in our part of the game. And each of these lessons teaches us a better way to be in every aspect of our lives.

If you are working with or raising people on the spectrum of autism you have the opportunity to be blessed. You have lessons ahead about being intentional and gaining a handle on your environment. You will have a chance to analyze it all and find what works. You will get the benefits of everything from baking soda and Epsom salt baths to garlic and algae to cleanse your toxins to a new appreciation for probiotics and the removal of candida-feeding sugars from your diet. You will learn to balance your minerals like magnesium for constipation or diarrhea. (I learned this only after much parental discomfort. First I spent a year and a half watching my son cry bathed in sweat and bearing down while he bled every time he had to pass an oversized, heavily compacted, dehydrated stool. Doctors offered me all kinds of laxatives and softeners, and after much rectal damage and almost two years of pain, all it took was a change in his magnesium supplements: cheap vitamins, easy solution).

It is because I have had so many years of discovery in relation to autism that I know what I know. And it is because I struggled so hard to gain this knowledge that I share what I've gained. Remarkably when I do that, I have the opportunity to watch as the kids and their families improve at a much faster pace than mine ever did. Again I say "and their families" because of the domino effect that improving one person in a group can have, but also because most family members have their own set of challenges. Remember that autism is influenced by one's genetics so it isn't surprising to find an assortment of disorders within the home. Maybe it can be deemed fortunate that the household disorders gathered together and grew until they became autism, which caused enough of a panic to cause everyone in the family to seek healing. So they (we) did something about it and everyone got better. Thank you autism.

Every time I watch a family change, the people inside say, "You've gotta write a book; you just have to write a book; you have to share these things you know." I wish that were possible: the sharing. The problem, as I've come to discover, with sharing the solutions I hold is that I don't really hold any, only problem-solving skills and experience. I get the answers in response to the questions that come up. That's why I am trying to share my approach and my experience instead: to teach you how to think about the problem without seeing it as a tragedy because devastation closes down creative thought and barricades you from the answers.

Following means letting the behavior speak for itself.

No matter how many times I explain the individuality of each person's brain, invariably I am asked to give an order of operations for how one goes about treating autism. At the very least they request a developmental model replete with approaches and techniques that will move a child from a to z as he passes through each stage in a sequentially satisfying manner. I watch speech therapists thwart development all the time because they need the sounds to follow a certain order of appearance. I see it with PT's, OT's and behavioral therapists. If what I see is truth, then autism doesn't follow a model. It just changes and grows because the brain is rerouting, according to its infinite wisdom, based on a need for homeostasis and using the information its sensory system gives it. We have no choice but to find the answers in the questions about the child

Follow, Follow, Follow!

My son Cash and I began a thing we labeled "walk and talks." He was about seventeen and still very challenged in regard to conversations. Each day we would head out on our walk and I would give him a choice of things to "sell me on." For example, get me to believe he should have a dog, or convince me that a Chevrolet is better than a Ford. Each subject came from an interest of his and so could be used at some other point when speaking with friends. On one particular day he had made a valiant attempt to convince me to take him for a driving lesson, but his logic had held no part in which I would benefit. I explained to him that to get people to do things there has to be something for them to gain. We walked in silence for a while. My mind was busy with all the lessons I still had to teach, errands to be done, and bills to be paid. I yanked myself back to an awareness of my son and thinking that he was mulling over the question I had put before him asked him what was on his mind. "It looks like they laid some new stones. I was just thinking about how thick the gravel is."

I am ashamed to admit that at first his answer brought a familiar thought to my mind, "Poor Cash is a simpleton." And then I caught myself thinking and realized how limiting that was. I never would have pondered over the rocks, but does that make pondering over them stupid? He was right, of course. The gravel was fresh. And it felt better to my feet. It was a nice thing to notice. The truth is a lot of people pay huge sums of retreat money to learn how to notice the stones. My son just did it naturally in the quiet of his head. So I tried to follow his lead. I quieted my mind and gained a moment of appreciation for my son's gentle ways.

Walk and talks were a special design based on Cash's interests. I had never done this as a regular part of anyone's program before but the privacy, being outside in nature, and using his motivation of wanting to work as a car salesman began the process. I followed his interests and got the idea. Cash learned more about how to communicate his wishes while simultaneously considering mine through this program than any other I had tried. In the year 2000 he turned eighteen and one year after this "notice the stones" day Cash got a job. He became permanently independent by the time he was nineteen at which point he bought a truck and a travel trailer to live in. I like to think that the walk and talks helped prepare him with the ability to negotiate.

As I have and will continue to explain, every time I work with a child, mine or someone else's, I design an approach that is based on the child's interests. This is because I want them to be interested. (As obvious as that sounds, very few special-education professionals use this technique.) Since the program essentially comes from the child, it is impossible to help your child by hearing what I did and copying me (or anyone else for that matter). It is, however, possible to learn from the reasons behind the choices.

Like when Andy looked at the preoccupied adults in the room, smiled, and squeezed his grandmother's breasts; we chose to stand as a barrier between him and his grandmother while explaining that breasts can be hurt this way. We dropped all energy from the subject matter and explained repeatedly. Even though this was how we helped Andy, when a different child squeezed his mother's breasts on the heels of squeezing every other squishy thing in the house, we chose to create a program of increasing the energy around squishy things. We engaged in an exploration wherein we categorized and searched for all things appropriate for squeezing that could be found in the home. We piled them up in the living room and then squeezed with all our might. This difference in our approach came from my perception about the reason behind the squish: reaction or sensation.

This type of analyzing the motivator for a behavior and then creating a response that will shape things towards a calmer end is the secret to any good program. And it is especially important when dealing with sensory dysfunctions, as there is so much acting out in regards to body parts, both private and otherwise. Thinking in a logical manner without pushing the panic button on thoughts of sexual deviancy around breast squeezing is much more useful than seeing sexual abuse everywhere and making faulty judgments based on comparing an atypical child with a "typical" one. It is a habit in our society to go for the sensational. That's why when facilitation created an avenue for stories of touching to be brought forth, everyone saw sexual abuse instead of sexual dysfunction, so they complicated the picture instead of helping to clear the issues.

Actually, anyone locked away in a broken brain of logical misunderstandings lives in a different perceptual world and not only behaves differently but draws different conclusions about what it means when the people in his world behave in any way at all. Even offering a glass of water to someone with a depth-perception issue who sees the extended glass as about to hit him in the face can be viewed as abuse in the eyes of the thirsty. There is a cute scene in the movie *Rainman* when Tom Cruise gets frustrated and puts his hand (firmly but gently) on the back of his brother's neck. It's an adorable interchange that easily illustrates the differing points of view between people about the event they are both involved in. Dustin Hoffman first moans "Uh oh" and then writes "squeezed and pulled and hurt my neck" in his "serious-injury list" notebook. Tom Cruise simply rolls his eyes.

Clashing concepts like these are often created when kids with a startle reflex caused by a visual processing issue wince because something moved too quickly in their peripheral field of vision. This reaction is not unlike our slamming to a stop when brought out of a daydream by the brake lights on the car ahead of us. But at least we can seek reassurance and companionship from the half-asleep person who was sitting in shotgun and experienced the situation with us. The startle-reflex-afflicted kid lives in a private world wherein he is being assaulted by the environment all on his own.

As previously stated there are several contributing brain problems that can cause a startle reflex. Some, but not all, of those can be a perceptual problem, a deep far-away focus or an over-firing amygdala creating apparently unfounded fear that overloads the sensory system. They can also be the result of abuse. Startle reflexes are just a clue to any number of possible problems. They don't necessarily mean that someone is hurting the child. But since that's one of the possibilities, all too often that is the conclusion people observing the behavior draw. Following behavior without preconceptions is necessary to do good work and not create bigger problems than are already there. The fact is if we assume dire home lives, our attitudes and assumptions put pressure on the caretaker to create a calm well-behaved kid. This pressure can contribute to the possibility that, due to a fear of being maligned or unfairly judged, such a home life will occur.

We truly can be the co-creators of what we choose to see. Whether it is stupidity, possibility, or abuse. I suggest leading folks not to panic but to peace because it is when we are at peace that we communicate. And when it comes to prevention of abuse, communication is key. In general, fighting leads to reactivity, which leads to fighting.

Like when my little friend's grandmother wagged her finger, furrowed her brow, and called Andy the breast squeezer a "dirty boy." True, she did so out of love and a desire to teach, but my cute little breast-squeezer client simply adored the drama of her response. It helped his brain to step out of its usual fog and focus. What fun! He reached out and gave her a really good two-fisted nipple pinch. The house came alive with action. Woo Hoo! He was thrilled by the dance. It was an awareness of his brain state and the fun such a response would bring that led me to choose the approach to drop your energy, become a barrier and explain, explain, explain. Had I seen him as a dirty boy, I probably would have felt the need to punish and upped the anti of his sensory delight. Such a response may well have taken this story down the path that leads to restraints and drugs for control. Instead, we chose to be more exciting when he didn't squeeze and his life moved along to games of Jenga and Gymnastics.

As you can see, though, there's no way to create the perfect environment—the environment really does matter. Recall that when a child has a foggy brain, excitement wakes it up, so this sort of child sees the world through snippets of clarity that they then string together to create a vision of their life. Think of it as a child in a dark room waiting for someone to flick on the lights so that he can glean a bit about his world. And then imagine that the lights are turned on by the big exciting moments. So all he ever sees is either intense anger or intense fun. Thus these children hold only the moments of exploding voices and action-packed adventures in the movie of their memories while the low-energy, regular-guy dad is never even heard. Be aware, though, that the over-anxious child does all this in reverse.

I learned the exciting-lights-on concept from observing my son. I remember realizing that Rye watched movies with an eye for excitement and that he only enjoyed the bigger broader bolder strokes of violence contained within even a commercial. These visions made him take notice. He was vacant during the plot driven, relationship and character-building in-betweens. Once I noticed this I watched him for a while and realized Rye also saw this way within his day to day.

It seemed that Rye only attended to his siblings when his brothers were freaking out and threatening to kill him. I noticed that whenever he was having trouble focusing enough to read, he'd do something to create this behavior in them. It seemed probable that he was using them to "wake himself up." He loved it when they would swear and chase and lose their tempers. He compiled a whole world of memories related to these indiscretions. Poor Cash was the older brother, so I insisted he handle Rye's behavior without too much of a reaction. This took the fun out of it for Rye so he tried to up the anti by putting his boogers all over the inside of Cash's pride and joy: his truck. No wonder Cash bought a travel trailer and moved away from home. (wink)

Well, whatever works, at least he is independent. Like I said, learning to lead your child to success is all about finding the right motivator. (wink wink)

And yes, most children are button pushers, especially in relationships with their siblings. However, though the desire to get a reaction is the same, with focus-challenged children the need is more extreme than just to annoy. With focus-challenged children, getting a reaction is like a form of self-medicating that they use to stimulate their brain. They are merely trying to help themselves by getting you to turn the lights on. But this behavior is also why their teachers often beg for Ritalin, instead of riddling. You can help your child focus by being a reactor. Just make sure to do it with intention and use behaviors you want him to copy. If your child is like this you don't need to shout to be heard; you can do comedy. A pratfall and a tickle that bring forth joy and laughter are equally as much of a brain wake-up, and have preferable long-term effects, to fist fights and explosions from which he strings together a picture that creates his world.

I tell the ADHD kids that I work with not to drink the poison and use me as the antidote because it locks us into a cycle and keeps us from making greater gains. I explain that I can use neurofeedback to help them understand and focus better, but that if they then choose to focus on the angry bits and pieces of life, what we are doing is making them better at seeing the violence. Whenever this is the case I spend a lot of time "antidoting those poisonous choices" and teaching them how to comprehend what they see. This is my role until they begin to choose differently on their own. This is true of autism as well. For families that lean on the neurofeedback to create the changes without restructuring anything in the environment, sometimes what they get is a child who is better equipped to manipulate but not necessarily in a user-friendly way.

THE ANTIDOTE: After twenty sessions twelve-year-old previously exclusive Dina began to look in everyone's eyes and consistently answer questions. She was also happy, though nervous, outside of the home.

THE POISON: called symptom management. Mom was a trained psychologist. She had a history of working in institutional settings with the behaviorally disturbed. She was thrilled at her daughter's response to therapy and satisfied by the changes achieved thus far. Due to her training she had a firm understanding of the challenges common to autism. As a means of diminishing the possible reactions these issues could bring about, she prevented people from taking her daughter into new environments. She made predictable the daily schedule and fired anyone who unexpectedly moved the schedule around. Dina's mom fought with her household staff. She was trying to ensure her child's comfort by explaining angrily that Dina was autistic and these things were too hard for her. Mom described the limitations in detail and she did so in front of her daughter. Dina soon began to scream whenever there were changes and new environmental stimuli.

I try to open up the possibilities by explaining that Dina was gaining greater cognition receptively and that if the people in her world continued to tell her what she couldn't do she would believe them. Thus, she could grow worse instead of better at handling the unpredictability of the world around her, simply BECAUSE she was getting better at learning how to become what was expected of her.

THE MIRACLE: After many, many attempts to believe in what was possible the family and caregivers changed enough to keep up with Dina's changes. Dina stopped screaming, looked in people's eyes, and made new "unpredictable" friends in new "unpredictable" environments. Dina is still autistic.

So I teach everyone how to make these changes until everyone can make them on their own. The fact is, as your child changes so must you. If your goal as a parent is to lead your son or daughter to independence, then you must always be just ahead of him or her. It is important to grow adept at following changes while leading the way to the new changes you will then follow. Remember to keep your eye on the goal of helping him/her live in a more socially comfortable and communicative place. I see this as much more important than math or science skills, though an interest in either could lead you to follow her to a place wherein you help her to embrace other science or math-minded friends.

Healthy social skills and ease of communication are your child's greatest challenge. Teach this through what is already there and the rest will follow.

There is no perfect environment for autistic kids; each one needs something different. I have suggested some kids leave school and others leave home. I've suggested the same child come out of school, then go in, and then come out again. We've designed segregated programs and inclusive programs, and always the ones that worked best were the ones where the choices were made as a result of understanding the style of the child in question at that particular time in their development. And always the ones that were the least effective were the ones where the choices came from the idea that the preexisting programs endorsed by the professional community know more about autism than parents do and vice versa. In my experience the only way to really make a difference is to do it as a team and get the autistic person's entire world to reflect acceptance back to them giving the experience of acceptance back to the people reflecting it.

One of my favorite examples of thinking outside the box and creating just such an environment comes from my own children's story. I had spent most of their growing up years wishing I could find a way to create congruency in their world and have everyone treat my children in a similar fashion. It was a frustrating undoable desire until the day I decided to take over and remove everyone from school. I had spent eleven years avoiding the job of teacher. I wasn't avoiding it anymore. My sons were in grades six, eight, nine, and ten. None of them could read, one couldn't talk, one couldn't talk sense, one couldn't talk with fluency, and the other couldn't stop stuttering and swearing. Two of my boys couldn't take care of themselves, nobody had math skills, language skills, friends, or an ability to control their tempers; and the way I saw it school hadn't led them anywhere but to special ed, detention centers, and court for foul-mouthed fighting and vandalism.

I needed a better plan.

I started with the concept of environment. I wanted my children to live in a world where everyone was happy and accepting. I was a single mom with very little money so there was no way to hire help, which meant if I was teaching one child the others would be out in the world getting feedback. I convinced my then twenty-two year old daughter to help me and came up with a plan. I would sell everything and buy an RV. Nine of us would travel from resort to resort. We would camp next to folks who were happy in their holiday homes and I would take turns teaching the kids. My daughter would oversee the basic running of the campground group games; and whenever my unusual children wore out the accepting smiles of the other vacationers, we would pull up stakes and set out for another resort full of fresh happy faces. Initially we seldom stayed longer than a day, but slowly the kids began to see the world as a happy accepting place and our trips began to stretch out and last, sometimes as long as a week or two. In less than a year I had four readers, three clear talkers, and three friend makers. My oldest, most challenged son merely learned to swim (also great considering the number of times I'd had to save his life). With each smiling face and each new friend (in a resort the number of friend choices is limited so my sons were constantly accepted as the best company available), my boys learned social skills and games like basketball, pool, shuffleboard, and mini putt. I watched my guys grow their self-esteem as every night we discussed how to improve on the opportunities the day had brought.

This was the first time ever that all of my spectrum children gained ground at a steady rate.

A small word of warning here: trying to follow your child's behavior and come up with ideas alone isn't enough because you are limited. You are only going to be able to come up with ideas out of the things you already know. Thus you must know more. You must be open to and actively seeking new information. I can't say this enough. Learn about the brain, the body, and the experiences of others. An autistic brain doesn't make sense of the mess in the same way a typical one does, so we can't use understanding of self in order to understand our child. Often an autistic mind shrinks from the cacophony of activity life presents and finds a way to focus on the singular in order to turn down the volume of family dynamics and societal noise. The concept of how to be noticed when your child is engaged in turning down your volume reminds me of the plot-driven Stephen King books I used to read. Each time I read one, the ride alone had me awake and ready to learn almost anything. Then he would plant a nugget, a singular bit of worldly advice, and I would hear it loud and clear. Since he had me on the edge of my seat, and since he only planted one or two nuggets of insight per book, it seemed I learned whatever he taught. Whereas when I read David Foster Wallace, I was asked to learn beyond my ability to focus. He was more than I could assimilate and I would lose touch with what I'd gained. Sadly, the David Foster Wallace approach was too overwhelming, even for him (he committed suicide).

So don't overwhelm. Teach your child one lesson at a time. Make yourself into the bright shiny object of delight that he can't help but see. Be like the Christmas tree impossible to ignore. But be only the tree, not the whole holiday.

Sometimes it is tempting to be the noisy crashing monster of demands. Many parents over the years have noticed that anger works to make their kids attend, at least in the short term. And since many of us are too tired to care or have no understanding of how to envision the - effects of our behavior, we can be fooled into thinking these techniques are the right ones. This is even more common to believe when dealing with autism. There are brain dysfunction reasons for this. Remember that autistic kids—like Dar on the run-way-no-car day— have been known to blurt out words or perform skills they couldn't otherwise say or do when placed in a state of emergency. And recall that this is possibly because fear focuses attention, and adrenalin slows down time enough to make putting the pieces together possible. Whatever the reason, observations like this have led many to be cruel in an attempt to be kind.

Several therapies have grown from this thinking. Some exist today. For example, I know of one that keeps the child in an emergency state by having him balance on a large ball while learning new skills. Using fear to increase focus works only in the moment and as such is a flawed approach. The flaw rests not only in the fact that such an idea loses the concept of quality of life, but also because the brain's reactivity to fear adjusts itself. Neuroreceptors shrink back and stop sending signals until we are desensitized to the stimuli that are no longer new. Thus to maintain the advantage that fear creates, teachers would have to up the anti and instill an even more threatening state of emergency. This is obviously a slippery slope headed straight for abuse and totally un-fun to enforce.

In addition, teaching a skill while scaring someone simply engages the amygdala to do the filing, and the amygdala is designed to file in a unique way. Its intention is to warn you when you are in danger, so it may file the ball and the outfit that the instructor is wearing and the smell of the room into memory and leave out the lesson altogether. It may also connect the lesson with fear and lead to a Post Traumatic Stress Disordered fear of learning and an inability to generalize anything but the fear itself. The amygdala fires and files with broad stokes that leave out most of the details to an event, so this approach could also theoretically teach the "big picture" concept of the lesson without an accompanying ability to remember the details. And finally, fear releases adrenalin, which is followed by a release of cortisol (stress hormone), and an overabundance of cortisol kills cells in the hippocampus, which causes memory damage.

Oh what a tangled web we weave, when first we practice to be mean.

So in conclusion: Don't drink the poison means, "Keep your eye on the life lesson!"

CHAPTER NINE

The Thing that Makes this Book Special Is

I Finally Figured Out What Helped My Children Change

light therapy, quantum feedback, exorcism, chelation, long-distance healers, b12 shots, carnosine, GFCF, hyperbaric, reiki, homeopathy, bio-meds, massage, cranial sacral, dolphins, horses, kefir, algae, probiotics, secretin, proteins, hormones, speech therapy, glutamate, occupational therapy, rebirthing, stem cells, Handel, desensitization, brushing, sensory integration, body ecology, isolation, ozone, prayer, and wishing wells

I did only some of these.

At every turn what I did, and still do, with or without neurofeedback depends upon the moment; it depends upon the child; it depends upon the family, the culture, the diet; it depends upon so many things that I can't actually write a book that answers this question. And yet now that I am deep into the writing of this book, it's a question even I would like to know the answer to. After all, I've already lived it. I should be able to look back and find a core reason, one singular thing that I can point to and teach everyone. What was it that I did so differently from all the parents whose children grew more autistic while mine grew less so even without neurofeedback?

Two of my children were violent and one even came with a "this kid is mean" warning label when I adopted him. (In fact, I suppose the social workers were right about this, since at five years old he beat and locked his crippled teacher in a closet. My other son just killed animals.) And yet, inch-by-inch, my dangerous children grew calmer and more loving (though admittedly neurofeedback sped up that process) while so many other people's children grew more violent. (This is not a small issue. Autistic children left unchecked have grown into adults responsible for their parent's death. I personally know of one woman who pulled her mother's eye out.) It seems to me that there must be some one thing that is uniquely different in my approach.

In search of the answer I've gotten together data and info and done hundreds of Internet and library searches. I've looked back over the details in my specialized approach to training and teaching and found bits and pieces and gems of obscure knowledge that should help me ascertain, why. So why? Why did five of the six family members I worked with (three sons and two grandsons) evolve out of their autism? Why? What is the one single most different thing about what we did compared to all the other homes I go into? What made our home with my adopted children and biological grandchildren so unique? And how did that uniqueness help them enough to lead them into becoming functional in the world?

It's a valid question. Especially since I chose a path so different from the advice of all the mental health professionals of the time. How did my sons become happy, living lives as hard-working, totally independent, tax-paying citizens solving problems on their own? I know it wasn't just the neurofeedback because for two of my sons neurofeedback came so late in the game of their healing and it wasn't even required for one of my grandkids. So though neurofeedback made things easily more attainable it wasn't really my secret. So how did it happen that so many differing types of autistic children grew healthy in my home without bio medical intervention or naturopaths or pharmaceuticals doing anything but getting in the way? I think I found the answer, the one single uniquely different thing that made us special. I think I've identified our group idiosyncrasy. It was the perfect partner to the benefits of the neurofeedback, that we didn't even use yet: The one common denominator that helped to get everyone (but Dar) most, or all of the way, off the spectrum. It was that:

I let them learn, while walking the line, oftentimes alone.

I know that sounds simplistic, and it is kind of, so let me explain. When my children were climbing I let them risk falling. When they were missing social cues I let them risk annoying the neighbors. When they were experimenting with food items I let them use their hands. Remember beautiful Mary, the naked centerpiece eating garlic and drinking anchovy oil? In this way I was much like her parents. I allowed. Sure, I insisted my kids make an honest attempt to do it "properly." but I also let them explore, and do, and fail, all in an independent fashion. Now when I go into homes and schools I see a variety of approaches. One is the over-therapied doer: from the moment the child wakes up to the moment his head hits the pillow there is a constant stream of therapies going on. The difficulty here is your brain doesn't learn to problem solve that way. If you don't have an opportunity to try to spontaneously use the skills you've been taught, and then learn from the success or failure of that attempt, then you don't actually gain the skill of generalization or independent performance because you don't have a chance to learn that you've learned it. The best approach is to be taught something, then go out and try it, be taught and go out and try, be taught and go out and try, until you make it your own.

Autism is a disorder that has trouble moving between theories and real life. Thus it is a disorder that learns better in an experiential design. Autistic people learn through doing. (Don't be fooled into believing that guiding her hand by placing your hand over hers is the same as doing it herself or that pretending to be in a store paying for candy is the same as being in a store paying for candy.) If an autistic individual has somebody constantly prompting and pushing and pulling and saying, "This is what you have to do next," then there is no opportunity for that person to learn what they themselves want or like. True, if that person is never given the opportunity to choose on their own how to behave in a given situation, then they can't fail. But they also can't succeed.

I have a family I work with that at present is afraid to let their son out of the house, even with a guardian, because he is stronger than them and can pull away from their hands. I understand the dilemma, but if he never goes out he will never learn to choose to be safe in the world. This is a solvable problem, but more important than the solution is the belief that every problem can be solved.

Another thing that happens in many of the homes or schools I go into is they do let the child choose. They let them choose everything. They don't want to mess with the autism or they are afraid of it or they are afraid of the temper tantrums or they are afraid of self-injurious behavior ("they" being the parents and the therapist and everyone surrounding the child), so they just allow the child to do whatever repetitious behavior the child chooses to do. This is different from what I did. I gave my children the freedom to explore and to learn and to try, but I still insisted that they try to do it in a relatively (relative to them in that moment) "normal" fashion. I always asked them to step up and try harder. Because—in my belief—my children weren't backward as a result of not wanting to learn or not wanting to be part of my world (as some were saying), but as a result of being different. And being different seemed to lead them to discomfort. So I taught them to be the same, only different. Since my children didn't learn how to do things by copying, simply modeling what was and wasn't typically didn't work. I had to teach them every step. That takes longer. So of course they were behind. But I figured that since we learn a lot of unnecessary stuff that we end up forgetting, if I just left all that out my kids could catch up because as long as they were using what I did teach they could remember it all.

I realized that if I wanted to teach them every step required for success, I would have to figure out what those steps were. I thought about it and decided that the steps I wanted to teach were the steps into our way of doing things: our way of being a society. So that meant that I would have to learn what our way was. Learning to analyze behavior in order to teach to it is the greatest benefit of having a cognitively challenged child. At least it is for me, every time I chose to learn, and then to teach. So I would choose to do things like let them ride a bike to the park on their own even when they still appeared uncertain of where the park was. I would then hide in the bushes and watch while they rode there. I was available to help them but only if and when they needed it. The biggest challenge here was to know when not to interfere. I stayed quiet and observed them as they learned to deal with people, even when they were yelled at for not looking where they were going, that is unless the yelling looked rewarding, or the not looking risked more than a scraped knee.

Sound easy? It's not. Not even remotely. But I think it is the difference.

We let our neuro-typical kids climb trees and risk breaking their arms because at some point we cease to look. We choose to trust and let them learn naturally. This transition requires a certain kind of believing in the child. Such a transition is necessary, even more so when your child is autistic. "Normal" kids can take a poll and ask their friends if Mom is being overprotective. Autistic kids get their beliefs about themselves solely from their disordered perceptions, and us, the adults in their world. So she needs us to see, in order to see, a normal child within. And it's our seeing a typical child just trying to figure things out that leads us to talk to her as if she is normal. And it's the "as if she is" that teaches her "to be." And it's seeing your child in this way that makes it seem right to explain conceptual things to him like the why of your choices as a parent. While it's knowing he learns slower, that makes it OK to explain and explain and explain again.

So you allow them to be their version of normal while you explain what normal is. Somewhere in between the explaining and allowing and explaining and allowing and explaining and allowing I believe is the magic that was different in my home. I have many times been recorded as saying that I have "tried it all" in respect to the therapies that have come and gone over the years for defeating autism. The truth is I just felt like I tried it all, because actually I have been in homes that have tried only half of all and that was way more than I even considered trying. So really at the end of the day it wasn't the therapies; it was the believing. I just believed, always, that they were children and that of course they would learn. I knew they were different, but that just meant to me I had to figure out how to help them learn, in their own way. It never occurred to me that they couldn't learn at all.

Of course I wasn't the only one in their environment.

Very often my attempts were thwarted by the well-meaning attitudes of others. I tried repeatedly to convince people (remember it was still a time when autism was blamed on cold-hearted parenting) that when Dar hugged with his face while holding his chest away it didn't mean he'd stopped rejecting us and was growing less autistic but that he was putting his face up close to avoid eye contact. I tried to explain that for him far away and too close up made him equally as invisible. I tried to explain that his autism wasn't about rejection but discomfort. I taught people to move him to a forearm distance away, look in his eyes, and sparkle theirs. This for Dar was real contact. And voila... we grew a therapy... which I now teach... all based on observing Dar's behavior. It was challenging because people believed autistic kids didn't like to get close up and personal (a total fallacy by the way). They wanted to be the one Dar chose to hug because it made them feel important in some way (despite the fact that Dar hugged anyone he couldn't get away from). The helpers who wanted to help mostly because they wanted to be seen as helping seemed to care more about being perceived as Dar's special person than about teaching him to see... the love in someone's eyes...when they looked at him...seeing love so he could then learn to see himself as lovable.

The other people, the ones that didn't want to hug him, seemed to see the face hugging (his head to their chest) as problematic and chose to teach Dar about "staying out of someone's personal bubble" instead of being thrilled he was reaching for contact and then using this motivator to shape the interaction enough to include their eyes. Still other teachers encouraged him to do his autistic behaviors so they could read a book while he rocked on the floor and looked at his fingers; "after all" they seemed to think, "he was never gonna learn anything anyway." The ones that believed he was capable of more learning than they had observed him do chastised, hit, and berated him. It was a difficult time with no consistency of approach. And still the majority of my kids managed to learn enough to maneuver the world, and engage in neighborhood play, fairly unsupervised.

Though I had all the same types of problems with the other boys, Dar's autism and early life deprivation were more extreme. Besides, I got him first, so he became my study tool. Dar was like a magnified version of autism, and because of this I was able to see what was underneath some of my other children's behaviors. One of the most obvious was that they all had a case of extreme performance anxiety whenever they were attempting to do anything someone else requested of them. Nowadays when an autistic person freezes in place while going blank in the middle of an activity, it is referred to as apraxia: that black hole of nothingness I explained to you earlier. At the time, when I watched my son it looked like fear and reminded me of how I would go blank whenever anyone was watching me try to learn something new. Since Dar only froze into fear when something was being requested of him, I saw his behavior more as performance anxiety than apraxia because apraxia happens with or without a request. This fear-based interpretation is why I chose to use fear eradicating "atta boys" and compliments more than prompts and verbal cues whenever my sons found themselves unable to move. With me they were cheered on and convinced of their ability, and with me they were quicker to perform new tasks and they performed them with greater ease. At school I was told to help them break out of this frozen state by touching their hand or using verbal prompts; these ideas were also useful, but when done without the cheers and hurrahs my kids seldom generalized the skill being taught and seemed stuck to the cue in order to act.

[For those who are revisiting the concept of trying to instill fear to get their child to behave or maybe even to stumble across that hoped-for word that fear has been known to pop out of autistic children's mouths, remember intimidation doesn't really work; it is simply an illusion. Because being statued with fear or enabled by emergency-state-driven adrenalin only enables the child when something other than the person doing the observing or requesting is the object of the fear. This is a concept well known to TV audiences of police programs everywhere. Whenever the officers want to make someone talk, the bad cop whips up the fear, but it's the good cop that gets the confession. This technique is called double-teaming. Getting confessions doesn't work as well head to head because people get locked into resistance. So don't go head to head. In fact don't even use the technique at all. The level of resistance to force or a loss of control is extreme in autism. And in autism, even double-teaming won't work because for the autistic individual to drop the frozen-into-a-statue state that was instilled by the "bad cop fear monger" takes time, lots and lots of time, as the chemistry in this challenged brain slowly tries to shift states back to a more comfortable place. So please don't scare the children, especially if they have autism. (Unless of course it's the only way to stop them from jumping out in front of a car. The truth be told, absolutely every rule has its moments of exception.)]

I learned all this from studying the techniques of others and from studying Dar. At first Dar ran from the room whenever you cheered him. Initially I thought this meant I had frightened him and should stop cheering. It was the very first behavior of Dar's that I ever tried to follow. At that point I was simply following the obvious with no accompanying long-term concept because I hadn't yet learned how to follow with intent and shape behavior. That most important component of following—know your goals, both long term and short—came shortly after I realized that by stopping the cheering I was taking the cheer out of both our lives. Once I figured that out, and since I wanted to help him be comfortable with and learn to enjoy approval, I reintroduced the cheer. I patted his back and used varying styles of compliments. I added explanations and energy fluctuations based on his reactions. And I loved and loved and loved and loved all the while hoping he could somehow tell how proud of him as I was.

Along the way I learned some tips and tricks. The main one being: Do what makes sense even if it means going against the grain.

I noticed that my children needed sameness so I became the sameness. I stayed consistent in my answers and approach but changed their room and their schedules constantly. I did this to keep them flexible enough to handle change and rooted enough to feel grounded. When they needed to rock their bodies I rocked their bodies for them because I wanted to help them see me as the means for soothing and gain a connectedness that wasn't coming easily. I played dumb when they gestured and moved quickly when they used words.

And then, when there were too many of them making noises for me to stay calm, I asked them all to sit against the wall (because mommy needed it, not because they were bad) and had a coffee.

Parents often ask me how did you pick what to teach when? I went by what I wanted most. Because not only did I follow my kids; I followed me. For example, I prefer flushing toilets to changing diapers. So I decided to potty train each of the kids at an early age. I figured it would benefit the boys as they learned to become aware of their bodies and follow a series of steps to achieve their goal. I also figured I would like parenting them better. We pretty much just moved into the bathroom until the skill was gained. Usually this was only a four-day sojourn. Even Dar learned within this time frame. Though after the alleged incident with his teaching assistant he began to withhold his bowel movements and became so constipated that his sphincter muscle was damaged. Then because of poor fine motor skills it was difficult for him to wipe his anus vigorously enough to compensate for his bodies inability to pinch off the stool. So in Dar's case I had to train him twice. Fortunately, neurofeedback seems to be helping his fine motor skills improve and the problem has moved mostly into the past. At present he is using his hands well enough to keep himself and the toilet mostly clean. I'm sure this must be a relief for him. I know it is for me.

Learning to hyper-focus on the lessons I wanted to teach—as in the four-day potty training bathroom campouts—was usually rewarded. But learning to factor myself, and my wishes into the "What to teach next?" question was the best learning of all. I knew it was me that would have to keep the kids going. Unless they are very, very, rich, it is always the parents who will be doing the work twenty-four hours a day, day after day, ad infinitum.

Perhaps it was because I had too many kids to actually do all the work that I established the style of allowing my children to experience and assimilate their learnings by giving them freedom. Of course this wasn't always met with great appreciation by my neighbors, who bit their lips anxiously while watching their property values drop due to the messy appearance of my kids in the eyes of the house-shopping passersby. As well, I must admit, very often the neighbors were more than just a little annoyed by my "outside the box" style. For example, one of my sons had a real strong desire to pound and twist and break things, especially if they were made of metal. So one summer I rigged up a surprise. I attached a vice grip to a foundation that I buried in my yard. I then vice gripped an upside down two-wheel bicycle into it. I said, "You can break this bike." Then I put rules to the task. "But you can't use any real tools or get any help. You have to just break it yourself using sticks and your hands." Every morning that summer I woke up to the happy sound of him Bang Bang Banging on that bike. I knew where he was and I knew what he was up to. AHHH!!! My version of Peace and Quiet!

What a wonderful summer, void of anyone yelling, "Mom, Rye broke th---." Too bad it was replaced by the sound of the neighbors shouting, "Can't you make him stop that &**%$ Banging?" Fortunately I didn't really expect the neighbors to like us, so despite the gossip and angry voices they often levied upon my kids I was happy because I was busy with the job of peacefully love-teaching my children. After all, Rye learned a lot about how bikes are constructed and we got a break from all that household breakage for the summer. It did, however, look weird to anyone walking by, and most of the people on our street would have preferred a rooster to Rye's alarm clock banging. So they started up a petition that asked us to move. We didn't. At least not right away.

So my unusual problem-solving choices continued to irritate the people around me even as they consolidated the skills within my home. Another example of this type of environmental challenge happened when, since all four of my children had different levels of life skills, there was a big argument between the principal and me about whether or not the kids could be bussed to school. He thought two of my boys could handle walking while two could not. I felt that this was a set-up for sibling cruelty and wanted either all four bussed or all four walking. And of course this was an enormous argument which, being the mom, I insisted on winning. So I refused the bus and taught them all to walk to school. I got an idea when I saw a bunch of kids at the day care all hanging onto a rope and I thought, "Wow, that'll work." So I went out and got this fancy rope and told the kids they all had to hang on to it as they walked to school. That way the more gifted ones could lead the more challenged ones.

It looked quite appropriate for about a day, but then we lost the fancy rope and Rye started asking me to tie him to his brother so he wouldn't have to hang on. We started finding sundry items like scarves and skipping ropes and things that didn't look nearly as official. It's amazing what a difference such a minor detail can make. Once again we were drawing a lot of attention from the neighbors. We were almost celebrities as Dar also found holding on too tiring for his muscles to maintain so he got tied too. I ended up with two brothers holding the rope and two tied to the ones holding the rope. Strangely enough, even though the teachers were also tying and untying at the other end of the walk, it was always only me that the fingers were pointed at. Oh well, my kids learned to walk to school. Then we moved.

They learned because I let them learn despite the opinions around me. Mine weren't the choices that most people would make. But then most people don't have the good fortune to have to, because most people don't have four autistic kids. However, that is quickly changing. Perhaps that (the growth in the numbers of children diagnosed with autism) is a good thing, upping the emergency status and forcing us to figure out how to help ourselves, and our families, instead of how to blame our neighbors for our discomfort. And if we do look to our neighbors, hopefully it's because we are generous enough to share our blessing and let them help. They just might have some good tips to offer, especially since it is becoming more and more likely that they will have some autism in their family too. For example, here's a tip from the mom in me: Autistic children learn better (in a way that solidifies and becomes more typical) in their biggest areas of challenge (language and social skills) from actual experience than they do from lessons. When experiencing the wholeness of an event—to the best of their perceptual ability—they are often able to grow the ability and then repackage it in order that it might be used appropriately in various environments. This is what it means to generalize a skill.

I knew this about my autistic children because I knew it about eccentric me. Thus, as I said, I let my children learn through experience. This is what made us special … I gave them room and let them "do" life in a very real way. Since they had to deal with the world and all its reactions to their unusualness, and since our people-populated world is unpredictable, they never knew what was about to happen next. This is a good thing. Despite the fact that many professionals say autistic children need sameness, in my experience, a few built-in surprises keeps them on their toes [(wink) pardon the inside joke, I just couldn't resist]. It's getting the right balance of freedom and support that is the trick. Too much unpredictability and kids shut down their sensory system so as to totally block us out and gain control over the situation, thereby experiencing nothing we have to offer. Too much sameness and they block us out because there is nothing new to notice and all people return to their own interests when under-stimulated by their surroundings. In the case of autism that usually means hyper-focused repetitive play. So my son roller-bladed everywhere, even though it didn't look as if he looked where he was going. It was his hyper-focused love of roller-blading that led him out the door. It was while he was out the door that he had the opportunity to learn. We were definitely different because in those days no one let their special children out.

Of course I dealt with the neighbors a lot. But that's OK because it ended up worth it. Though I don't think it was my crazy out-of-the-box choices on how to problem solve the reactions of other adults so that my kids could parade the neighborhood, so much as the fact that I was willing to trust my own ideas, that helped my children improve.

I know I have already written bits and pieces of this story, but for the sake of chronology I am going to repeat myself, again.

Eventually I got to the point where six of my kids had grown and gone and I only had two who were still living in my lap. Both of these children were still really struggling to handle the world at large. The other two autistic boys had learned and changed and come off the spectrum. However, even though they were independent, they were not really comfortable in their own skins. They experienced bouts of depression, had sleep disturbances, slow thinking... stuff like that.

And so even though they were considered "off the spectrum," there was still lots of room for improvement all the way around. That's when I found neurofeedback.

Neurofeedback has been the most amazing therapy I've ever done with any of my children or myself or my family members or the world at large. I say this because at no time have I come across a person that does not respond to this treatment and is not made remarkably better in their ability to handle their emotions, settle their sensory system, steer their body, and cognitively improve their understanding of how the world works.

Anyway, I started using it on my children and within two years number three was off the spectrum. As you know, Dar, who is still extremely disabled, was so badly damaged before I adopted him that I'm still not sure how far he can get, though I am open to seeing him get far. Dar has serious issues beyond just autism; part of his skull never formed and some of his brain matter hardly shows any brain-wave activity. He also has nerve damage in the brain stem. This makes controlling his tongue extremely difficult. I guess we'll just have to wait and see, but I do know that since by age twenty-three he couldn't talk, whereas with the addition of neurofeedback by twenty-seven he could, anything is possible. Quite frankly, hard to understand or not, I would call that a miracle!

Another part of what really worked for my family was that since we were such a large group, I had to be very organized. I had to insist upon things and run the house with a kind of strictness. To compensate for that orderliness, I gave them a lot of freedom, a lot of room to try things, kept things flexible, and covered them with compliments. This was doable because I was also very clear on what the rules were, and what they were about. I made sure everyone knew how they had to behave in the house and what they had to do for chores. An example of how I created the choices for their behaviors can be found in the fact that, since a lot of autistic children have eating disorders, and mine were no exception, I analyzed the reason. Three of my children vomited religiously, but two of the three were doing it because they wanted to. One of my sons liked to throw up because—before I adopted him—he got out of eating that way—and for him eating was an uncomfortable thing to do. The other son just liked the steamy warm sensory sensation of it. Often when he was just hanging around doing nothing, he would do this thing in his throat that would initiate a spasm and he'd throw up ever so gently. Whereas my other son who couldn't help the situation would projectile vomit, the two who did it on purpose just kind of oozed warm gelatinous liquid out of their mouths and all over their front. It was quite horrid to watch, actually, but they seemed to enjoy it.

Maybe it was the sensory the warmth or the wet pungent smell that tickled their senses. At any rate, it didn't tickle mine. I just wouldn't have it—because obviously the food needed to stay in them; also there were just too many kids for me to cater to two people's inability to choose to keep their food down. So I just said, "Well you can do that if you like, but if you do that onto your plate I'm just gonna wash the vomit off and hand it back to you"—and then did—once each! They very quickly decided that this wasn't the response they were after.

Important to note here is that I wasn't upset, I wasn't angry, I wasn't saying things like "Shame on you." I reacted without judgment, anger, or energy. I simply washed it off and handed it back. I think some of that is why my children simply reacted to my reaction with a shrug and a change in behavior. It's as if they were given a chance to discover that "Oh, I guess I don't get to have a food issue." Not judging the behaviors you ask people to change is not a little point. The difference—is the difference. Had his vomiting upset me or seemed "bad" in any way, my approach would have simply been cruel and may even have reinforced the behavior as their resistance to my resistance grew.

As always, what works for one doesn't necessarily work for another. This third child, Dar, had a problem with his digestive system and actually had outbursts—seemingly unrelated to his diet or emotional state—of spontaneous oral ejaculations. He'd just be walking along with his usual hippity hop bopity bop dippity dop gait. He would suddenly and without warning projectile vomit, then continue on his way without missing a single dip or dop. His situation wasn't the same as the other two—this behavior wasn't intentionally done—at least it didn't appear to be—so it was more confusing for me. He had a lot of food issues and would often leave his food in his cheeks for the whole day. And though he looked like a cute little chipmunk saving for winter, I decided it was important to teach him to swallow.

At first I tried to understand the problem by using a psychological profile. I thought, "Poor thing, he was starved and seriously malnourished before he was adopted; maybe he is literally being a chipmunk and saving his food for later." But then when I watched him I discovered he was having a lot of difficulty chewing, which made anything other than liquid a challenge. It followed that he couldn't swallow many things while the look, smell, and/or texture of certain foods bothered him. At the time I had no knowledge that it was his brain stem tongue nerve lesion complicating the issue, but I did know he had to eat. So I began to manually teach him how to chew and to swallow. I would help him to move his jaw appropriately and to reposition the food with his tongue. I gathered all kinds of foods and introduced one after another in order to desensitize him to certain textures. And though mastering all this took over a year—one step at a time for Dar was really one step at a time—it still never occurred to me to say, "Oh, he has trouble with certain kinds of foods so he doesn't have to eat them. Let' s just give him mush."

The lesson here is that most children can learn to overcome even some of their biggest challenges. However, blindly choosing their biggest challenge isn't always a choice made with the child's best interest in mind. In my defense, I had not yet learned to follow. And as a result I fed him the same food as everyone else in the family, food that wasn't actually good for him because he had a leaky gut. Thus, as a means of self-protection his body was evicting a lot of what he was eating because it was stunting the growth in his brain and making it harder for him to learn. I share this to demonstrate that, yes, you can learn from my life; and sometimes what you'll learn is that mine was not necessarily the right approach. It is, however, the approach I took. I just taught him to chew and said, "There's no option here; everybody eats this for breakfast; everybody eats this for lunch; and if you don't eat what you're given, you wait until the next meal." When you have eight kids, those are the kinds of rules you make. And so my kids learned to chew and swallow and keep down a whole variety of grocery choices. They ate because I said so. And for three of my boys that proved to be a good thing. For one, it would have been better had I let his body take the lead.

Slowly I learned to be a better observer, and eventually I realized that my projectile vomiter was having digestive difficulties whenever he ate something with dairy in it. Not only did I learn to be a better observer but I also learned not to do the Semmelweis reflex dance and deny my complicity in the creation of his undernourished body because of my own guilt. And since I was growing more and more willing to see my mistakes in order to help my children, my mistakes began to serve us. For example, since Dar didn't really have any choice in the chewing and the swallowing of what he would and wouldn't eat, I was able to stand back and see where the patterns lay. And since I wasn't doing guilt once I saw the pattern, I had the energy to take action on finding a solution. I researched non-dairy diets and we became macrobiotic. His vomiting stopped. Interestingly enough, even though our new diet helped him improve, schools at that time saw milk as a fundamental need for children and believed me to be making a negligent choice with regard to his nutritional needs. Milk was still a religion and it was virtually sacrilegious to suggest any harm could come from drinking it. So they gave him milk even though I asked them not to and the vomiting resumed. Not one of the people I spoke with in the school's employ would listen to my observations or honor my requests about this without a doctor's note. Unfortunately the doctors I spoke with at the time agreed with the teachers rather than with me. In fact, even the neurologists I talked with just (figuratively) patted my hand and told me I was grasping at straws. Nobody was even willing to give my son an MRI, let alone test for allergies, because no one wanted to believe that milk, the perfect food, could be affecting my son's cognition. Besides he was autistic and "Who cares?" seemed to be the prevailing attitude.

I never did win this long and upsetting battle with the authorities on autism. It wasn't until Dar was sixteen and I took him out of school that I was able to permanently stop the vomiting—at which point I watched him grow—as big as a house.

I think some of the reason I never won that battle until I removed him from school was because my biggest dilemma raising special-needs kids was the question of "Who to believe?" I kept getting lost in the confusion of uncertain thinking: "Wow, all these teachers, all these therapists, all these people—they all believe very strongly in what they are doing and they all want very much to help my child. They all think they know more than me and they all disagree with me. Maybe they're right, but they also all disagree with each other. How am I supposed to make my way through this? And who the hell should I listen to?" I figured I wasn't supposed to listen to me but the problem was, I was the only one I could ever really hear. My search for the all-knowing professional was to be forever unrequited because none of them thought my children could be healed. And in my mind that meant they didn't know.

This belief in my children was the fundamental difference between me and the people teaching them; it was a fundamental difference that was never rectified. Every once in a while I would try to take on the popular beliefs and approaches of the time, but because we weren't coming from the same intention we were satisfied by different events. Their teachers tried to give them coping techniques and a handful of skills. I was playing detective and trying to solve the mystery while marching them headlong into independent life skills. For example, when I noticed in my middle son a need to have structure and a need to be part of a team in order to combat his low self-esteem by gaining him some self-perceived social envy accompanied by very "black and white" thinking, I began to direct his learning toward gaining the skills necessary to enlist in the army. I headed him towards this life choice even though, since he was such a great jazz dancer, I would have preferred he stay safe and simply dance for Disney World. But what can I say? I was a good mom. I set my needs aside in order to honor his. [pat pat pat on my own back (wink)]. Fortunately for me, as I looked deep enough to find my children's fundamental core, I learned to do the same for me. Thus in my attempt to find ways to teach my children to teach themselves, I taught me. As it turns out, I have been blessed both by autism and everyone I've ever disagreed with on the subject.

I was never in concert with their teachers though I learned a lot from them.

In fact, I learned a lot from every approach I tried with my kids, including all the different things that different therapists asked me to try at home. Sometimes what I learned was that we were treating my children with ugliness, and sometimes it was the ugliness that illuminated the beauty. Sometimes I would see gains from repetition of play; sometimes I would see boredom set in and regressions begin. Mostly though, I spent a lot of money at the dentist for all the raisins that got stuck in my young men's teeth. In the end the only thing that really helped to raise my children from their respective disabilities, the only thing that really made the difference, was me, believing it into being.

I believed in my children and in myself enough to take them out of school and say, "Fine, I'll do everything. I'll do the job I've been avoiding and hoping that someone else would do. I'll be their teacher (and eventually their therapist) too."

I mentioned this moment of acceptance before and I mention it again because it was the turning point that I have watched many parents avoid. And yet if I'd made the decision sooner my kids would have come through sooner, and then they would have had a much longer history of fitting in.

Sooner is better than later, though later is MUCH better than not at all.

Once I took on the job of teacher I did what I have been telling you about. I looked at each of my children and thought the questions, "OK, what are this one's interests that I can help him grow from; what can he already do that when magnified will put him into the world in an independent fashion? How do I also help him to fit in and make friends? And what skills other than the ones he is already motivated for will he need to pull that off?" Once I had a list of answers I discarded all the peripheral learning kids are forced into and taught mine only the things they needed to know.

One of the things they didn't need to know was how to get along with other kids. They were going to be adults much longer than they were going to remain children. In many ways adults are easier for autistic children to deal with so I figured befriending those much more predictable adults was a more useful skill to acquire. Thus we ignored other kids and began learning how to be grownups. [The truth is I think we learned this one together. (wink)]

Because a life was not something an autistic person ever actually got, I added long-range vision. This way I could think in terms of "not autistic" so that some day they could get a life. Instead of asking myself how to teach my kids to cope with their disability or how to help them not stare and stim for quite so long—as if a little less staring was a useful life goal—I asked myself, "How do I help you to not stare so long so that I can teach you something that may interest you more than staring? Then you will be busy so you will stare even less and stare even less and stare even less until eventually you've acquired so many interests and behaviors that what you stare at is understandable to me and you are not diagnosable as autistic anymore?"

Because I had bigger questions I got bigger answers. I so believed my children capable of achieving independence that I spread the idea to them. And in my opinion, them believing in themselves was the biggest component to their changes in the direction of success.

So in the end nothing worked until I rolled up my sleeves and taught them myself. [Hopefully I have said this seven times. (wink)]

CHAPTER TEN

Section One Summary
Tools of the Trade

Sometimes I get sick of hearing about me. Often I write or lecture or perform or speak on the subject of me. It makes sense to be engaged in this activity given that I have been working unofficially with autism since 1983. (That's when I first began adopting my four children who were *at the time* on the spectrum of autism, though *at the time* they didn't know there even was a spectrum.) That my story can be of some use to others seems likely, but I've already lived and learned from it so writing it down or talking about it can seem, well, rather retro. It's like a nostalgic walk into my past on an overused path for me, but maybe we can gain something from it. Ironically, since it is my job to do so, I look back a lot even though I am a person who lives in the present and as such am not all that interested in looking back. I am that person who never reads her notes or regrets her decisions, who seldom watches home movies or looks at photo albums. So here I am surprising myself by gleaning the value of retroactive learning.

I have just read over *MIRACLES ARE MADE: A Real Life Guide to Autism* in order to edit its pages, and while reading I realized that my life is incomprehensible, even to me. In fact, now that I have raised my kids I have only the vaguest idea of how I did it. I do know it was a lot of work.

As I look back over my journey I see why people are so flabbergasted and understand just how much I bit off when I chose this path full of differently disabled folks to raise. In fact, I am still chewing on a little piece of it called Dar. As you already know, he remains challenged, maybe because he is the oldest and therefore the one I learned on or maybe because he was the most disabled in the first place. Regardless of why he remains behind or how the rest of us got through, I do know that I do not really know how we made it to here. Except to say that I was smart enough (or dumb enough) not to believe in the odds. And by rereading my own manuscript I relearned to believe in limitless possibilities, especially for Dar. Somewhere along the way I think I had forgotten that. I think this because I read between the lines of my words and heard myself believing in the speed-of-change limitations my still-autistic man-child and his disorder were predestined to have. It is time to let that go.

As Gomer Pile would say, "Gawwwleeeee!" It turns out that telling my story of raising this mix of two biological and six adopted children into lives of independence and mental health is actually an inspirational one—for me. Cool! I hope it gives you as much permission to love what you gain from your mistakes as it does me.

So it is my experience of floundering around and trying to help my children while making many, many mistakes in the process that really qualifies me to help others, because I learn from the floundering, from the successes, and from the failures. And then I tell you. I learned that what worked for one child wouldn't necessarily work for another. So, I would have to learn how to choose between the choices of what was right for whom. I learned how to follow the clues my children laid out for me and, as soon as I learned that, I learned more. I learned that the real key to healing a loved one lies in the commitment of the relationship created between you. Very early in the process it became obvious that forcing skills upon my child made both of us unhappy, and that forced skills don't generalize, whereas ones that are coaxed from within through laughter and play do. Therefore, I went to where my children were and behaved like them until they were willing to behave like me. One step at a time we grew together until eventually, all but one, were healed enough to pay taxes and have careers, apartments, friends, cars, and socially acceptable hobbies.

During my journey of learning I added professional training and certifications to my toolbox. In 2003 I was the only professional from the Autism Treatment Center of America that was certified in two modalities:

Mentor Counselor and Child Facilitator. Then in 2004 I added neuro-feedback to the list of ways in which I could help to heal the brain. To date I have helped hundreds of adults and children using a combination of neurofeedback, playroom, Socratic dialogue, and family dynamics counseling. And, using all the same therapies, I have also helped myself.

I have been the parent, the professional, the student, and the client using neurofeedback. I have used all my skills on myself in order to heal my own sensory/social integration disorder. It is the knowl-edge that I have gained from living with and seeing autism from every perspective that I have tried to share. Hopefully through my sharing you have been relieved of the need to reinvent the wheel the way I found myself doing.

Here are some reminders: Most autistic children are trying to stabilize themselves so you have to help them—if you don't help them they'll help themselves, and if they are left to help themselves they are probably going to choose something perseverative (repetitious). In order to help themselves they will have to perform this repetitious behavior so hard and so fast and in such a hyper-focused manner that it'll be hard for you to work your way into getting them to pay atten-tion to you. So, you want to respond to every sound, every movement, and every moment of connectedness that they give you. And you want to do this in an approving, adoring, exciting, engaged fashion. Sound exhausting? Trust me; it's not—not in comparison to responding in a judgmental, teachy, forcing manner. It's much more energy-giving to smile at your child and say, "Holy cow, I love that sound!" Think about it. Think about a time when you were in public, on a plane perhaps: Everyone goo goo-ed and ga ga-ed over your child and everyone on the whole plane, including you and your child, smiled and slept soundly. Now remember a time when you heard someone trying to control their child in order to not disturb others. But they controlled them with "Don't! Stop that! Cut it out or I'll spank you!" and everyone got off the plane edgy, angry, and extremely tired.

The trick to remember is you get back the energy you put out.

If you are doing this: Pushing aside their sounds because they're not saying what you want them to say and asking a million times and they're answering something a million times more until everyone is exhausted...

DO THIS INSTEAD: If your child makes a "daw" sound, say the first thing that comes into your head, such as: "Wow! That sounded like dog!" Then take action and make it into something real by running and getting a toy dog. Get out of the circle of frustration and help your child see that communication is fun!

Help them balance their brain waves by helping them choose what they focus on by being the most exciting, most awesome, most fun thing in the room. And then you will be. Think of them as a blind person because in truth they do have a type of blindness; they have developed a way of feeling the room like someone who can't see will do—they feel your energy—they feel your presence. Because of that, if you pretend that you think they are great, but you really think they are a drag, they will know! Trust me on that one: If you want to have the desired impact, you have to "buy in" first. So do it. Look at what they are doing and think it's the most adorable, cutest thing you ever saw in your life. Now do what you do for all your kids—that you perceive as the cutest most adorable thing you ever saw in your life—teach them how to grow up.

Know that there is somewhere you want to take the moment. For example, let's say you have a seven-year-old child that is making a babbling sound. OK, if your child was a baby and babbled, you would listen to it and turn it into language—no mystery; no need for training. Just do what you did when the child was two, but does it longer and many more times. So what if you thought s/he would learn faster; worrying about that just makes it go even slower. You'll have the energy if you're having fun, and it's fun when the child likes it, so work with what your child likes. Think about the little girl who said "pup;" there's nothing inherently fun about that to grownups. But she liked it so we did too, over and over and over again.

Think of it as beautiful, adorable, delightful, and cute. When we find children adorable, we love doing what they do; we love entertaining them—so when your children babble, get excited; turn it into language or copy the sound and say, "Wow! That's a fun sound. Here's mine!" and give them a fun sound back and then maybe throw a sentence in. Don't worry if they ignore you; do it anyway. Then notice that they ignored you and try a different noise level or style of response. The point is the more you judge them and tell them that what they are doing is bad, the more they are going to hyper-focus into their ritualistic behavior in order to escape your judgment and escape your negative energy. In fact, you'll have to do the same because nobody likes the feeling of being in negative energy. And that's when it will be you who stops looking at them.

At some point in our lives every one of us has avoided looking in someone's eyes to avoid seeing a judgment, either coming at us or reflected back.

Once you stop looking you increase the distance between you. And this chasm can grow until the gulf becomes seemingly insurmountable. So my suggestion is this: Put the brakes on that behavior and turn it all around. Start teasing and tickling and laughing and hugging and if they say, "No, go away," then you say, "Oh WOW! GREAT! I LOVE that you said 'no!'"—and stop. Then explain, "If you don't want me to hug or tickle you, I won't, Wow! I'm so glad you told me; I had no idea!" Give their words power: "Any time you want me to stop anything, you just say 'stop,' and if it's safe to stop, I'll stop," so they are OK with you when you take control: "Sometimes I have to do things like hold your hand to cross the street, but if it's safe to stop, I'll stop." And then always, always, always do what you say, even as you are saying it. DO NOT HOLD ONTO THE CHILD AND FORCE HIM TO HEAR YOU FIRST BECAUSE THEN HE WILL NOT HEAR YOU AT ALL! [Oops! Sorry. Was I shouting? Did you hear me? (wink)]

Your actions must reflect your words. Be mindful.

Recently I saw the cutest little animated film, *Kungfu Panda*. I was watching this movie with my grandchildren, which of course made it extremely fun. Anyway, there's this Panda who really wants to be a Kungfu hero but he really sucks. He's fat and can barely make it up a flight of stairs. He seems completely inept with a foolhardy dream. That's when his master discovers that if there's food hiding somewhere, Mr. Panda can do the most phenomenal feats of gymnastic prowess in order to get it. I was hysterical with laughter because this is exactly what my autistic twenty-seven-year-old son is like. And possibly yours!

Answers come from everywhere: In the movie the master realizes that the way to train the Panda is to use his motivator to teach with: the same goes for us. We must embrace the motivator, not try to extinguish it, because it is the motivator that will show you the way to teach. It's a good movie. Go watch it—even if you already have. It's fun and it's silly—but it's also right. Think about the way that the teacher changes his approach when he realizes that he has to follow the motivation of the student, and then go home and observe your child and figure out how to do the same.

My experience has been that at the end of the day it is always the parents that guide the children into healing—even if the healing is done at the hands of a particular clinician or therapist—because it was the parents who saw something in their child that said the healing was possible enough to bring that therapist into their lives in the first place. Because of what they saw, at least one of those parents continued to look for the magic key. They followed the path presented by their child's needs in conjunction with their family, and trusted themselves enough to find the things that matched them and their particular child's learning style.

So what I do—because I see that as true—is just share the concepts. I share the concepts of the tips that I've learned. And teach the lessons from along the way of living my life. I share with parents and professionals around the globe. And then, though I continue to guide from a distance, I leave it in the hands of the parents, and inevitably they change their children's lives for the better. In the end they assimilate what I teach and become a much greater expert than me on their child and his disorder.

I've heard a lot of people say what I just said. In fact, many of the therapies that I followed and trained with and tried to learn from over the years attracted me because they said that they viewed me, the mom, as the expert. I've heard therapists say this, but they've never actually treated me as if they believed it was true. Hopefully I am the professional whose behavior reflects these ideas because I truly believe that—though I may have some techniques and therapies to share—it is the parents who are the experts in regard to their child. When I was not listened to, I had a tendency to not listen as well, and very often it was years before a good idea that some clinician had shared burrowed its way into my brain and became something I could use. Hopefully I can help prevent some of the missed opportunities and disillusionment that such a collision of communication creates.

Remember parents, you know your child better than anyone else. You can do a better job of helping him or her than we can. You only need to understand some of the things that I, and others like me, have come to know.

CURE BY COMPLIMENT:

At one point I wanted to call this book *Cure by Compliment* because I think that's the main thing that I learned with regard to how to help people worldwide, not just autistic children and autistic adults: Compliments cure both the giver and the receiver.

Most people want to feel good and they want to do well and they want to fit in and they want to be comfortable in their own skin. (Let me clarify my definition of the words "fitting in:" they want to fit into the world in a way that makes it easy to maneuver). When people are not achieving these goals, usually the reason is that they don't know how to. Unfortunately when they seek to find the way—especially if they are a cognitively and emotionally disabled —most often they are given directions by being told what's wrong with them. This generally results in an even lower sense of self-esteem and reinforces the problems they are trying to solve while giving no clear answers on how to find their way out of their discomfort. It's especially bad if a person is told, "Don't do that!" without at least being told, "Instead do this."

But if you tell them how great they are at the things they are doing right, they will at least know which pieces to keep in order to improve; and their feeling of self worth will grow big enough to begin the process of feeling comfortable in the company of another. This is so much better than feeling wrong in comparison to everyone else. That just increases the desire to shrink away, from society, and especially from everyone who is trying to "help."

Complimenting absolutely everything a person does that is moving in the general direction of "fitting in" shows them the way to grow. I see us—the therapists, teachers, and parents—as being the lighthouse warning inexperienced travelers of the dangers in the terrain and guiding them to a place of safe living (aka comfortably communicative behavior and self-motivated learning that increases social acceptability). If we do not show them the way to "normalcy." then how will they know what it looks like and what is preventing them from getting there? I liken this process to the story of Hansel and Gretel: Someone has to be smart enough to drop some rocks and make a trail that shows the way. And just to make sure those rocks get noticed, someone has to translate the concept into obvious clues that illuminate the path like, "Looking in my eyes the way you do is so smart. Now I know you're talking to me!" in order for the person to be comfortable and interested enough to look out instead of in. So show what it is about them that does or doesn't "fit in" by complimenting what does. We all need help seeing our own challenges because nobody—autistic people included—knows what it is that we do not know until someone (or something) helps us to know it.

Remember to keep in mind that each of your lessons is a pebble going somewhere, so make sure you know where it is you are wanting them to go.

If one of the things you are hoping for is your child's independence you might consider this: In some ways the autistic child is so fiercely independent that s/he seldom embraces learning the things that are necessary in order to become our version of what that means. So because of the child's desire to be on his or her own, they end up dependent. The good news is that we can use this hankering for "doing one's own thing" as the motivator that gets the child (or adult) to follow your pebbles into society. In this way we turn the whole thing around and the desire to be independent makes them so.

The way to make this u-turn is by looking at the skills your child already has and complimenting the heck out of them, while at the same time marrying these compliments with emerging skills. For example, "You are so good at holding a paintbrush; let's use it to brush your doll's teeth." Remember that "emerging" in the case of autism can be even subtler than that. It can be as simple as responding with joy upon hearing a rounded sound next to the usual sharp sound. But making a u-turn is always a variation on the same thing, a compliment. "Oh my gosh! What a beautiful round sound—ouuuuuu—that sounds like shower. Shhhh! Here come my fingers for a showerrrrrr!" And with each compliment illuminating their path like a shiny pebble on the ground showing them the way, they build and they build and they build themselves into someone that can do some approximation of what you're trying to help them do.

Try talking as if your child understands you. Anything less is condescending and nobody responds well to that. Remember though, he or she only understands when he or she is focused enough to hear you. Though more pronounced with autism, such behavior is not unique to the disorder. That's how people are. For example, you will only understand what I write when you are focused enough to take in what you read. That's why both of us must package the same thing differently over and over and over again until we "get it."

Stay cognizant that your kids process at a different speed than you—so if you ask them a question, wait for the answer. (This waiting period can be as long as two minutes!) After all, if you're asking you must want to know; right? So wait for it. Use a pose of gentle expectation so that your little one feels no pressure or disappointment for how long it might take to bring the words out.

Beware the rhetorical question for it is worse than useless; it teaches one to not answer since no answer is expected. Begin now to erase these from your speaking style and laugh at yourself as you discover how hard a task that actually is.

Teaching language works in a similar fashion as laying out the pebbles in order to gain social skills. For example, if your child speaks but doesn't answer questions, try this: Ask, "Do you want to go to the store?" Now wait for the answer. If no answer is forthcoming, then guide the child by supplying some possible choices. In this case we asked a yes or no question, so guide them with some yes or no choices. Simply say, "You can tell me yes or you can tell me no." And then wait. Give it a minute this time. If you still don't get a response, then say, "Well if you don't tell me the answer, then I'm going to have to guess what you want and I might guess wrong so…" Now repeat the question and the choices. If you still don't have an answer, repeat the explanation but add, "OK. I'm going to guess that your answer is no (or yes). You don't want to go to the store. I guessed that mainly because I don't really want to go and since I don't know what you want I'm usually going to guess what I want. That's why it's better to talk. You have way more power that way." HINT: Kids love power!

In many cases giving choices is just a way of nudging while informing what comes next. Variations on this technique are useful along the way to building relationships and communicative language that's interactive. You're not just asking for words and labels like the pieces of an unrelated puzzle … but offering communication and the ability to gain control in the world—a big motivator for these kids. Understand that requested speech comes from different processing than spontaneous… Most therapies put all the value on requested and responding speech. Personally I value spontaneous words a little more because a spontaneously sharing individual with his own ideas and interests is the definition of independence. And besides, if it's never spontaneous it means it's never been generalized. But don't throw the baby out with the bath water here. Requested speech is harder for an autistic child than spontaneous speech and as such represents processing challenges much in need of healing. (Requested speech is not to be confused with echolalia which is simply the act of habitually repeating what has just been said). Thus each time speech is requested a child gains an opportunity to succeed and this exercises even more than speech. It also works much needed social-skill sets like cooperation and compliance.

And so we learn from doing.

Learning in order to know—in order to gain a skill—is very different from learning in order to prove that you know. In many ways it's inferior and in many ways it's superior. For example, when I followed the chain of the need to know neuroanatomy I learned neuroanatomy. I didn't also have to learn history because it was a prerequisite to getting my degree—I wasn't going after one. I didn't worry about whether or not I would have enough credits for a particular degree. I just got to the point of knowing what I came there to know. There was just too much to do to waste time rounding out. So in my career I did—as all parents of autistic children are forced to do—a lot of learning outside the loop of PhD's. Once I decided to become a neurofeedback specialist, I took the required course and then audited the remaining classes in order to gain the rest of what I needed to learn. I audited neuroanatomy classes and pharmaceutical classes and various aspects of biofeedback and all sorts of things related to emotional and mental functioning. I audited because then I was able to pick and choose what I was learning. This is why I know so much about my chosen interests.

On the flip side I ONLY know a lot about MY chosen interests, which is not nearly as good—if I want to prevent Alzheimer's in my old age—as a more eclectic education is. Fortunately, I am not very worried about Alzheimer's (wink). Besides, I sidestepped the checks and balances making it so that there was no policing of what I did or did not know. Since I was not after a degree there could have been no one to make sure I understood the lessons the way I was meant to. Thus I could have been confused by what I'd learned and proceeded erroneously. Fortunately, Dr. Burke, my boss at the time, was not only brilliant on the subject of neuroanatomy but he was also merciless at insisting I convince him that my protocol choices were based in hard science. Thank you Dr. Burke for teaching me how to think on the subject of how we think. And thank you for not holding my hand but instead insisting that I be vigilant as I kept my eyes open for evidence related to the accuracy of my understanding. Fortunately for the people I work with, my children, and me, staying aware of the evidence by observing behavior is my expertise.

Not that errors are always a bad thing. Errors are a part of learning. I don't mean just a willingness to be wrong but the error itself. Erroneous thinking is a recognized source of discovery for the headstrong and such a path is common in every kind of science. The sundial was created and based on the thinking that the sun revolved around the earth. Once we paradigm shifted to believing that the earth revolved around the sun, we treated the old concepts as if they were so foolish that they were never considered real science in the first place. However, many a textbook was written to teach otherwise. Many advances in behavioral medicine have also been based on erroneous thinking, advances like joining in an autistic child's repetitious behavior. In the beginning the parents that started this therapeutic approach had no understanding that our socially necessary mirror neurons would be stimulated by copying. They just saw the child as living in his own world and wanted to join him there. As we learn more about the science behind why a particular treatment works we can perfect it, little by little, learning by learning. Fortunately, in the absence of perfection, many therapies work, even without our knowing why.

This is a great comfort to me. Because early in my training one of my professors said, "We don't really know what a brain wave is, not completely." And I remember thinking, "Well at least we know they're important, because when they stop it means we're dead." Fortunately the bottom line for most of us is "Does it work?" And the answer I've seen is "Yes!" So as long as that's true I can continue to help people and not worry so much about whether or not we know it all. Fortunately I have the binary code belief system to operate from and neuroanatomy to guide my choices.

In fact I so want to redefine how we as a culture approach training, education, and information gathering that, in order to stay ahead of the curve, I have decided to call myself a social therapist. After all, improving social abilities within social environments is one of the biggest aspects of what I do. And since there's no such thing as a social therapist, if I become the first one then the training path that I define is the training path required. I kind of like that. (wink)

Just as I like the enormous success I am having with the people I help. In my world I do not define success as "calmed down" because often that looks like "so calmed down we got them drunk on their own brain waves." Instead, I define success as *meeting major life goals like going from mute to verbal regardless of age.* And, as I have said many times, I'm not the only practitioner seeing these results. The field of neurofeedback is full of them, regardless of style.

I am also not the only parent to educate myself to save a child. In fact, the way I approached it is pretty much the way we all approach it. As parents of autism we are in a kind of emergency "need to know, need to act" situation, so we suck up knowledge like a sponge, assimilate and apply it. For me, such a vacuum-like approach to learning is congruent with who I am, and who I was, even way before I got autistic kids. For example, when I was single parenting two babies and wanted to learn jazz dancing but couldn't afford the classes, I wrote a letter to the community center. I said something to the effect of, "Hey you know I've taken jazz, so I want to offer to volunteer as an assistant in one of your classes." And it was true. I had taken jazz. But I was only five years old at the time. The administrators didn't ask for the details so I didn't tell. But I did learn—in a hurry. Since I was the assistant instructor, there was no time to think about or question what the teacher had just modeled for everyone. I just had to know how to do it—so I did.

What that experience taught me was how easily and quickly I learned whenever I removed my self-doubt—and resistance. The minute there was no room for "Can I do it?" and I was left with "I have to do it," I did. That's why so many parents of autistic children are such enormous fonts of information, knowing more about their child's disorder than the professionals whose advice they are seeking do—because the parents have to. Parents understand autism from a twenty-four hour a day lifelong vantage point, from the behavior of their particular child and from within their own family dynamics. I repeat: The parents know more about the child in question than we (the autism specialists) do. They are simply hiring our little piece of the programming pie, our little slice of expertise. Thus, if when the parent asks, we give our expertise openly while not needing the parent to agree with, or even use, our particular specialty—then we become a team.

In the world of mental health parents are often blamed for their children's behavior just as doctors are often blamed for their patients' illness. This is an unfortunate reality. In many ways the practitioner is at a great disadvantage with his/her patient because he/she is caught in a one-sided relationship. In the role of therapist great care must be taken to keep client confidentiality. Not so for the client however. Thus, though the therapist cannot share the confessions of the client, clients can and do tell story upon story, revealing their version of the events, that took place in the clinician's office. These mental health patients will say what they say according to their present state of mind and seldom worry about the long-term effects of slandering their doctor. In addition, they often share their version of the truth in an attempt to manipulate the listener and gain support. Thus, for the health professional, telling an irrational client they are being irrational oftentimes ramps up the emotions and leads to angry irrational clients, spreading slanderous untruths because they are intent on avoiding the advice they have just paid to get. In a way the reaction proves out the diagnosis. Generally, a rational client will just role his or her eyes and change practitioners, or join a gym. However, regardless of the pitfalls, it's the irrational clients we are there to help. So we risk our reputations and show them the definition of irrational while putting their face in the picture.

Helping people is risky business and can be almost as bad for one's reputation as raising teenagers. (sigh) Working with parents, though extremely rewarding, is no exception; in fact, it's especially challenging. Because many parents have half bought into the concept that their child's challenges are their fault and as a result they are quite defensive. This makes them hard to guide and easy to offend. Which is scary because when parents are mad they use chat rooms to globally ruin a reputation. And while it's important to share information about your practitioner, it's equally as important to take some deep breaths and clear your thinking first. I consider myself very blessed. I go into people's homes and see how they live. For the most part they drop their defenses and show me their lives in the hopes that I might help their child. Because they have to they trust me. It's very brave of them.

I think its brave because, though in general gossip is the parent's tool of retribution, the law is the practitioners. Sometimes they report parents out of hand. There are volumes worth of stories wherein this sort of damage has been done to loving parents for being different. Unfortunately the legal system believes in the expert and hasn't yet learned that the expert is the parent... though that does seem to be improving... Thank you Jenny McCarthy!

However, the problem is still a reality to be understood and worked within: Since the "health practitioner" remains stuck in this one-side position, some of them lose their compassion and become the manipulators as they break that respectful code of silence by involving the law, even when they shouldn't. Everybody, regardless of position and status, is fallible and human: buy their advice knowing that. Always, always, always follow yourself.

At any rate the majority of mental health workers don't behave this way. And if they are struggling with mental health field frustration, their reaction is usually more insidiously disguised as benign. Generally, when they need to vent, professionals gather in groups and share how difficult their anonymous patients are. Since names are left out stories can be redesigned to suit the purpose. When the clients are kids, invariably the parents are discussed. And before you know it, this anonymous world of parents as a group is being slandered albeit with big words and lofty expressions. I say this from experience because I have personally stood up and chastised many a conference gathering of practitioners for saying things like: "Parents are the issue. If I could, I would treat the child and never talk to the parent." In these face-flushed spontaneous lectures I have stated over and over that helping is our job and we can't do it well until we accept that Mom and Dad are the final word on their child. I believe it is a necessity to accept this truth because only then will we stop competing for the position of highest authority and get on with the job.

The possibility of real brainstorming and information sharing is lost whenever any group perpetuates the us-against-them mentality. In my opinion we must engage in teamwork instead of oppositional sides vying for position because it takes a team to do this job faster and better than we are doing it now. This attitudinal adjustment is something that has to happen; otherwise the chasm grows bigger and we model anti-social behavior for our anti-social autistic kids.

So let's relax and talk. Most of us, parent and professional alike, really are, just trying to help. Case in point: I was recently at a seminar wherein one of the women got some difficult news: her grandson had died. In the midst of sharing and searching for a ride to the airport I was gifted this story:

The baby had been born premature and very sick. There was no way to know if he would live or die. The odds were against him. This grieving grandmother's eyes welled up with gratitude as she told me of the amazing life her now dead eight-day-old grandchild had lived:

Right after he was born medical professionals and parents joined forces and began to use their talents to create possibilities and seek a beautiful quality of life for this one-pound baby boy. First child and parents were flown to a special hospital with a nesting room for preemies. The entire family was welcomed by the staff and given an opportunity to live with their life-supported child. Music, special lights, movies of inspiration, and pictures of heaven on the ceiling were all in evidence, creating a visceral feeling of support and joy. The nurses made signs and even created a special breathing chart upon which the parents would put stars whenever their son managed an unassisted breath. Best of all, every day, parents and staff celebrated life. Every day they brought in cake and blew out candles indicating another milestone in the journey of this frail little boy. I was hearing about a death and smiling about a life. Personally I think it's beautiful to imagine that every day was celebrated just because he was there! A day-to-day birthday party celebration of love! We should all live this way.

This sweet soul was operated on, resuscitated, and kept alive for all of those eight birthday party days by the expertise of the doctors, the skills of the nurses, the love of his parents, and the community of the group, which included paramedics, helicopter pilots, and cleaning staff.

As she told this story I was in awe of the teamwork. I was reminded of the many times a doctor, nurse, or paramedic has saved me and/or someone I love. We all have a role to play, and when we play it together everyday is a celebration. Living in harmony and solving problems just because they are there puts joy in the journey. And living like that makes it so we no longer need to seek the answer in the outcome because we hold it in our hand.

Hopefully this book will help illuminate the value of us all, even if we are a little autistic. (great big huge sun-blinding smile)

SECTION TWO

RESOURCE ME

I have been impressed with the urgency of doing.
Knowing is not enough; we must apply.
Being willing is not enough; we must do.

—Leonardo da Vinci

CHAPTER ELEVEN

Autism Basics

For those of you who are reading Section Two before Section One I will tell a story I've already told. A long time ago a social worker told me that my four-year old autistic son needed immediate help as he had "the worst" social skills this man had ever seen. He then said that he couldn't help immediately because there was a yearlong waiting list to get any help. He continued to explain that unfortunately early intervention was the key to success so by the time that year has passed it'd be too late because my son would be beyond the age that fell into the definition of early intervention. Not to be stopped I jumped straight into problem-solving mode and asked what they would do to change him. He said he couldn't tell me that because he didn't want me to do it myself. Can you say "Catch 22?" That's the way it was back then. And because so many doctors half spoke and hid their information from parents, we got many skewed ideas about the disabilities of our children. I remember a time when one doctor asked if my son could alternate his feet walking up the stairs. He never explained anything to me, other than that it would be important. So I spent three months teaching my son to alternate his feet thinking that this alone was all it would take to cure his autism. I know it was naïve of me, but I saw my son as a normal albeit nonverbal kid with some weird challenges, so I figured erase the weird challenges and normal is what he would be left with.

I was wrong. A person can only be added to, grown out of what is, because when you erase you end up with nothing.

But it was 1985, back when they still believed autism was caused by not giving your child enough affection, and several places were trying to make up for that by using ammonia jets and cattle prods on the children. In my show I say, "Of course you could only use cattle prods at school; if parents did it at home it would be abuse." Now that I've told you about the social worker I guess you can see where that joke came from. The truth is the techniques they would have used on my son had he been accepted into that school, well, nowadays we call that abuse.

Fortunately we have come a long way since then, and every year we get better at working together to enable our children. But we are only just "getting" better; there is still an enormous distance to travel in regard to keeping everyone informed. Parents are often frustrated. That's what this book is intended to help. However, keep in mind that there's a constantly growing body of knowledge, which translates into loads of wonderful work. There is an enormous learning curve ahead for everyone, parent and professional alike.

Never count on your doctor for all the answers. It's unrealistic.

In all fairness there is too much to know to know it all, even if you are a doctor. I hold lots of information in my head. I know things like, four times as many boys as girls are diagnosed with autism and that that is partially due to the size of the corpus callosum (highway transporting information from one brain hemisphere to another) and partially due to the genetic differences that come into play with regard to chromosomal abnormalities in disorders like Fragile X. I know that late onset of autistic symptoms often correlates with mutated migrations of neurons into the left hemisphere during the years when this part of the brain is shaping itself for logical processing, and that early onset correlates with mirror neuron migration and myelination missteps. Sound impressive? Well sounding impressive is a lot easier than being impressive.

Fortunately, in order to be impressive and make a difference in this population, I don't have to know any more than what does and doesn't work. I don't have to understand why it's happening, I just have to interrupt the errant brain development and set it to changing in a new direction. This is because my personal therapy of choice is neurofeedback. And it uses information to let the expert (in this case the brain) fix itself. And as such it is like teaching the family to heal from within. Neurofeedback is based on hard science and has been healing and improving brain functioning in seizure disorders since the early sixties. There exist many good quality studies and lots of evidence for the efficacy of using neurofeedback on a variety of disorders. And yet when your child was diagnosed, most of your doctors just suggested behavior conditioning and a drug or two for psychosis, sleep, and focus.

In this world of quickly changing information overload, there's no way to avoid confusing old news with new news. This is true of everything that pops up on our computer screen when we do an Internet search, but it is especially true of information on technology and the brain. We are just learning too quickly to keep up. In fact, in the last three weeks while I've been writing this book two new treatment approaches and one new biological discovery have been brought to my attention. (JOIT process, a therapy that teaches the child how to relax in order to attend; the off label usage of an available acne drug called minocycline, which is being used in Canada to reverse Fragile X symptoms; and the exciting discovery that in many autistic people, genes which respond to experience weren't missing, as previously believed; they were just stuck in the "off" position. This last bit of information helps to explain why neurofeedback is so effective in helping heal spectrum children). So by the time this is published much of what I say will be old news and much will be missing. However, there is a whole lot here to get you started. So dig in and become more informed.

Become more informed because the number one most important thing I can tell you (over and over again) about raising a child with autism is this—the parent must become the primary expert. The more informed you are the easier it will be to decide whether or not you are dealing with an Autism Spectrum Disorder in the early stages. Once decided, it is information that will help you pick and choose where to put your time and energy. Knowing the world of autism is what will guide you as you seek which professionals and what therapies are best suited to you and your family to help you reach your goals. (Autism Spectrum Disorders are whole-brain developmental disorders. Different people respond differently to different solutions).

And while learning and teaching yourself so that you can teach your child, try to build a commitment to also heal your child in order to heal yourself. Knowing and accepting that we are a genetically connected part of the picture and should apply many of the therapies to the whole family can prevent the creation and reinforcement of what diagnosticians sometimes call "Sick Person Personality" in and around the child in your house.

After all, if everybody is healing, nobody is engaged in the act of being sick.

And though this section's primary purpose is to help you ferret your way through the multitude of questions that came to mind the minute you began wondering if your child was autistic, it is my sincere desire to share something even more valuable: confidence, hope, and the absolute joy of meeting the challenges presented when dealing with autism.

Getting Familiar with Autism

This chapter is designed to introduce you to all of the new terminology, medical jargon, and even slang that you will begin to hear as you immerse yourself in the world of Autism experts. I say autism "expert because whether you are a teacher, professional, parent, grandparent, sibling, or friend of someone with autism, if you are going to be involved in the caring of an autistic child in any way shape or form, you are going to have to understand the disorder inside and out to then begin to understand this child. To that end I have peppered the book with personal stories that give reason to and make a practical application of the information you are ingesting.

First and foremost, this child is a child. It is important not to lose his or her individuality within the diagnosis. While autism is a major aspect of your child's personality, it does not define him or her as a whole, and it is going to become increasingly important as you develop a program for this child that you identify his/her unique interests, thoughts, feelings, and talents because it is his/her unique thoughts, feelings, interests and talents that create the doorway in—to gaining his/her cooperation as you ask him/her to build and grow. After all, autism aside, all children grow greater when we focus on and build upon the things they love the most. This becomes even more paramount when teaching autistic children. Many therapeutic approaches are aimed at expunging behaviors. This effectively shrinks children to less than what they already were. I prefer to build upon and make functionally inclusive all their self-stimulatory behaviors. This approach is not only more user friendly but it is also a more beautiful way to be with and see your child. So while this chapter is going to identify the signs, symptoms, possible causes, and methods of diagnosis of autism spectrum disorder, it is also going to attempt to do so it in a way that does not lose sight of the child as an individual.

Let's start with the most fundamental question of all…

What Is Autism?

Autism Spectrum Disorder (often termed "Autistic," "Autistic Disorder" or "Classical Autism") refers to the most common condition in a group of pervasive development disorders. Autism typically appears in the first three years of life, though onset has been known to occur as late as the age of four. It is a complex neurological whole-brain disorder. Autistic individuals may present with a wide variety or spectrum of symptoms, the severity of which ranges from severe to mild. However, they all suffer from some combination of the following: language delays or other communication problems (like echoing speech or using gibberish), poor or limited social skills (like an inability to comprehend cause and effect or question and answer), and a propensity to engage in repetitive behaviors or severely limited activities and interests.

One should keep in mind that autism is a spectrum disorder, and depending on the individual one or more areas of the brain may be affected; the degree of that effect varies person to person and brain area to brain area.

What Causes Autism and Can It Be Prevented?

There are many theories and suppositions ranging from television to genetics, but excluding Rett's Syndrome, there is no verifiably known cause for autism spectrum disorders. However ASDs often occur among people who have certain other medical conditions, including Fragile X syndrome, tuberous sclerosis, congenital rubella syndrome, and untreated phenylketonuria. Some harmful drugs taken during pregnancy also have been linked with a higher risk of autism, specifically the prescription drug thalidomide.

While scientists aren't certain what causes autism, it's likely that both genetics and environment play a role. Autism tends to run in families. Studies have shown that identical twins, who have the same DNA, are much more likely to share the diagnosis of autism than fraternal twins, whose DNA is different. Recent studies strongly suggest that some people have a genetic predisposition to autism. In families with one autistic child, the risk of having a second child with the disorder is approximately five percent, or one in twenty. This is greater than the risk for the general population. Researchers are looking for clues about which genes contribute to this increased susceptibility. In some cases, parents and other relatives of an autistic child show mild impairments in social and communicative skills or engage in repetitive behaviors. Evidence also suggests that some emotional disorders, such as manic depression, occur more frequently than average in the families of people with autism.

That being said, as of this writing, though a variety of chromosomes have been implicated, there is no known cause for autism. Many anatomical or physiological peculiarities have been found (e.g., cerebella abnormalities, temporal abnormalities, oversized head, overgrowth and late pruning of neurons in the early years of development, overactive brain-wave activity, deficiency of dipeptydal peptidase; low levels of oxytoxin, IBD, dermorphin, sauvagine, opioids, secretin, free sulphate, too much lead, mercury, pollution, allergies, even TV and cell phones have been implicated). Other studies suggest that people with autism have abnormal levels of serotonin or other neurotransmitters in the brain. These abnormalities suggest that autism could result from the disruption of normal brain development early in fetal development caused by defects in genes that control brain growth and that regulate how neurons communicate with each other. While these findings are intriguing, they are preliminary and require further study. The majority of researchers believe that most cases of autism begin before or shortly after birth.

Scientists are working hard to make sense of all the data, and many theories have been put forth. None of these theories have proven to be universal to all autistic children or have allowed a given individual to be identified as suffering from a particular spectrum disorder with a specific cause. Nevertheless, many spectrum individuals have been helped through a variety of approaches. Autistic children are extremely complex. They have chemical imbalances, nutritional imbalances, hormonal imbalances, physical abnormalities, and learning/behavioral deficits. Helping them requires a willingness to look at all the various possibilities while still not becoming overwhelmed and put out of action by the multitudinous possibilities. You have come to this writing for information. That makes you part of the puzzle. Revel in the challenge, partner with professionals in the field, and begin. There is no known way to prevent autism. The theory that parental practices are responsible for autism has long been disproved.

What Are the Odds that My Child Is Autistic?

Once considered a rare disorder, today autism affects as many as one in every 110 children (though the figure can vary slightly dependent upon the source). That means around every twenty minutes a new case of autism is diagnosed. Males are four times more likely to have autism than females.

The diagnosis of autism is typically not made until three to four years of age or later. However, some early warning signs of autism appear in the first year of life, and it can be detected as early as eighteen months of age. This is a significant amount of lag time. (Actually the youngest child I ever worked with was five months old. He had begun twisting his body to avoid eye contact and turning his head away with great force. His intervention was begun at such a young age that his brain completely assimilated the changes and no diagnosis was ever made). Research has shown that early identification and intervention can make the critical difference for children with autism. Although your child is never too old to be helped, the results of that help are definitely affected by age and the subsequent hardwiring of the brain.

If you suspect your child may have autism, do not wait—intervene. Begin by encouraging eye contact and rewarding touch. Compliment and celebrate every sound your child makes. Then begin looking for help. If you still have questions after reading this book, go to the web or the library. Get comfortable with the fact that the various sources of information may include incongruence about treatments, therapies, and prognoses. Since autism is still not completely understood, and keeping up with all the research is a staggering proposition, much speculation and many opposing views remain in the field. We—the professionals—are still finding new and better ways to help these children optimize their skills.

By purchasing this book you have already begun to tunnel through the cornucopia of treatments and beliefs about autism, ranging from traditional to alternative or holistic approaches. My advice is to relax. Though creating a treatment plan is an important step you will want to make fairly quickly, it is not an emergency. Your child is simply, wonderfully special and not in danger of dying. Take your time and make it an adventure. Otherwise, the search can be quite overwhelming.

What Are Some General Age-Related "Signals" You as the Parent Can Use to Help Identify if Your Child Is "On The Spectrum?"

4 Months of Age:

Your child avoids eye contact, does not react by looking at you when you make social sounds such as humming or clapping, does not show as much interest in people as objects, or does not smile back when you smile at him/her (without being tickled or touched).

12 Months of Age:

Your child does not combine eye contact with smiling, does not babble or the babble does not represent speech, does not follow your gaze to look at objects, does not try to engage other people in what she/he is doing, does not respond when his/her name is called, does not point using the index finger, does not show caring or concern when you cry, or does not wave hi or bye.

24 Months of Age:

Your child does not attempt to share her/his interests with you or others, does not imitate common activities such as driving the car, does not develop pretend or make-believe play, or does not use two-word phrases in an appropriate manner.

What are the Common Signs and Symptoms of Autism?

Regardless of where your child fits on the spectrum, most of the treatment modalities will be the same. Therefore, it is often easier to understand for parents if we just lump them all together under one big umbrella of autism. Simplifying the way a child is diagnosed can help curb the feeling of overwhelm the parents experience and help them move on to individualizing the treatment itself. So, with that in mind, individuals with autism usually have at least half of the traits listed below.

Varying in intensity these symptoms can range from mild to severe.

- Apparent insensitivity or oversensitivity to pain
- Echolalia (repeating words or phrases instead of normal language)
- Chooses to be alone or has an aloof manner
- Uneven gross/fine motor skills
- May resist cuddling
- Spins, swings, or lines up objects
- Non responsive to verbal cues; acts as if deaf
- Problems interacting with other children
- Resists changes in routine
- Does not point
- No real fear of dangers
- Little eye contact
- Sustained odd play and unusual body movements
- Inappropriate attachment to objects
- Difficulty in expressing needs
- Noticeable physical over activity or extreme under activity
- Tantrums; may display extreme distress for no apparent reason
- Unresponsive to normal teaching methods

Self-Diagnosing an ASD

Your son or daughter may not have developed language and/or social skills normally in the early months of life. Even if he/she did develop such skills, she/he may have lost some or all of these skills. Your child may have begun using some type of repetitive body movement (e.g., hand flapping, spinning, rocking, head shaking). Perhaps your little one stares at a book, feels the shag carpet, or listens to the sound of the dryer for many, many minutes each day. Possibly, when you change things (e.g., buying a new blanket, replacing a favorite broken toy with a new one, redirecting the way a toy is used), your child pulls away, has inconsolable tantrums, or hurts himself / herself. Maybe she/he is overly sensitive to texture, lights, sounds, smells, or tastes. He/she may have delayed motor skills (e.g., walking, riding a tricycle, chewing). Maybe she/he prefers to play alone or maybe he/she just doesn't interact with peers the way you thought she/he would. Possibly he/she is too busy lining things up, putting them in order repeatedly, flicking lights on and off, or opening and closing a favorite door. In addition she/he may display unusual motor behaviors (e.g., peering at things from the corners of his/her eyes, walking on tip toes, walking with an unusual gait). Finally, maybe your child's enjoyment of affection has a strange quality to it as if love and affection were only accepted or enjoyed in an idiosyncratic manner designed by your child. As you can see, autism looks different depending upon the individual child and his/her particular "recipe" of perhaps two scoops of social, three scoops of repetitive, and one scoop of language challenge.

How Is It Clinically Diagnosed?

Autism is diagnosed most often through the use of a questionnaire meant to gather information about a child's development and behavior. Doctors rely on a core group of behaviors to alert them to the possibility of a diagnosis of autism.

According to the The DMV-IV—the little book that defines all known medical disorders for the purpose of diagnosis—those behaviors are divided into six characteristics of ASDs.

To qualify for a diagnosis a person must have six or more issues from 1, 2 and 3.

At least two of the issues must come from 1: social interaction.
A. Marked impairment in the use of multiple nonverbal behaviors, such as eye-to-eye gaze, facial expression, body postures and gestures, failure to regulate social interaction, or a failure to develop peer relationships appropriate to developmental level.
C. Lack of spontaneous seeking to share enjoyment, interests, or achievements with other people (e.g., by lack of showing, bringing, or pointing out objects of interest).
D. Lack of social or emotional reciprocity.

At least one issue from 2: language as used in social communication.
A. Delay in, or total lack of, the development of spoken language (not accompanied by an attempt to compensate through alternative modes of communication such as gesture or mime).
B. In individuals with adequate speech, marked impairment in the ability to initiate or sustain a conversation with others.
C. Stereotyped and repetitive use of language, or idiosyncratic language.

At least one issue from 3: symbolic or imaginative play.
A. Encompassing preoccupation with one or more stereotyped and restricted patterns of interest that is abnormal either in intensity or focus.
B. Apparently inflexible adherence to specific nonfunctional routines or rituals.
C. Stereotyped and repetitive motor mannerisms (e.g., hand or finger flapping or twisting, or complex whole-body movements).
D. Persistent preoccupation with parts of objects.
E. Lack of varied, spontaneous make-believe, or social imitative play appropriate to developmental level.

Some screening instruments rely solely on parent observations; others rely on a combination of parent and doctor observations. If screening instruments indicate the possibility of autism, doctors should ask for a more comprehensive evaluation.
A comprehensive evaluation requires a multidisciplinary team including a psychologist, neurologist, psychiatrist, speech therapist, and other professionals who diagnose children with ASDs. The team members should conduct a thorough neurological assessment and in-depth cognitive and language testing.

Autism varies widely in its severity and symptoms and may go unrecognized, especially in mildly affected children, or when more debilitating handicaps mask the disorder. In addition, since hearing problems can cause behaviors that could be mistaken for autism, children with delayed speech development should also have their hearing tested. After a thorough evaluation, the team usually meets with parents to explain the results of the evaluation and present the diagnosis. It is hoped that everyone involved with a diagnosis would have significant experience with ASDs, their diagnosis, and their treatment.

But of course that is not always the case, and since parent information carries a lot of weight with regard to diagnosis, sometimes the professionals involved are confused by the details being presented. In addition, the preexisting medically held belief that autism is an unchangeable state muddies the ability of some diagnosticians to see clearly. For example, when my son Rye was diagnosed the doctor was thrown by the fact that Rye had improved enough to point at things and listen to directions right after I adopted him. So the doctor "invented" a diagnostic phrase "Infantile Autism—Improved." And when Dar, my other son, showed signs of emotional connectedness to me within weeks of leaving his very abusive previous environment and coming to live as my child, several doctors refused to diagnose him. Dar ran around their offices constantly grunting; he rubbed his face on the carpet, stared at their rubber mats, and flapped his hands. He sure seemed autistic to me but they wanted to wait another year—at which point he would be beyond early intervention age—before diagnosing him. They believed his behavior might be emotionally based due to his mother rejecting him—an old completely erroneous idea about some forms of autism. It actually took two years before my son got his diagnosis—our obvious bond confused doctors so they chose PDD and UNEDUCATABLY RETARDED as his label, because "autistic kids don't care about their mothers."

The idea that autistic children don't love their parents is a commonly held misconception on the part of many… a better way to say it would be "autistic kids often don't display their emotions in a manner that we can understand as an expression of love."

Like my affectionate son Dar, now-a-days children with some symptoms of autism, but not enough to be diagnosed with classical autism, are often diagnosed with PDD-NOS. (Not Otherwise Specified) Children with autistic behaviors but well-developed language skills are often diagnosed with Asperger syndrome. Children who develop normally and then suddenly deteriorate between the ages of three to ten years and show marked autistic behaviors may be diagnosed with childhood disintegrative disorder. Girls with autistic symptoms may be suffering from Rett syndrome, a gender-linked genetic disorder characterized by social withdrawal, regressed language skills, and hand wringing.

What Does an Autism Diagnosis Really Mean?

A diagnosis of autism indicates that an individual has significant difficulties in three major areas: communication, socialization, and behavior. These impairments may become noticeable immediately after birth or in any of the years after that but before the age of three. Most individuals with autism also have some degree of inability to interpret sensory experiences and to know that people have thoughts different from their own (mind-blindness). Some people with autism may be severely challenged in all these areas while others may be mildly affected or have combinations of mild and moderate impairments. It is estimated that fifty percent of people with autism test as having mental retardation. Unfortunately though, most standardized tests are insufficient in that they do not make allowances for language or motor skill deficits accompanied by non-compliance or—better said—inability to comply.

Since autism is a spectrum disorder, symptoms can vary widely between individuals. Many individuals with autism will develop a seizure disorder at some time in their lives, commonly at the onset of puberty. Often two people with the same disorder look very different from each other. In general, people with the diagnosis of autism are considered to be more severely affected than those with PDD-NOS or Asperger Syndrome. (This is obviously not written in stone since the only child I had that was labeled PDD-NOS was the only child I had that was so most severely affected.)

Some individuals with autism never speak; some only echo those around them while still others may be adept at word acquisition but have difficulty with the give and take of normal conversation. Some may have intense social challenges and become completely withdrawn from other humans while others simply seem self-absorbed or eccentric. The stereotypic movements of autism like rocking, flapping, or toe walking are not universal to all ASD individuals and neither is the rigid need for sameness. Though many individuals with autism will engage in these behaviors, a goodly number will perform less obvious repetitive behaviors such as repeating phrases, performing ritualistic sequences or small, hard-to-notice rhythmic movements.

Many doctors, teachers, and other professionals are uninformed about autism. It is not unusual for diagnosis to take many years due to the fact that the majority of physicians are unfamiliar with the many manifestations of autism. Many doctors may advise parents to take a "wait and see" attitude; however, this is absolutely the worst approach for an autistic spectrum disorder. Early intervention is the key to a good outcome. Thus, the earlier and more intensive the intervention, generally the better the result.

Autism and the MMR Vaccine

The MMR vaccine protects against three different diseases (measles, mumps, and rubella) through one shot made up of three separate vaccines. The shot is given twice during childhood. Before the MMR vaccine was given to children, there were about 400,000 measles cases reported each year in the United States but in 1999 there were only a hundred cases reported. From these figures alone it seemed obvious that the MMR vaccine was doing good work.

Why is There Concern about the MMR Vaccine Causing Autism?

A small study in London in 1998 first raised the possibility that autism is linked to the MMR vaccine. While the study did not prove that MMR vaccine causes autism, it did increase the level of concern of many parents. Since England was where the controversy began, let's look at some figures from that country.

The MMR immunization was introduced in the UK in 1988 with the first dose aimed at children of twelve to fifteen months, a second at three to five years. It works to protect against measles, mumps, and rubella by stimulating the immune system to produce antibodies against the three different strains of virus. It was well received by both parents and doctors and over ninety per cent of children were being immunized by 1992. Most children received the vaccine with no obvious serious side effects, but it grew increasingly apparent that some became seriously ill within a few weeks. These children began behaving strangely, stopped talking, and became socially withdrawn, staring into space for hours on end. Many developed a raging thirst, bizarre eating habits, multiple food allergies, hyperactivity, and sleep problems. This was usually accompanied by abdominal pain, bloating and bowel disturbances, and some became incontinent of urine or feces. They did not simply fail to develop but lost what they already had: Thousands of children—even as old as thirteen—who had all developed normally until receiving the vaccine, became very unwell with a remarkably similar pattern of events after having the MMR shot. The behavior these children showed was similar to autism, but since it had such a late onset it was termed "autistic regression."

Most of the parents felt sure that the cause of these devastating changes in their children was the MMR vaccine, but if they mentioned this concern to their doctors it always met with dismissive reassurance that it must have been a coincidence because the MMR was safe. One doctor, instead of dismissing the possibility of a relationship with the MMR vaccine, listened to the worried parents and studied some of the affected children. Dr. Andrew Wakefield, from the Royal Free

Hospital in north London, published a paper in February 1998 in the medical journal *The Lancet* suggesting that the MMR vaccine could be the cause of the children's autism and bowel disturbances, which he calls "autistic enterocolitis." Dr. Wakefield was vociferously attacked for causing unnecessary worry in parents and the MMR vaccine was vigorously defended as being "highly safe and effective."

Does the MMR Vaccine Cause Autism?

After reviewing all of the studies, including the study from London, which raised the possibility of an association between MMR and autism, the Institute of Medicine found that the evidence suggested "no link at the population level between MMR and autism." The committee does believe, however, that the studies they reviewed do not rule out the possibility that in some rare cases, autism might be associated with the MMR vaccine. The IOM recommends further research in order to investigate this rare possibility and to understand better the causes of autism in general.

Chief Medical Officer, Sir Kenneth Calman, also felt confident enough to say, "I have concluded there is no link between MMR immunization and autism." Questioned in Parliament in 1997 on the possible link between MMR and autism, then health minister Tessa Jowell reassured MPs that: "No vaccine is issued in the United Kingdom unless it passes the highest standards for quality, and parents should have confidence that the vaccines that are provided are both safe and efficacious." However, those safety trials on the MMR followed children up for only three weeks. This is alarming for a vaccine aimed at millions of healthy children.

In 1999, a study by the Committee on Safety of Medicines released the results of a study that England's Department of Health claimed "reinforced the conclusion that there is no link" between MMR and autism. The first, by the Committee on the Safety of Medicines, involved examining questionnaires sent to the parents who had suspected MMR as a cause for their child's autism—1200 questionnaires were distributed and 126 examined in detail. The study concluded: "It is impossible to prove or refute the suggested associations between MMR vaccine and autism."

Obtaining precise figures for the number of children affected with autism has in the past been quite difficult because the government does not keep records. But the second study cited by the DOH looked at one area—north London—and found an alarming increase in autism there. The incidence was running steadily at between four and eight of the children born there each year between 1978 and 1985. Then came a dramatic increase to just under 50 of the children born in 1992, the last year studied by Professor Brent Taylor and colleagues at University College London. Even so, they concluded: "Our analyses do not support a causal association between MMR vaccine and autism."

Dr. Andrew Wakefield, the doctor whose research triggered the health scare over the MMR vaccine in the UK eventually moved to Texas and founded an autism center called the Thoughtful House. In February 2010 he resigned from the center following disciplinary hearings at the General Medical Council in London. The hearings ruled that he had acted callously, dishonestly, and irresponsibly over the 1998 paper in the Lancet medical journal, which claimed to have found a link between the MMR, bowel disease, and autism.

Recall that it was Wakefield's research that prompted a slump in the number of children administered the inoculation for measles, mumps, and rubella.

However, despite the UK's position as of this writing (2010) at least one case of vaccine-related autism has been verified by American courts. US Assistant attorney General Peter Keisler's ruled in November 2008 on one of three test cases into the MMR-autism link. In his conclusion Keisler said, "Compensation is appropriate."

The case involved a child who when she was eighteen months old received nine vaccinations, two of which included thimerosal, the mercury containing preservative which was in vaccines until 2002. Within days the girl, who had previously been healthy, suddenly stopped responding to verbal direction. She suffered a loss of language skills and eye contact. She began to suffer from insomnia, incessant screaming, and back arching. Seven months later a diagnosis of autism was confirmed.

The US government defended itself by pointing out that the girl had a pre-existing mitochondrial disorder, which was aggravated by the vaccine. The US court concluded that—in some cases—the MMR (measles mumps rubella) vaccine can cause autism. The question that remains is: are they only referring to old vaccines containing thimerosol or does the danger lie within the vaccine virus itself. Lots of kids with autism have mitochondrial disorders. In fact, probably many more than we are aware of, because children with autism are diagnosed and tested based on behavior. Very few children—autistic or not—have their mitochondria checked.

Perhaps Wakefield's rash "speaking out" about the vaccine / autism link led the way to accidental discovery or perhaps it led the way to erroneous believing; neither is easy to ascertain.

Interestingly, according to most media reports, since the American ruling of medical complicity in the mitochondrial case, which was one of 4,900 cases being considered for compensation, the situation instilled fear in many health officials that this finding could open the floodgates for even more claims. And it did. However, at the time (coincidently) of Wakefield's ruling most were overturned or had already fallen away. This Wakefield ruling, instead of closing the door to the issue of vaccinations, reopened the floodgates for renewed debate. Some advocates of the link between MMR vaccine and autism have changed position in light of the developments over the past year. For example, Alison Singer, a senior executive of Autism Speaks, who resigned from the group in January 2009, urged it to use its resources to look elsewhere for answers because "looking where we know the answer isn't is one less dollar we have to spend where we might find new answers. The fact is that vaccines save lives; they don't cause autism."

Other groups remained loyal to Wakefield and began campaigns of accusations that the new findings were a cover up.

For example, The National Autism Association posted this response only hours following the General Medical Council's decision: "Parents of children with autism around the world are calling the findings against Dr. Andrew Wakefield in the UK's General Medical Council unjust and a threat to researchers investigating autism as a medical condition." In addition this quote, posted on the Age of Autism Web site by Hollywood couple Jim Carrey and Jenny McCarthy, shows the adamants of many parent-driven organizations "It is our most sincere belief that Dr. Wakefield and parents of children with autism around the world are being subjected to a remarkable media campaign engineered by vaccine manufacturers reporting on the retraction of a paper published in The Lancet in 1998 by Dr. Wakefield and his colleagues." (Despite the fact that I stand on both sides of this fence, I feel compelled to point out that only parents are educated in the patterns of their children's lives. And though it would be considered "proper" to then also point out that scientists hold the science information while parents hold the lived history of the child, the truth is parents aren't locked out from what the medical professionals know whereas the same is not true in reverse. Parents can discover cures as readily as scientists can—evidenced by the story of Lorenzo's Oil—by investigating what the scientists know and applying it to what they have lived out. This is even easier now than it was at the time of Lorenzo's parents search for answers because what the scientists know has become infinitely easier to access. The same is not true for what the parents know about their child. Parents live with rather than document about the moments in their child's life, thus parental knowledge must be lived out to be accurately gained: It just may be that the solutions will be found in the hands of the parents with the best observational skills.)

For his part Dr. Wakefield remains steadfast on the subject of his innocence: "The allegations against me and my colleagues are both unfounded and unjust, and I invite anyone to examine the contents of these proceedings and come to their own conclusion."

Civil War era lawyer, orator, and philosopher Robert Green Ingersoll once said, "Science built the Academy, superstition the Inquisition." But science also created therapies such as blood letting for migraine headaches (there is some actual science logic here but no actual benefit). Since all fields or groups when found to be misinformed generally engage in cover up and denial, we can only hope that a flexible open-minded approach to embracing scientific proof and not superstition or financial or guilt-ridden fear drives the future of the debate in the relationship between childhood vaccines and autism.

For my part I deal with the fallout. The MMR debate led to large numbers of children being vigorously chelated as their parents tried to remove mercury from their over-laden children's brains. Given that many of us grew up with the expression "mad as a hatter" which referred to the mental illness caused by the mercuric chloride (mercury), Hatters were exposed to when making hats its not hard to comprehend the reason for the worry. After all, the devastating effects of mercury is not a secret; it's a poison we've written fairy tales around and one doesn't have to fall down a rabbit hole to be driven mad by this metal.

So I understand the logic behind why the parents chelate, but in general I hate the effects of chelation in the children I work with. Understand though that my lived experience is biased because if the treatment worked for the child and the child got better, then I am not called in to treat them. Thus I only meet the kids who weren't helped by chelation even though the parents often continue to do it. So my experience and subsequent opinion are somewhat tainted by the people I see. Perhaps Wakefield's ruling even the playing field and curb the MMR fear somewhat. However, perhaps it shouldn't.

How about if, instead of our medical community fearing the possible financial repercussions of the mitochondrial decision, we celebrate the possible health solutions that such a finding could lead to? Regardless of the fact that the mitochondrial girl's findings support Dr Andrew Wakefield's suggested link between vaccines and autism, even if he did gain the evidence for that link in an undesirable fashion. Perhaps the issue should be examined not from the question of how did we find out or what will it cost us or who does it offend but is it accurate? What if we stopped inoculating all children for five years? Would the numbers go down? Would the rate of autism drop from one in every seventy boys to one in every one hundred? In my opinion that would be definitive. But that is only my opinion, because in science there is always an out, as regards this sort of data: In science you will often hear "Correlation does not prove causation" and "If he got better it must have been a misdiagnosis." Strangely it seems often more palatable for medical professionals to accept their diagnostic flaws than it is for them to accept misinformed blame. It is called the Semmelweis Reflex and is much explained in Section One. The history of "is or isn't the MMR to blame" reminds me a little of that Semmelweis Reflex hand-washing question.

Personally, I don't think vaccines cause autism any more than dirty hands cause childbed fever. I just think that since the cause or complicating factor could possibly be on the dirty hand or in the contaminated needle one should clean it off, or out, or avoid it altogether. But then, that's just me. (wink)

My beliefs are not based on conspiracy theories but rather on the fact that …

**History has a way of repeating itself until
eventually we come around to the same issue enough times
to learn something new from it.
(Lucky number seven???)**

The widespread use of medical mercury in order to mass produce, cut costs, and increase profit margins, as well as the ensuing disagreement and denial of medical or government responsibility even to the point of accepting that there is any danger to be responsible for, is not a new debate exclusive to vaccines.

Way back in 1819 when an English chemist named Bell combined silver coin shavings and enough mercury to form a paste, dentists—eager for filling alternatives—embraced the new amalgam and labeled this fifty percent mercury compound that hasn't changed its composition much in the last 180 years "silver fillings." This cost-effective compound took dentistry out of the hands of the wealthy by giving patients who were previously stuck choosing between an expensive gold filling or a pulled tooth something affordable with which to repair their disintegrating enamel. In 1832 a couple of brothers brought the amalgam into America. They spread the paste and seeded the poison. In fact the term "quack originated as an abbreviated expression that referred to unconcerned dentists pouring mercury into mouths: In Europe, mercury is known as quicksilber. Any dentist who would place mercury fillings was called a quacksilber or quack for short.

The debate over mercury fillings is long and involved and has been going on since 1843. Dental associations were born and died over the issue of "to quack or not to quack." Groups were divided and dentists' licenses were pulled, while rules for and against quacksilber were written and rewritten to create pressure dependent upon the tides of the financial times. Eventually as the overbearing arm of the amalgam company grew stronger, dentists were forced to choose mercury over mental health. In America today dentists and consumers alike still choose to keep the money in their pocket and the mercury in their mouths as they put approximately fifty tons into their teeth each year. This is unfortunate given that human and animal studies have found a direct relationship between the level of mercury in the brain and the number of fillings in the mouth.

Mercury is very volatile. Vapors are released when the compound is agitated, compressed, or exposed to an acidic environment or increased temperatures. Thus, our acidic mouths are a perfect place to create these vapors as we grind, chew, and ingest especially hot food and beverages. In fact, mercury release increases approximately fifteen times when you introduce anything hot or acidic, when you chew, and even when you brush. But don't stop brushing because corrosion also releases mercury. (Kind of a Catch 22 mercury mayhem of the mouth.)

Once it is released into the mouth, mercury flows into the body, by either inhaled vapor or ingested particles. As vapor, it may pass into the bloodstream for quick absorption and distribution to body tissues or travel to the brain and central nervous system. When mercury particles are ingested, mercury chloride can be formed in the stomach; many of the bacteria there can transform it into methyl mercury, an even more poisonous form of the maddening metal.

Symptoms of mercury poisoning from dental amalgams are not limited to mouth problems like bleeding gums, white patches, metallic taste, burning sensations, ulcers, gum disease, and/or blackish purple discolorations. Mercury also affects the brain, causing depression, anxiety, hallucinations and mania. In the digestive system constipation, colitis, diarrhea, and cramps can develop. The thyroid is easily damaged by mercury as the endocrine and cardiovascular systems are compromised. Mercury often leaves the immune system weakened and vulnerable to secondary diseases and infections. In addition, the central nervous system shows symptoms such as chronic migraines, convulsions, dizziness, epilepsy, loss of fine motor coordination (especially in the hands), muscle paralysis or twitching, arm and leg numbness, tremors and tingling in the hands, feet and lips. Diseases such as multiple sclerosis (MS) have been indicated as a possible outcome of the toxic overload one's dental work can create.

Since studies show that mercury passes through the placental membrane in pregnant women and into the brain of the developing child, it is plausible to consider that autism might be just another disease of the mouth. Thus, mom's dental amalgams are a complicating factor when considering mercury toxicity in autistic children, especially given the increased odds of diagnosis when the toxicity happens in utero. Worst of all scenarios is to expose your fetus by having dental work done during pregnancy. However, even if Mom diligently waited to have her teeth fixed until after her baby was born but then breastfed (out of love and a desire to keep her baby healthy), she might still unknowingly increase the risk of damage because unfortunately mercury is also suspected of passing into infants via breast milk.

The point is, the issue of mercury and government responsibility does not begin and end with vaccines. Nor does that responsibility fall merely on the shoulders of the government: consumers, medical professionals, and big business all share a piece of this problematic pie. The fact is regardless of how the children become toxic many are. And since, when working with and observing autistic individuals, all of the above symptoms can be seen in some, some symptoms in all, and none with none, it is necessary that we work together to clean up and become informed if we wish to end the suffering. It is interesting to me that every time I give a talk, there are so many who throw their hands up in despair and ask why the autism figures are climbing. Truly, with such a toxin-filled environment wherein our carpet and furniture-filled homes, our clothing, our air, our water, our food, our electric fields, our background radiation and radio waves have all been tapered with, the healthy babies are the ones to be perplexed and amazed by. But don't be overwhelmed by progress. Be benefited by it. We are lucky. We live in an information accessible world. It is up to us, the individual, to become knowledgeable, responsible, and willing to make the moment-to-moment choices that will cause big business to create cheaper less toxic solutions as we attempt to survive and raise and satisfy our families. Remember, big business isn't a thing; it's a group of people running a thing, and they get autism too.

It is easy to fill oneself with the passion of blame and avoid actually fixing anything by turning our pointing fingers into fists of rage, but that doesn't generally help the child at home. It can, however, dilute the effectiveness of scientists and therapists who have to watch their back instead of your children's brains. This blame infused Semmelweis Reflex type behavior splashes everywhere as medical doctors flat out disbelieve the lived experiences of parents who describe watching their children disappear in front of their loving eyes when the inoculation-induced fever passed. Many medical professionals deny the lived experience of the parents because it doesn't fit into the literature they subscribe to, and often as a result the parents then turn their backs on the doctors skill and experience just as the doctor turned his back on them and theirs.

I, along with many other neurofeedback specialists, deal with a goodly amount of fallout from this knee-jerk behavior. Even as we hold out our sensor-filled hands offering help to parents and professionals, both of these groups often refuse to investigate the evidence we present them with. They simply disbelieve our experiences as we report on this amazing therapy and the healings it has facilitated. Perhaps this is because having things be so simple —as some beeps from a machine teaching a brain to improve seizure thresholds or let go of stress in such a way that it changes that person's pursuant behaviors—doesn't fit into most people's previously held idea of hardworking sufferer or lifelong disorder. Strangely it is the role of hardworking sufferer and lifelong disorder that many people prefer to live with, hold on to, and embrace. Ironically, as it turns out, believing in easy is very often hard. But we should choose to believe in easy anyway because then it is easy.

As it turns out a world of people grabbing pills and people disdaining pills—all based on emotionally driven ideas rather than experience and information—is a problem perpetuating one. Unfortunately, in a society such as ours many people stand in different camps pointing righteous fingers of superiority at each other. Thus the various groups argue about non-useful criteria for credibility like degrees being valued before lived experience and lived experience being valued before degrees. The arguments are heated with passion and a great excuse to not actually look at the issues we say we wish to solve. Hence it is that many, or possibly even most, people live in a world of "talk to the hand I don't want to listen" because they might have to change something and take action upon themselves once they hear what the other camp has got to say".

It is our resistance that slows down our progress and reinforces the disabilities in our kids. If you think about it, when we behave like this—running around with our fingers in our ears and looking at only the issues we are comforted to see—we are modeling autism.

I realize how broadly based this book is. That is on purpose. It is my intention to inform you and then ask you to use that information with your child or client or area of study... find solutions and then bring that information fearlessly out into the world to swim in the pool of what is already known as we search for and gather answers. It is my intention to ask each of you to embrace the expertise of the other.

Last month I attended a symposium. I listened to the evidence of scientists who had worked with minute attention to detail investigating viruses, bacteria, and antibodies in the blood of ASD individuals. (Note: I assume that they were supported at least in part by government funds and that their ensuing success was in part due to the responsibility the government takes, especially when it wants to find something besides mercury as the cause for this pervasive developmental disorder. All problems have a silver lining.) They had been searching for answers and found PANDAS (Pediatric Autoimmune Neuropsychiatric Disorders Associated with Streptococcal infections). This is a condition caused by an immune reaction triggered by the presence of Group A Beta-Hemolytic Streptococcal infection.

Various strep bacteria produce toxins as part of their infectious nature. The immune system responds in an attempt to neutralize and eradicate the toxins. However, this immune-toxin reaction creates immune complexes that are deposited in various tissues of the body. If these immune complexes land in the kidneys there is an immune reaction called post-streptococcal glomerulonephritis; in the heart it is called rheumatic fever, and in the brain PANDAS can ensue.

The autoimmune reaction in PANDAS is directed to the Basal Ganglia area in the brain. This area has been associated with disorders such as obsessive-compulsiveness (OCD), strange body posturing/movements called chorea, and the typical TIC movements (quick jerking or vocal tics) associated with Tourette's syndrome. Thus, though having PANDAS doesn't equate with having autism, since these symptoms are often part of autism, having autism often correlates with having PANDAS.

According to the scientists at this symposium, though PANDAS (especially the OCD aspect) responds quite well to a long-term course of Penicillin, the best treatment is intravenous immunoglobulins (IVIG), which is aimed at short-circuiting the autoimmune response. Another treatment option is plasmapheresis, a blood-cleansing process performed to help diminish the immune-toxin reactions. These treatments (like many things related to autism) are both expensive and controversial. In fact, even PANDAS itself is challenged as a diagnosis, likely because it is still diagnosed via a history of symptoms and therefore the influencing "strep" factor is elusive to find with certainty. Thus children with PANDAS are easy to pass off as just another child with Autism Spectrum Disorder. Therefore, if you go to your neurotherapist for help with your child's OCD symptoms, you are unlikely to be offered IVIG or plasmapheresis or even penicillin though a prescription for antidepressant may be readily handed out. Be informed! If you think your child has PANDAS and you want to try the treatment, ask.

So there I was, just another conference attendee, listening to the separate camps on the issues of "is it real or is it not" when the oft-flung arguments against inoculations and antibiotics came to mind. I thought of all the parents who wish to blame the vaccines or the anti-biotics prescribed to their children in the early years before the autism showed itself and realized that, not just the mood-enhancing prescription pad pusher but, they themselves, would likely miss this information in order to believe that it was doctors rather than viruses that were to blame. (It's just plain hard to point your finger at a virus.) I found myself again thinking about all the groups with beliefs sending them searching for answers, like parents and doctors who wish to find and redesign the illness causing genetic anomaly and so will likely miss the truth of how mercury might precipitate the disorder: All the different groups pre-deciding what to look for and then finding it. Most likely, they find it because all the answers are correct, as everyone holds a part of the answer. "'If we want to know it all we would do well to hear each other," I thought and then, laughing to myself, realized I'd been daydreaming. I tuned back into the lecture as these wonderful doctors described their very difficult, very precise, very successful (during the study) treatment.

For me it is wonderful to know that these people exist: Working and working and working to find the cause. Their skills are not mine. I cannot do this type of work. Though I am relentless at teaching to the brain, studying blood is beyond my interest. Hopefully, their skills will mix with mine. Parents and educators will know how to respond to behavior and doctors and therapist will know how to heal. Hopefully my job will become obsolete. For that I would be eternally grateful.

Don't misunderstand; I love my job. I love autistic children and I no longer bemoan their condition. I just dig in and help. But that doesn't mean I don't see how much it hurts, how difficult this epidemic is for everyone it touches, even if the silver lining does shine like a diamond glittering in the sun. Still, I would love to be out of a job. Especially where Dar is concerned.

So Are the Inoculations Ever to Blame? And now that Thimerosol is (apparently) Out of the Vaccine, is the Vaccine Safe?

Well, let's consider what a vaccine is: A vaccine is the introduction of a weakened virus in minute amounts. This introduction is meant to cause just a little illness that will teach the body how to fight the virus and create immunity. It is a great idea that has saved millions of lives, but it is an idea based on the theory that the person receiving the vaccine has a healthy immune system. If your child has a toxin-laden or damaged immune system—something of which you may not be aware—then getting him/her vaccinated is probably not a good idea. No vaccine is one hundred percent safe (even if your doctor doesn't bother to mention this.). And the controversy surrounding the MMR makes that vaccine even more dubious.

In the case of the MMR question ,not only the mercury containing preservative used (until 2002 and possibly about to be reintroduced) to keep the vaccine fresh but also the measles virus itself have been implicated as contributing to the rising levels of autism. At present most researchers believe that autism is a genetic disorder with a predisposition to being unable to handle toxins, allergens, and heavy metals like lead and mercury so prevalent in our environment. But many naturopaths and complimentary medical professionals believe it is also related to the measles virus found hiding in the gut of autistic children: An interesting correlation since the gut of an autistic child is rarely, if ever, entirely healthy. Vaccines—the injection of the illness you are trying to avoid—has always been known to cause minor side effects such as fevers or rashes and sometimes serious life-threatening conditions. With that in mind, and since the start of the recent increase in autism can be traced back to children who were born in the mid 1980s in Britain and the 1970s in the United States, (these were the first children to receive the MMR vaccine) and since the question is complicated by the present-day fact that these kids have high levels of mercury and the thirmerosol has now been removed from the vaccines, but not from the environment, to date, the question of safety is not an easy one to answer.

What Are the Risks of Not Vaccinating with MMR?

Four years ago measles caused over a million deaths in children around the world, mainly in countries without widespread vaccinations. A decline in the number of children who are vaccinated could cause an increase in the number of measles, mumps, and rubella cases and sickness (such as pneumonia and brain damage which ironically is what autism is) and much death in the United States. For example, before measles vaccines were introduced, one to two children died out of every one thousand children who got measles.

Perhaps the only way to truly address the controversy will be to change the immunization habits of the population and then study the results. At any rate the present danger to not immunizing your child is minimal given that the majority of children are still being vaccinated effectively reducing the number of carriers. And added to that is the fact that those large numbers of children who died before vaccines were introduced were living at a time with fewer medical advances. At present we are much more likely to see the children safely through any measles-related illness. Thus the numbers from then should not be thrown about and related to what the numbers would be now.

Should I Not Have My Child Vaccinated with MMR until more is Known about the Risks of Getting Autism?

This is a question for each individual to answer based on their own opinion of the situation. However, in light of all the families I work with, their case histories and the case histories of my own children, if I did choose to vaccinate anyone again I would do it like jumping off a cliff—with my eyes closed and praying for safety. Why? Because though there is not likely any risk of getting autism from the MMR vaccine, it is clear that when combined with a preexisting condition the vaccine can trigger onset. And since the preexisting condition would be invisible to me or I wouldn't be considering vaccinating in the first place, I'd have to close my eyes and pray.

Admittedly, even after evaluating the scientific evidence, many committees still support the advice of pediatricians that people should continue getting their children vaccinated using the current recommended dose schedule. But fortunately many also don't.

The Hippocratic principle is that doctors should "first do no harm." So my thought is that at the very least parents must be told of the concerns surrounding the MMR vaccine. Doctors should obtain "informed consent" when offering any medical intervention, especially when the "patient" is not ill to start with. That means discussing the risks as well as the benefits.

Would it be Better to Vaccinate My Child with Separate Measles, Mumps, and Rubella Vaccines Rather than the MMR Vaccine?

I would consider either using the vaccines singly, vaccinating only for rubella (to prevent birth defects during pregnancy), or not vaccinating at all. It may be safer for healthy children to catch these illnesses rather than run the risk of immunization. My opinion here is a little biased because Dar—the son who is still autistic—was vaccinated repeatedly as a result of our moving from one country to another while each country had different school enforced inoculation rules to comply with. Each time he was inoculated we lost some more of his hard-won functioning. By the time I was informed enough to have stopped this the—possibly coincidental—damage was already done. In retrospect, I don't believe that Dar's inoculations caused his autism. I do, however, think they were a contributing factor to his inability to heal in a more profound way.

CHAPTER TWELVE

Autism Spectrum Disorders Defined

There are several pervasive developmental disorders, and even within one particular disorder (e.g., autistic spectrum disorder), individuals differ in the spectrum of symptoms. Your child may even fit into more than one of the disorders as defined by different diagnosticians. In addition, due to the creation of a spectrum of choices many experts still disagree as to whether a particular disability belongs as a PDD or an ASD though ASD is becoming the more accepted term. This is because there are common elements to all the disorders. When searching for a label the diagnostician relies heavily on how you, the parent, represent your child. Thus, since there are some subtle differences among the disorders that become important when designing a treatment protocol, you become an integral part of your child's healing process every step of the way.

What are the differences among the various pervasive developmental disorders?

The five disorders under PDD are:

1. Autistic Disorder
2. Asperger's Disorder
3. PDD-Not Otherwise Specified (PDD-NOS)
4. Childhood Disintegrative Disorder (CDD)
5. Rett's Disorder

Autistic Disorder (Originally called Early Infantile Autism or Kanner's Syndrome) There are three distinctive behaviors that characterize autism. Autistic children have difficulties with social interaction, problems with verbal and nonverbal communication, and repetitive behaviors or narrow, obsessive interests. These behaviors can range in impact from mild to disabling. The hallmark feature of autism is impaired social interaction. Parents are usually the first to notice symptoms of autism in their child. As early as infancy, a baby with autism may be unresponsive to people or focus intently on one item to the exclusion of others for long periods of time. A child with autism may appear to develop normally and then withdraw and become indifferent to social engagement.

Children with autism may fail to respond to their name and often avoid eye contact with other people. They have difficulty interpreting what others are thinking or feeling because they can't understand social cues, such as tone of voice or facial expressions, and don't watch other people's faces for clues about appropriate behavior. They give the appearance of lacking empathy.

Many children with autism engage in repetitive movements such as rocking and twirling, or in self-abusive behavior such as biting or head banging. They also tend to start speaking later than other children and may refer to themselves by name instead of "I" or "me." Children with autism don't know how to play interactively with other children. Some speak in a singsong or monotone voice about a narrow range of favorite topics, with little regard for the interests of the person to whom they are speaking.

Many children with autism have a reduced sensitivity to pain; many are abnormally sensitive to sound, touch, or other sensory stimulation. These unusual reactions may contribute to behavioral symptoms such as a resistance to being cuddled or hugged.

Children with autism appear to have a higher than normal risk for certain coexisting conditions, including Fragile X syndrome (which causes mental retardation), tuberous sclerosis (in which tumors grow on the brain), epileptic seizures, Tourette syndrome, learning disabilities, and attention deficit disorder. Sometimes autism is the secondary diagnosis and the core disability is something else—like my adopted son Cash who had fetal alcohol syndrome accompanied by "Autistic-Like Mannerisms." (This is an old term meaning PDD that is never used today.) For reasons that are still unclear, about twenty to thirty percent of children with autism develop epilepsy by the time they reach adulthood. While people with schizophrenia may show some autistic-like behavior, their symptoms usually do not appear until the late teens or early adulthood. Most people with schizophrenia also have hallucinations and delusions and these are not known to be found in autism.

Asperger Syndrome is a separate developmental disorder that does not meet the criteria of other pervasive developmental disorders. Features of Asperger's are severe and sustained impairment in social interaction; the development of repetitive patterns of behavior, interests, and activities; and significant impairment in social, occupational, and other important areas of functioning. Interestingly, though boys are four times more likely to have autism than girls, boys are eight times more likely to have Asperger's than girls within the pervasive developmental population.

Individuals with Asperger Syndrome often appear on the surface to have normal language skills and, in fact, often appear to speak as though they are college professors or very intelligent or eccentric people. This sometimes masks the language deficits they do possess in the area of pragmatics (the give and take of conversation). However, the greatest difficulty people with AS have is their profound difficulty in relating in acceptable ways to other people, particularly to same-aged peers (i.e. children). While those with autism may be aloof or withdrawn, many times individuals with AS seek out other children but in very awkward or rigid ways that other children find strange. Individuals with AS, particularly as they grow and develop, are often teased about their odd ways of relating to others and about their unique ways of communicating.

Individuals with AS also display ritualistic behaviors, although many do not exhibit the stereotypic motor movements so commonly thought of as autistic behavior. Instead, these individuals pursue with a vengeance very particular topics of interest that can be as simple as cartoon characters or as unusual as water towers, or amassing facts about the migration patterns of the brown bear. It is the quality of these obsessions that is unusual. An AS person's obsessions usually engulf the majority of that individual's time and thoughts, often to the point where it dominates their conversations and activities.

Many individuals with Asperger Syndrome exhibit academic skills that fall into the superior or genius range, although some individuals show characteristics of learning disabilities as well. Quite often, these latter individuals most commonly exhibit a particular type of learning pattern known as a non-verbal learning disability. This entails poor grapho-motor and visual-perceptual skills combined with immense difficulties in math calculation skills. They also often have difficulties with tactile sensory issues (touch). Additionally, some individuals with AS also possess delayed fine-motor skills and are often described as quite clumsy.

There is great disagreement among experts about whether AS is an interchangeable term with High-Functioning Autism or whether it is a distinct, separate diagnostic category. However, in general, individuals with AS often have better outcomes if they are given the appropriate supports. Finally, it is highly important that individuals with AS not be pushed too hard. Often, educators as well as parents may be blinded by their strengths and not fully realize the amount of effort and energy it takes for these individuals to make it through the day. As such, individuals with AS are at very high risk for developing secondary emotional disorders such as anxiety and depression if they are not fully supported while learning in their own unique manner.

Pervasive Developmental Disorder—Not Otherwise Specified (PDD—NOS) is a non-specific diagnosis, which in general, means that the clinician didn't feel that the individual had enough characteristics of another more specific diagnosis (usually autism) to qualify for that diagnosis. However, in practice, what PDD-NOS often means is that the clinician or educational team didn't have enough expertise in autism spectrum disorders to make a specific diagnosis. Additionally, some clinicians don't feel that a family can accept the diagnosis or feel that the family might give up on the child if the clinician or educational team gives an autism diagnosis.

Many professionals with expertise in autism feel that PDD-NOS is a "non-diagnosis." International authorities such as Dr. Bernard Rimland of the Autism Research Institute in San Diego, CA feel that PDD-NOS is merely another way of saying, "I don't know what is wrong with your child." Currently, there is universal disagreement as to what degree of impairment constitutes the difference between an autism or PDD-NOS diagnosis, and it is likely that if a child has received the latter, the family will hear many different terms used to describe their child over the years.

In general, however, individuals diagnosed with PDD-NOS will have the same difficulties as those diagnosed with autism, although perhaps to a lesser extent. The interventions for PDD-NOS are the same as those for autism, and early intervention is still one of the most important aspects of treatment for any child with an autistic spectrum disorder. Nevertheless, it is important to remember that any intervention should be geared toward the individual needs of the child. That said, it should be noted that any available information related to autism will also be useful and applicable to a child diagnosed with PDD-NOS.

Again, the label may depend more on the expertise of the clinician giving the diagnosis as well as the geographic region where the child is diagnosed than on the actual characteristics of the child.

Childhood Disintegrative Disorder is—as the name implies— a disorder of disintegration of previously held skills. It occurs in children age three to four who were typical until age two. Over several months, a child with this disorder will experience a loss of intellectual, social, and language functioning.

Doctors sometimes confuse this rare disorder with late-onset autism because both conditions involve normal development followed by significant loss of language, social play, and motor skills. However, there's a more dramatic loss of skills in children with childhood disintegrative disorder and a greater likelihood of mental retardation. In addition, childhood disintegrative disorder is far less common than autism and has a later age of onset.

Childhood disintegrative disorder is also known as Heller's syndrome after the Viennese educator, Theodor Heller, who first described the condition, which he initially proposed be called dementia infantilis. It has also been named disintegrative psychosis and pervasive disintegrative disorder.

As far as treatment and prognosis go, there is no real reason to differentiate between childhood disintegrative disorder, autism, and PDD-NOS. No cause is known for any of them and treatments are the same. As for prognosis there is so much individuality in all of the pervasive developmental disorders that essentially we come down to the same answer over and over again: Early intervention is the key.

Rett Syndrome is a rare disorder that affects one in every 10,000 to 15,000 live female births. It occurs in all racial and ethnic groups worldwide. It is usually included as a Pervasive Developmental Disorder because there is some confusion with autism—particularly in the preschool years. Otherwise the course, cause, and onset of this condition is much more fully understood than autism is.

In people with Rett syndrome very early development is normal. Head growth then slows. It is a childhood neurodevelopmental disorder characterized by normal early development followed by loss of purposeful use of the hands, distinctive hand movements, gait abnormalities, seizures, loss of speech, and mental retardation. It affects both males and females but the males die shortly after birth so it is considered a female only disorder.

There are four stages of Rett syndrome. Stage I, called early onset, generally begins between six and eighteen months of age. Symptoms at this stage can be somewhat vague, so parents and doctors may not notice the subtle slowing of development. The infant may begin to show less eye contact and have reduced interest in toys. There may be delays in gross motor skills such as sitting or crawling. Hand wringing and decreasing head growth may occur, but not enough to draw attention. This stage usually lasts for a few months but can persist for more than a year.

Stage II, or the rapid destructive stage, usually begins between ages one and four and may last for weeks or months as purposeful hand skills and spoken language are lost. Some girls also display autistic-like symptoms such as loss of social interaction and communication. General irritability and sleep irregularities may be seen. Gait patterns are unsteady and initiating motor movements can be difficult. Slowing of head growth is usually noticed during this stage. The characteristic hand movements (wringing, washing, clapping, or tapping, as well as repeatedly moving the hands to the mouth) become obvious. Hands are sometimes clasped behind the back or held at the sides, with random touching, grasping, and releasing. The movements persist while the child is awake but disappear during sleep. Breathing irregularities such as episodes of apnea and hyperventilation may occur, although breathing is usually normal during sleep.

Stage III, usually begins between ages two and ten and can last for years. Though apraxia, motor problems, and seizures are prominent during this stage, there may also be improvement in behavior, with less irritability, crying, and autistic-like features. An individual in stage III may show more interest in her surroundings; and her alertness, attention span, and communication skills may improve. Many girls remain in this stage for most of their lives.

The last stage, stage IV—called the late motor deterioration stage—can last for years or decades and is characterized by reduced mobility. Girls who were previously able to walk may stop walking. Generally, there is no decline in cognition, communication, or hand skills in stage IV. Repetitive hand movements may decrease, and eye gaze usually improves.

Rett syndrome is caused by mutations in a gene, which is found on the X chromosome. Scientists identified the gene—MECP2—in 1999. Because the MECP2 gene does not function properly in those with Rett syndrome, insufficient amounts or structurally abnormal forms of a protein called methyl cytosine are formed. The absence or malfunction of the protein is believed to cause other genes to be abnormally expressed, but this hypothesis has not yet been confirmed. This is an incurable (at present) lifelong disorder. Life expectancy is shortened though many people live well into their forties. Because it is a rare disorder little is known about what can and can't be expected or even hoped for within an afflicted woman's lifetime.

Autism (Autistic Spectrum Disorder) is a disorder of social, communicative, and repetitive behaviors that are sometimes accompanied by severe fears, phobias, tantrums, overly-sensitive sensory systems, retardation, special talents (autistic savant), self-injurious behavior (e.g., head banging), an inability to creatively fill leisure time, and skill sets that can be learned and then forgotten on a repeated basis.

Atypical Autism (late onset) is different from typical autism in that it is often diagnosed as having had an onset after three years of age. It also has an increased dual diagnosis of retardation or low IQ scores. My son Chance received this diagnosis only after he had been diagnosed with so many learning, sensory, and logical processing challenges that eventually the various disabilities were all gathered up under one umbrella and renamed Atypical Autism. This type of reasoning may be responsible for some of the rise in the numbers of children diagnosed with ASD today. Additionally, your child may receive this diagnosis if he/she only meets two of the three social, communication, and repetitive diagnostic criteria of autism. Thus, since IQ deficits are typically easier to teach to than social, communication, and repetitive disorders, this means that atypical autism may be easier to treat than autism.

ASD Statistics or Prevalence of Autism

Autism is the most common of the Pervasive Developmental Disorders, affecting an estimated one in 150 births (Centers for Disease Control and Prevention, 2007). Roughly translated, this means as many as 1.5 million Americans today are believed to have some form of autism. And this number is on the rise.

Based on statistics from the U.S. Department of Education and other governmental agencies, autism is growing at a startling rate of ten to seventeen percent per year. At this rate, the Autism Society of America estimates that the prevalence of autism could reach four million Americans in the next decade.

Autism knows no racial, ethnic or social boundaries. Family income, lifestyle, or education levels are not factors. It can affect any family, any child.

And although the overall incidence of autism is consistent around the globe, it is four times more prevalent in boys than in girls.

Are There Disorders that Accompany Autism?

Several disorders commonly accompany autism. To some extent, these may be caused by a common underlying problem in brain functioning.

Mental Retardation:

Of the problems that can occur with autism, mental retardation is the most widespread. Seventy-five to eighty percent of people with autism are mentally retarded to some extent. Fifteen to twenty percent are considered severely retarded, with IQs below thirty-five. (A score of one hundred represents average intelligence). But autism does not necessarily correspond with mental impairment. More than ten percent of people with autism have an average or above average IQ. A few show exceptional intelligence. And many are simply not testable. (Thus these numbers are highly suspect, especially considering that some clinicians probably report untestable clients as testing in the retarded range instead of simply stating "not testable.")

Interpreting IQ scores is difficult, however, because most intelligence tests are not designed for people with autism. People with autism do not perceive or relate to their environment in typical ways. When tested, some areas of ability are normal or even above average, and some areas may be especially weak. For example, a child with autism may do extremely well on the parts of the test that measure visual skills but earn low scores on the language subtests.

Seizures:

About one-third of the children with autism develop seizures, starting either in early childhood or adolescence. Researchers are trying to learn if there is any significance to the time of onset, since the seizures often first appear when certain neurotransmitters become active.

Since seizures range from brief blackouts to full-blown body convulsions, an electroencephalogram (EEG) can help confirm their presence. Fortunately, in most cases, seizures can either be completely eradicated or seizure thresholds lowered through the repeated use of neurofeedback therapy, a high-protein diet and flax oil. This treatment can be complimented by medication where necessary.

Fragile X:

Fragile X is often confused with autistic spectrum disorder due to the large number of fragile X individuals that also have autism: One third of all fragile X individuals have autism. Fragile X is a hereditary/genetic condition and one of the most common causes of genetically inherited mental impairment. Its effects range from subtle learning disabilities with normal IQ scores to severe retardation, autism and "autistic like" symptoms. Fragile X syndrome has been found in about five to ten percent of people with autism, mostly males. This inherited disorder is named for a defective piece of the X-chromosome that appears pinched and fragile when seen under a microscope.

People who inherit this faulty bit of genetic code are more likely to have mental retardation and many of the same symptoms as autism along with unusual physical features that are not typical of autism. Since many families are completely unaware that they carry the defective chromosome, it is always a good idea to have any autistic diagnostic include testing the individual in question for fragile X.

Tuberous Sclerosis:

There is also some relationship between autism and Tuberous Sclerosis, a genetic condition that causes abnormal tissue growth in the brain and problems in other organs. Although Tuberous Sclerosis is a rare disorder, occurring less than once in 10,000 births, about a fourth of those affected are also autistic.

Hyperlexia is a remarkable disorder that is sometimes considered a subset of Asperger syndrome and is sometimes considered a disorder of its own. Hyperlexic children have a precocious ability to read words far above what would be expected for their chronological age or an intense fascination with letters or numbers. However, they have significant impairments in verbal comprehension, in social skills, and in interacting appropriately with people. They may listen selectively, appear deaf, echo what is said to them (echolalia), or rote memorize commercials or passages from books with no apparent understanding of the meaning: Difficulty using pronouns correctly and comprehending "What…Where…Who…Why?" questions. Like Asperger's individuals, hyperlexics can be very literal thinkers with difficulty comprehending metaphors. The hyperlexic child is best helped with a program of intensive speech therapy that focuses on language and comprehension skills and uses the child's reading skills as the primary teaching tool. ** Teaching that uses a child's interests and already-established skill sets and that builds on those skill sets using positive reinforcement is the most effective way to teach any child, on or off the spectrum. **

Scientists are exploring genetic conditions such as Fragile X and Tuberous Sclerosis to see why they so often coincide with autism. Understanding exactly how these conditions disrupt normal brain development may provide insights to the biological and genetic mechanisms of autism.

What Research Is Being Done?

Eight dedicated research centers across the country have been established as *Centers of Excellence in Autism Research* to bring together researchers and the resources they need. The Centers are conducting basic clinical research, including investigations into causes, diagnoses, early detection, prevention, and treatment. Investigators are using animal models to study how the neurotransmitter serotonin establishes connections between neurons in hopes of discovering why these connections are impaired in autism… researchers are testing a computer-assisted program that would help autistic children interpret facial expressions…a brain imaging study is investigating areas of the brain that are active during obsessive/repetitive behaviors in adults and very young children with autism...other imaging studies are searching for brain abnormalities that could cause impaired social communication in children with autism... clinical studies are testing the effectiveness of a program that combines parent training and medication to reduce the disruptive behavior of children with autism and other ASDs.

Researchers are investigating the potential for autism to develop in utero. It is known that contracting rubella during pregnancy and Strep when very young can, in rare cases, cause autism. This is referred to as PANDAS- Pediatric Autoimmune Neurological Disorder Associated with Strep. Slowly but surely science is finding the way... by studying everything imaginable...

Like: The now famous fruit-fly research wherein scientists discovered that a protein called neurexin may be a genetic risk factor in autism because it is required for nerve cells to form and function properly. This research became a much-talked-about item when Sarah Palin, John McCain's running mate in the 2008 Presidential election, spoke out against it as a waste of money while simultaneously promising to fully fund programs in support of special needs children. Oops!

Research can be done in a laboratory or hospital or on a trends sheet. Globally we are attacking the problem from all sides. In my field positive outcomes have been found in studies designed to establish efficacy with neurofeedback as a treatment for autism and more of these control-group studies are underway. But even before reaching the level of double-blind-control-group study, any preliminary investigation can give us clues to help shape our choices and behaviors. For example, a preliminary study out of California reviewed long lists of products used from a few months before conception until the child turned one. Out of their 500 children (some autistic, some not) 138 of the children with autism were twice as likely to report using pet shampoos, bug sprays, and other products containing pyrenthin than the parents of the neurotypical children were. So read the label and don't buy the pyrenthin.

My ears perked up when I read this report because it reminded me of my two biological grandsons who both displayed symptoms of autism. They were my daughter's youngest two. These children were born during our bug-spraying spree: our newly purchased home was infested with roaches. So we sprayed and sprayed and sprayed. The roaches died but maybe so did some of the children's brain cells. Of course there were other markers for those children, other demons to blame for their symptoms: Like the fact that the youngest was a part of a short-lived group of children that got his vaccination just after birth shortly before leaving the hospital. So the bug spray is just one of many possibilities. At present, just as we've come to see cancer is a gene that is turned on by toxins of many different forms. With autism there are no clear culprits and the picture is always complicated.

Much as we'd like to know who the bad guy is so we can incarcerate him away from our children, very often there isn't just one. We are challenged on who to blame and, rather than incarcerating, we end up educating, both our children and ourselves. Fortunately we don't need to know why to do that. In my house we stopped spraying and taught the grandchildren. At present they are "off the spectrum."

Is There Reason for Hope with Autism?

Once thought of as "untreatable" or "incurable," discoveries of genetic factors and chemical imbalances offer much hope for families of children with autistic spectrum disorders. But hope doesn't have to be held in wait for the next scientific breakthrough to come trumpeting in with the "cause" of the disorder. Hope for recovery exists now and is the reason behind the words "early intervention." One of the best interventions I have witnessed and/or worked with in the field today is EEG biofeedback for the brain (neurofeedback). It is a most exciting scientific advancement. Neurofeedback is a holistic approach that does not rely on medications and that can make observable changes for the better in the individual being treated. The changes are both comparatively rapid and permanent in the majority of cases.

Even without neurofeedback there is a lot already in place and available to families. Some examples of family-based behavior and cognitive therapy play programs are as follows: Son-Rise®, RDI, Greenspan aka Floortime, TEAACH, Miller Method, Response Training, Discrete Trial Training, ABA, Lovaas, and Growing Minds. Also available are speech therapy; sensory integration techniques; and visual, auditory, and vestibular retraining programs. Though for the most part medications have been found ineffective in the treatment of autism, sometimes symptoms of the disorder (e.g., hyperactivity, self-injurious behavior) can be eased through the use of medication. Also many clinicians have reported success using a variety of "alternative therapies" like homeopathy. And despite the overriding "professional" opinion that autism is a lifelong disorder, there are many, many stories of children overcoming their diagnosis after having had interventions from play programs like Floortime, or therapies like neurofeedback, or diets like the GFCF, or miracle discoveries like the off label usage of the hormone Secretin, or all of the above at the same time. One of our celebrities, herself a mom of autism, Jenny McCarthy has been making a lot of good noise while sharing stories of families around the Nation wherein she, and all those other moms, have made a real difference in the symptoms of their child. Truly the question is no longer "Is there hope?" but rather "What am I hoping for?"

My answer is "The next step. I am always after the next step. And since that's not so far to reach I always get there." I have my own way of looking at things. For example, I call my kids "off the spectrum" once they are completely independent, mostly happy, and a little bit quirky. For me that's normal enough. You'll have to find your own definition.

CHAPTER THIRTEEN

Treating Autism

Ok, so now is where the fun begins. Unlike many disorders, treating autism does not have one particular suggested therapy that you will do once or twice a week, and then just cross your fingers and hope that weekly progress turns into emergence from autism. Instead, treating autism will become a way of life. Continually researching new modalities and deciding whether they are right for your family and your child will become second nature. Having a positive and loving attitude is about to become the most important part of your therapy; not only will your attitude play a huge role in your child's progress but it will also decide what your experience of raising your autistic child is like. You will be tailoring a program to suit your individual child, utilizing many of the therapies/treatments out there and changing therapies as your child changes, progresses, and grows. Yes, treating autism takes work, hard work, but it is not without its benefits. In my experience every family that abandons their feelings of despair and takes on an attitude of proactive parenting not only begins to see big changes in their child, but their entire experience of raising their autistic child and living their lives becomes a positive and mind-expanding one.

To reiterate from Section One I will take a little digression here. In case you are reading Section Two first I want to give you a snapshot of what my experience with treatment for one of my sons

has been like. Dar is my oldest and definitely most autistic son. In fact, after raising four boys on the spectrum of autism, two grandsons on the spectrum, and working with countless families with children with autism, my son Dar is still the most severely autistic person I have ever met. (My other three sons and two grandsons no longer meet the criteria for a diagnosis of autism.) As such, Dar has been the catalyst for a large part of my autism education. I have tried many things with Dar. I have done ABA, Son-Rise®, auditory training, a myriad of supplements, secretin, bio meds, blue green algae, and the gluten-free, casein-free diet you name it I've tried it, or at least it feels like I have. And every single one of these things helped—some a little, some a lot. But where Dar was concerned none of these glorious effects ever lasted. In fact, though the GFCF diet and the introduction of some essential supplements (that will be listed in detail later) has been essential to two of my sons' progress, it wasn't until I discovered neurofeedback therapy that I finally saw the greatest and longest-lasting (still going strong) changes in both of them that I had ever seen. I quickly became a professional practitioner of this modality, if at first for no other reason than to learn as much about it as I possibly could for my son.

Dar began as my first patient. He was twenty-three years old. He was easily frustrated, non-verbal, self- injurious, and occasionally violent. When not in a fit of sensory overload he was totally sweet. Dar was one hundred percent dependent on others. His hands were mostly closed; he could manipulate very few objects, and he had an intense tremor whenever he would purposefully reach for something. I'd done everything I could think of to help him and still he was truly the most autistic man I have met to date. Then Dar did neurofeedback. By the time he was twenty-six he was talking, **yes, talking!!** Others could understand him a little. He could use his CD player and help fold clothes. He continues to improve every day. At present, I have quit all other therapies and use only neurofeedback to facilitate this constant progress. At this point my family coexists in harmony with him and the neighbor kids occasionally invite him along. Best of all, he doesn't hit anyone, not even himself (well sometimes he uses a good clunk on the chin as an expression of "so there"). Dar requests neurofeedback if he feels stressed, though we don't always understand his request because neurofeedback is hard to say. According to Dar neurofeedback makes him "always feel better."

And that's enough for me. But for you, you will want to explore many of the treatment modalities and pick the ones that seem to apply to the individual needs of your child.

Various Treatment Modalities

Therapies and behavioral interventions are designed to remedy specific symptoms and can bring about substantial improvement. The ideal treatment plan coordinates therapies and interventions that target the core symptoms of autism: impaired social interaction, problems with verbal and nonverbal communication, and obsessive or repetitive routines and interests. Most professionals agree that the earlier the intervention, the better.

NEUROFEEDBACK—BIOFEEDBACK FOR THE BRAIN— IS THE MOST EFFECTIVE TOOL IN YOUR PROGRAM.

EEG Biofeedback (neurofeedback) uses operant conditioning to alter brain waves so that a client's brain can achieve more flexibility and stability. In addition, it can help decrease or prevent excessive arousal or anxiety and assist the client with attention and motivation. Neurofeedback can be done at home under the supervision of a clinician and is most effective when combined with family dynamics counseling and play therapy.

Find a clinician experienced in ASDs who will oversee you every step of the way as you implement an at-home always-available treatment plan. I cannot say it enough: neurofeedback is amazingly effective. I have seen loads of apraxic kids begin speaking. Neurofeedback is non intrusive and uses the brain's own feedback system to elicit change.

It may seem unrelated but the recidivism rate for addicts goes from eighty percent (the norm for programs such as AA) to twenty percent with the inclusion of neurofeedback. The connection between the disorders is that there is a lot of brain similarity between the person addicted to drugs and the ones addicted to behaviors and foods such as casein and gluten. With the right environmental support, changing the symptoms of autism can move just as dramatically and be equally as permanent. This exciting therapy treats and makes permanent physiological changes in the brain.

Immediate Responding Basics

The minute you begin suspecting that your child has an ASD, start encouraging eye contact with great excitement and fun. When and if the child pulls away, respect his or her discomfort and offer a new choice of perhaps back rubs or foot squeezes. Always reposition for eye contact and respond to touch and sound with joy. Your child's brain is malleable so if you show it which way to grow it will. Seek help from professionals who believe in change and see your child as beautiful. A quick personal story:

When my grandson at age five months began twisting his body away and repositioning his head to avoid eye contact, no one in the family hesitated. We immediately began passing him around (since he was still a babe in arms this was easy to do) from person to person (one of many advantages of a big family). We would call his name and ask him to look at us. We played and played with the usual "goo goo goo, aren't you beautiful!" affect that people use with babies. The difference between raising him and raising another child his age was we seldom set him down, and when he looked away we just turned his body to face us again. When our arms tired we passed him on. Since the neurons in his left hemisphere were still migrating into position, we chose to light the way down the path we wanted them to follow with our love and attention. This child returned to his previous desire to play with us and is symptom free.

Don't shy away from your child simply because he shies away from you.

Floortime™/DIR (Developmental Individual Differences)

A DIR program often includes interactive experiences at home that may range from two to five hours a day. A comprehensive program also includes interactive speech therapy (three to five times per week), occupational therapy (two to five times per week), and consultation to parents for Floortime interactions and family support. DIR programs are presided over by trained consultants. For the most part a Floortime program incorporates play and interrupts the child's repetitive games by inserting roadblocks into the play. It is a very environmentally inclusive approach. During the preschool years, an important component of such a program is an integrated preschool. The preschool should be composed of one-fourth of the class of children with special needs and three-fourths of the class of children without special needs. The preschool should have teachers especially gifted in interacting with challenging children and working with them on interactive gesturing, effective cueing, and early symbolic communication. This intention is to enable children with special needs to interact with children who are prone to socially extending themselves through game building and speech. Dr. Stanley I. Greenspan has written several books that are readily available and can be consulted for a more detailed description of his approach.

Applied Behavior Analysis aka ABA

A relatively new sub-field of Psychology, ABA, has been around since the early 1960's and was largely influenced by scientists such as Ivan Pavlov (1849–1936), Edward Thorndike (1874–1949), John Watson (1878–1958) and B.F. Skinner (1904–1990). Over the years ABA has evolved and adapted away from the very controlling style of the earlier version designed by Dr. O. Ivar Lovaas and sometimes referred to as Behavior Modification. Thus, as is always the case with changes in learning, the field of ABA therapists and their approaches are highly varied. A present-day program should respect the child's age and functioning levels enough to identify his/her comfort. In general, ABA refers to a style of teaching, which uses a series of trials to shape a desired behavior or response. Skills are broken down to their simplest components and then taught to the child through a system of reinforcement. Prompts are given as needed when the child is learning a skill. As the child begins to master a skill, the prompts are gradually faded until the child can do the skill independently.

The program should be very positive with the child being set up for success by starting out with easier trials, reinforced, then moved on to more difficult tasks. A high-priority goal is making learning fun for the child. The child's progress is documented on a daily basis so that the therapist can track what the child is learning and whether the teaching approach is effective. The program is intended to be more than just behavior management. It should be a step-by-step approach complete with curriculum that teaches the following: language skills, social skills, play skills, fine-motor skills, self-help skills, as well as academic knowledge needed to successfully mainstream these children into normal classroom settings.

The Son-Rise® Program

Originally created by parents of an autistic son (their story was a made-for-television movie in the early seventies), The Autism Treatment Center of America and their techniques have grown into an organization with stories of success from around the globe. Their son, who was completely healed of severe autism, has just recently taken over as CEO of this large not-for-profit organization.

The treatment plan itself places parents as the key teachers. They are taught how to direct the program from the safe and nurturing environment of their own home (a specially designed room is advised). Parents learn how to train volunteers and/or paid help whose job it will be to play with their child. An integral part of the Son-Rise® Program is the technique of joining the child and copying his aberrant behaviors in an attempt to stimulate mirror neuron growth, discover motivations, and encourage respectful bonding. The "helpers" join the child and watch for "green lights" indicated by eye contact, touch, or sound. The minute they get any of these behaviors, they jump into action with excitement and joy.

The Son-Rise® Program values above all else a non-judgmental, loving, and accepting attitude of the child and his/her behaviors. They follow the child's motivation and teach through interactive play. Electronic self-run non-interactive toys are discouraged.

Relationship Development Intervention aka RDI

Relationship Development Intervention (RDI) is a parent-based clinical treatment for individuals with autism spectrum and other relationship-based disorders. RDI is based upon the model of Experience Sharing developed by Steven E. Gutstein, Ph.D. As its name suggests, the primary goal of RDI is to systematically teach the motivation for and skills of what is termed "Experience Sharing interaction." According to the RDI model, deficits in Experience Sharing have been found to lie at the core of autism spectrum disorders. Certified clinicians serve as facilitators to parents to help them implement and customize the program in accordance with the individual and his/her family's needs.

RDI claims that its methods are based upon extensive research in typical development as well as scientific studies of individuals in the autism spectrum. They begin by challenging at the edge of each person's current capability and carefully, systematically teaching the skills needed for competence and fulfillment in a complex world.

Applied Verbal Behavior Analysis aka AVB

Applied Verbal Behavior Analysis views language as the key feature of intervention with autism. Language training is incorporated into all activities, and there are a large number of daily trials that include discrete trials and natural environment trials. Discrete trials can be defined as teaching activities to a child at a table setting. Natural environmental trials can be defined as teaching a child in a natural setting such as at the drug store, while folding laundry, dressing for school, etc.

It incorporates the use of reinforcement when teaching or using intervention with a child. The reinforcment (raisins, toys, whatever your child likes and wants) is used to encourage the child to continue trying. This will also involve fading the reinforcment once the skill is mastered.

Occupational Therapy

OT is a health care service concerned with an individual's ability to function in everyday life activities and occupations that provide meaning to the individual's life.

Children are assessed in terms of age-appropriate life tasks. Occupational Therapy addresses areas that interfere with the child's ability to function in such life tasks. OT may be provided to children in the form of play activities, which are used to enhance or maintain play, self-help and school-readiness skills. This may be accomplished through the maintenance, improvement, or introduction of skills necessary for the child to participate as independently as possible in meaningful life activities. Such skills include copying skills, fine-motor skills, self-help skills, socialization, and play skills.

Occupational Therapists use a variety of theories and treatment approaches when providing services. Such approaches may include: developmental theories, learning theory, model of occupational performance, sensory integration, play theories, and others. The choice of therapeutic methods depends upon the specific needs of the individual child and the Occupational Therapist's background. Many OT's choose to employ a combination of approaches to meet those specific needs.

Sensory Integration Therapy

Sensory Integration Therapy is a type of occupational therapy that places a child in a room specifically designed to stimulate and challenge all of the senses. During the session, the therapist works closely with the child to encourage movement within the room. Sensory integration therapy is driven by four main principles:

1. Just Right Challenge (the child must be able to successfully meet the challenges that are presented through playful activities).
2. Adaptive Response (the child adapts his behavior with new and useful strategies in response to the challenges presented).
3. Active Engagement (the child will want to participate because the activities are fun).
4. Child Directed (the child's preferences are used to initiate therapeutic experiences within the session).

The vestibular/auditory/vision therapies integrated into the Bolles Sensory Learning Method are also occasionally termed Sensory Integration. This therapy is done over a two-week period (with the vision light portion sent home and extending beyond the office portion). The child or adult lays on a moving bed in complete dark with headphones on and a light of varying colors over the face. The brain-improving theories are complicated, but essentially the idea is to integrate the three senses into their correct pathways through the use of sound, light, and movement. My own personal experience taking my son through the Bolles Sensory Learning method is that he became happier and more interested in trying new things. However, the effect seemed to wear off within a month. On the other hand, one of my clients achieved the beginnings of language from this method. Her changes were long lasting and continued to accrue over time.

Speech Therapy

The belief in Speech Therapy is that proper structure and function of the oral areas is necessary for speech and correct sound production. Thus, often intervention to improve the coordination, strength, movement and placement of the lips, tongue, jaw and cheeks is required.

For the apraxic child with autism a speech therapy approach called "Prompt" seems to be the most effective, as it utilizes external prompts which remind the child how to move these fine-motor portions of the oral system. Unfortunately, for children with autism speech therapy often requires that the child be available and focused enough to try to follow direction. Since the therapy generally has to happen on the therapist's time frame, it is often discarded as ineffective. A speech therapist that employs the use of parents and teachers is of the most benefit to this population.

Which Behavioral Approach Do I Use?

I use them all. I can't stress enough the importance of designing a program based on the needs of the entire family. Some parents gravitate better to task-oriented learning for their children while others want to hug them into health. A mixture of everything that is available based on the learning styles, energy, and financial options of the entire group is the most likely to meet with success. Generally, I use neurofeedback, family education about brain functioning and how that impacts the emotions and behaviors of the group, and basic parenting skills as the foundation of a program for my clients. Then we adapt and create dependent upon child and familial results and reactions. I know this is kind of a non-answer answer; but truly, following the family—even if it's yours—is the only way to approach such a monumental task with any hope for successful healing. Such a realization is liberating. It means that you can be doing the correct thing even if it's different from the correct thing someone else is doing. Once you are informed, you can focus on the needs of your child and your family. Trust yourself. Gravitate to what "feels" right, harmonious, and good to do. Everyone in the home must be considered.

Managing Autism Naturally Diet, Nutrition, and Exercise

A healthy diet is always a good idea whether it is for you, your child, or your spouse. However, just what a "healthy" diet is and how to get your spouse or child to eat one are questions that become even more challenging when dealing with an autistic family member. Many autistic individuals choose colors or textures or special food groups and eat only those. Some ASD individuals eat everything they are given but don't know when to stop. Still others don't know when they're hungry. Some have difficulty chewing or swallowing and are challenged to eat at all. Experimentation, creativity, information, and observation are the necessary ingredients to solve this puzzle.

For example, imagine that your child only eats white food, and you read that some children are negatively affected by casein and gluten and that all children with autism should go on a GFCF diet (gluten/

casein-free). That's the information piece. Now you experiment by removing these items (grains and dairy) from your little person's diet. You already know white foods are more readily eaten. Therefore, be creative by finding white specialty breads, cut up white chicken breast, or grind up white blanched almonds to coat everything and magically make all colored food white. OK. Last step. Time to observe. If after three months the change in diet has no effect on your child's well-being or behavior, then this is not a necessary change for your family. However, by engaging in the experience, you will have still benefited; you will have learned about the choices your child is willing to eat. Voila! A healthier diet.

One more example; this one regards exercise. You just heard that some autistic children have too much serotonin while you also heard that serotonin increases one's ability to sleep. Your child doesn't sleep, and so you dismiss this idea. However, then you learn that serotonin is stimulated by movement and realize that your child often runs back and forth for hours at a time. You don't know if there is a connection, but you do know that research has found that exercise increases deep sleep, decreases stress reactivity, increases self-esteem, and increases such chemicals as BDNF (brain-derived neurotropic factor) that actually "heals" the brain. Therefore, you decide to do some experimenting. You let your child be your teacher and start taking him for long walks in an unpopulated area every day for a month. You make the walk fun by singing or clapping or whatever he/she likes, and by the end of the month you discover that you feel better though you're not sure about your child. You try it out for another month, mainly because it feels good. Then maybe you start to notice a greater bond between the two of you, an increased calmness in your child and also in you. Subsequently, even though your child's sleep hasn't improved, you keep the walk as a part of your child's program and smile a little smile every time you put on your one-size-smaller jeans. Ironically, one day you change the routine with trepidation and take him for a walk in a highly stimulating area. Eureka! He sleeps and you have discovered that in your child's case stimulation is the key.

The GFCF diet

If you are like many people, you've decided that you want to start using dietary intervention in an attempt to reduce symptoms of autism/PDD in your child. Most of us, however, do not know how to go about doing this in the most effective and safe manner. Obviously, as in any new treatment, some preparation must be made prior to beginning. I am including in detail an effective plan to implement the Gluten-Casein Free (GFCF) Diet, in hopes it will ease your transition to this type of treatment.

Starting a GFCF Diet

One of the first things to remember in beginning this diet is that your child's body is not used to the change. Many researchers and groups supporting the GFCF Diet feel that the need for foods containing Gluten and Casein act much like an opiate in the child's body. They become addicted to it, and therefore will go through a period of withdrawal when the diet is changed. Take it easy and start slowly, eliminating foods gradually to help ease them through this transition.

Begin by changing the diet one meal at a time. Breakfast is a good place to start. There are many gluten substitutes on the market that can be used for baking, etc., and these will make excellent meals such as pancakes, waffles, biscuits, and other breakfast items that will satisfy the taste and yet begin the process of weaning the child off of the gluten-based products. Cereals based on rice or corn also work well in place of wheat-based breakfast foods. Then add on other meals as appropriate until all meals are included in the diet.

Start the diet by removing dairy products (casein) from the diet. Be sure to check the labels on products you use around the house for products that may contain dairy as secondary ingredients. For example, many products contain lactic acid. All lactic acid does not come from dairy products. It can be produced from potatoes or cornstarch. Make sure if the product has lactic acid listed on the ingredients that the source is not from a milk product.

A short (reiterated from Section One) note about my son Dar: When he was a child way back in the early eighties, I heard through a friend of a friend of a friend that a child had been cured of PDD by removing milk from his diet. Not one to leave any stone unturned, and since I had already observed a milk addiction in my son, I stopped feeding my son milk. Initially he was upset, but after a few weeks I did notice that he seemed to tantrum less and was more emotionally steady. Unfortunately, milk was the most believed-in food product of the time, and so I was the only one who stopped. I fought with family members, school officials, and doctors. Eventually, I decided to put my energy towards the battles I could win and dropped the "milk issue." Cut to: my son and I living in an apartment alone for six months. I removed dairy from his diet. He seemed a little more clear-headed but nothing too dramatic. Until I put it back in. He drank his milk voraciously. He was hysterically happy for about forty-five minutes. He began laughing and running around the living room. And then he stopped. He began to turn red, sweat, moan, and punch himself in the face. It was like he was coming down off a drug… and indeed he was. Of course I still had to fight with friends and relatives to keep milk out of his diet. But at least I knew I was right. Trust yourself.

Foods to Avoid

Next remove gluten from the diet. Gluten is found in wheat and other cereal grain products. Again, be sure to check for gluten that is hidden in other ingredients that you might not think would contain it. For example, caramel colorings may contain this substance, as may such things as malted vinegar and many meat products, which could contain grain as a filler. It may even be included in products such as raisins, as a drying agent. Also avoid foods which contain "natural ingredients," since this term could actually mean anything. The consumer does not know what those ingredients are, so better safe than sorry. Keep in mind something that could "sneak up" on you. Often a product will say "New and Improved" and the change in the product may be the addition of the very ingredients you are attempting to avoid. The important thing to remember is that careful analysis of ingredients in products will help prevent including the very products you are wanting to eliminate in the diet inadvertently. The list of foods that could contain gluten is almost endless, so be sure to check carefully.

Once the diet is converted over to a GFCF diet, closely observe the child for signs of reactions to any of the products that you are using. The range of things that children can have reactions to is endless, so keep a close eye as you substitute, especially if you are using foods they haven't tried before. For example, foods containing peanuts or peanut oils may cause severe allergic reactions. Caution is the word when dealing with these products.

In considering the GFCF diet, consider the things that need to be done in order to successfully implement the diet. Some advanced planning can help you put this diet in place with a minimum of difficulty and help to ensure that your child makes a successful transition to it.

Gluten-free Flours

Generally speaking, you should avoid wheat, rye, barley, and oat flours. There is some debate as to whether spelt, kamut, buckwheat, and millet also contain gluten. Common flours used in this diet are brown and white rice, potato starch, and tapioca flour/starch. Other flours available are quinoa, soy, chickpea, and sorghum. They tend to be more expensive than the other flours, and have stronger flavors, although they can be substituted in small amounts for other flours.

Using Xanthan Gum to Replace Gluten

Xanthan gum comes in a fine powder. It is used to enhance a smooth texture, and to act as the "glue" in baked goods when gluten is removed. It helps to keep gluten-free baked goods from getting too crumbly.

When using xanthan gum, be sure to mix it with another flour before exposing it to liquids, since it does not mix well with liquids. (And if you spill it on the counter, wipe it up with a DRY, not wet, towel).

Guar gum is a similar replacement but is rumored to be linked to intestinal difficulties.

Casein Tips

Casein is milk protein. It is difficult to avoid, particularly since many "dairy-free" products (whipped toppings, creamers, etc.) contain casein. It is helpful for me to watch for the "Kosher" symbol on foods, making sure that they are not followed by a "D" indicating the presence of dairy. In addition, check ingredient lists and avoid butter flavor, buttermilk, casein, caseinate, cheese, cream, curds, custard, hydrolysates, lactalbumin, lactoglobulin, and lactose.

Reactions to the Diet

Some parents choose to go "cold turkey" by removing both gluten and casein from their child's diet simultaneously. Withdrawal is possible for those who have an intolerance to these proteins.

It is important to monitor what a child is eating, since other foods can prove to be a problem once the gluten and casein are removed. For example, my son Rye had a fixation for raisins (the very food reward that the behaviorists in his school were plying him with and that was rotting his teeth and causing him to get a mouthful of mercury in the form of fillings—the reality of these dental toxins was something I hadn't yet learned). As it turned out Rye had an intense yeast condition—evidenced by all the gas our family had to endure—and yeast loves sugar. Hence Rye craved raisins, and lots of them. The school was happy to comply. During this phase of Rye's childhood, he was too busy enjoying the sugar rush to remember any of the skills he had used to get the raisins. He just mimicked what was asked of him, opened his mouth, and got another hit. He generalized very few if any of the skills he gained from this approach. Rye's reaction to sweets isn't an unusual story. Often it becomes apparent that a person is also intolerant to corn, soy, eggs, yeast, sugars, food dyes, etc., and just as often that intolerance is displayed in the form of a craving. Keeping a diary or journal of the foods being consumed, along with behaviors observed, can be very helpful. Some fruits (Rye's raisins, apples, bananas, and citrus such as oranges) have the same effect on some children as gluten and casein do, causing difficulty with focusing and paying attention, and more frequent obsessions.

In fact, Rye has been so helped by a change in his diet that recently he called to tell me he'd been sad and was perseverating—it's very cool when your no-longer-autistic son calls you from his own phone, in his own apartment, on his day off from working highway construction, and says, "'Hey Mom, I figured out I'm still allergic to gluten cause I had a piece of cake and started to perseverate (meaning he was thinking about something over and over again).

Many parents report a dramatic change in their children once they begin—or go off—this diet. Others become discouraged when they do not see much of a difference. This may be due to their child's genetic make-up, age, the strictness with which the diet is followed, and the severity of their autistic behaviors (if the diet is being used with a child with ASD). It is generally felt that once implemented, the diet should be followed strictly for three months before determining results.

Knowing how long to stay at an approach is determined by more than the body's needs, though. It is also a question of family, child (adult) psychology and environmental factors. For example, when Brent—my lousy husband, terrible father, awesome friend, fantastic grandpa, rejuvenated lover, and terrific assistant—was diagnosed with terminal cancer we (my children and I) all took a step back and re-assessed what was important to us. As it turned out "diet" was not on the list. However helping Brent maintain his commitment to survive until the birth of his twin granddaughters was. We strengthened ourselves with humor and often joked that Brent was so amazing it would take two brand new souls to replace his old and learned one.

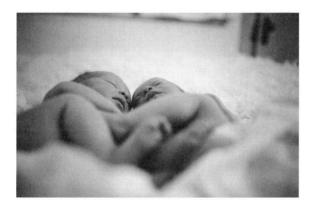

In January 2010 Malaea and Tsara brought my grandchild count to ten. For Brent it was almost as many though we only shared eight.

Brent was too weak to hold more than one at a time but at least he was alive.

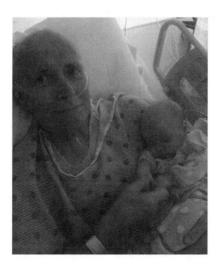

In April of 2010, four days after the above picture was taken, Brent died.

Two days before falling into a medically induced coma he looked into my eyes and said, " I fell in love the minute I met you." (I was sixteen. He was twenty-two) "So sorry I resisted feeling it most of the time." I brushed it off with "No worries" and walked away tasting my tears as they streamed down my face. In the words of our once autistic grandson: *I hope you do good in heaven.*

James Brent Leach May 27, 1951 – April 9, 2010

After Brent died a heavy existential sadness consumed me. Day after day I woke up feeling angry and resentful wondering what the point to his life had been. Then one early morning I woke up to something different. It was the sound of Dar crying. This man who hadn't cried for twenty-five years, this man who had been blocked from sadness and diverted into head banging ever since that "Go! Run Way! No Car!" long-ago day, this man was moaning out a newly acquired word in his bed. I opened the door to his plea "DAD!!!" and knew I was helpless. Dar's tearless eyes begged me as his throat moaned for Brent in an animal-like wail. For a minute I was motionless and then his body became racked with huge man sobs and I ran to embrace him. We held on that night, hour after hour, trying to sooth away the loss of this companion who had become everyone's father friend. And I began to glimpse the point of his existence.

Brent's imminent death brought an upside for the house. Life was suddenly too dear for me to waste any of it policing my children. I had never wanted my overzealous helping to lead them to see themselves as flawed and in need of fixing. However, while Brent was slipping through our fingers it occurred to me that I had been teaching Dar exactly that. Thus, I made some changes in the house. Since Dar had become something of a milk and bread thief his nieces and nephews had come to dislike and resent visiting him. This was because in order to minimize the risk of food contamination in Dar's diet, Dar's diet became their diet whenever they were at my house. However, the shortness of Brent's life was causing enough of a paradigm shift in me to gift me with a new perspective on why Dar's thievery had evolved in the first place: Perhaps it wasn't because he was addicted to the foods. Perhaps it was simply because he felt left out? I had seen plenty of evidence that Dar was being kept at arm's length by those he loved because his favorite foods were considered unhealthy. So maybe I was onto something. I gave Dar full access to the kitchen. I announced to the family and to Dar that he could eat anything he wanted as long as he "handled" how the food made him feel without getting angry, eating my walls, or losing established skills.

Initially Dar underwent many behavioral adjustments that I could have attributed to allergies or addiction but after several months of me reminding him not to act out and promising that the food would stay available as long as he calmed down, Dar's speech, self help, self confidence, social connectedness, forethought, afterthought, and consideration for other's, improved dramatically. (Of course he was fatter but fortunately he was also self-initiating the treadmill.)

By the time the twins were born (Happy note: they are the first babies in the family for whom Dar will always be a talking man.) Dar was an independent self-helper (good thing too; twins are an amazing amount of work even for Dramma's). And by the time Brent died Dar was a new man with a new attitude making strange concoctions in the kitchen. Maybe that freedom to be, to do, to fail, to succeed, to give up, or to just try is what made it possible for Dar to cry. And now that he can cry maybe he will no longer have to hide sadness in apathy and/or anger. We shall see.

Since dropping the gluten-free casein-free diet, Dar has became more of a participant in the family... more loved and appreciated by his nieces and nephews... sharing and talking better than ever before, possibly because we are treating him as someone who can be trusted to make the healthier choice. And maybe just possibly because Brent's death taught him (and us) that life is precious so partake of it.

Since that time I have seen greater development via trust and teaching than restriction and control on many occasions, for many people as they dropped the GFCF dietary restrictions. Is it because most of the children I refer to were on the diet first and their guts had already healed? Or is it because the diet is less powerful than the need for freedom of choice??? The fact is I don't know because if the subjects in question weren't on the diet first then I have nothing to compare their behavior to. I do know that over-controlling people and/or their environment sets them apart and makes them special (needs).

So is the diet worth it??? Not if it is at the cost of feeling connected to family and friends.

On or Off the Diet, Here are some Foods to Include

Meat, the many varieties of fruits and vegetables, some legumes and beans, nuts, white rice, herbal teas, and foods that make your children happy.

Dietary Supplements and Autism

Tips For A Successful Supplement Regimen

As a default, it is believed that most Autistic spectrum children NEED the Recommended Daily Allowances (RDA) of supplements missing from their body because the foods are not being eaten, or the nutrients from the food is not being absorbed.

A few hints:

1. When following a gluten-free / casein-free diet supplementation is important.
2. Proper eating—a balanced diet needs to be a part of the process. This is an on-going battle with ALL children. We as parents need to strive for balance with protein, carbs, sugars, veggies/fruit for our kids' good health. I know this doesn't sound easy, but work on it everyday and it will become easier over time.
3. Do your best to eliminate or control these items in your child's diet:
    * Yeast
    * Refined sugars
    * Dyes/natural flavors
    * Excessive intake of carbohydrates
4. Test for what supplements are missing from your child's body.
5. Work with a qualified doctor (DAN—an acronym for Defeat Autism Now. DAN Doctors is a worldwide group of Doctors that many of my clients use. But the world of doctors is not limited to this group. There are also many other Doctors gaining notoriety as specialists working in the field of autism. Also I must confess here that I don't actually follow this advice myself, I just Google and go, from learning to learning. But this is because I have the kind of mind that can make sense out of the mayhem. If you do not, then grab yourself a professional who can make sense of it for you.)

Some of the most commonly believed supplements to be missing and needed for children on the spectrum are:

- Calcium
- Zinc
- Magnesium
- Cod liver oil (make sure it is tested and MERCURY FREE)
- Essential fatty acid (EFA Powder)
- Selenium
- Probiotics (ProBioGold, Culturelle, Biobeads)
- TMG or DMG or SuperNu Thera (the B6 family)
- Vitamin C, Vitamin E, and or CoQ10 (antioxidants)
- L-Gluthathione (supplement or topical cream)
- Taurine or other amino acids
- Folic or Folinic acids

(In this section I am sharing common beliefs and ideas, though my personal approach is much less stringent. Once I discovered neurofeedback, I was able to ease up on most of the above points.)

Starting a Supplement Regimen

A reputable company making products that many autism spectrum children use is Kirkman Laboratories. They make a wide variety of supplements that are hypoallergenic, GFCF, and some with no artificial flavors. For more information please see: www.kirkmanlabs.com because they work primarily with kids who have special needs.

Now, with all good things are rules. Parents need to follow directions given by supplement manufacturers and their doctors.

Other Supplement Suggestions are as Follows:

1. Do not overload your kids. Give them the RDA for their weight and age per a doctor.
2. Because most of our kids have a leaky gut, these supplements will not absorb properly. If it is appropriate for your child, then sticking to the gluten-free / casein-free (GFCF) diet will help repair the gut over time (one year or more).
3. Add one supplement at a time three weeks apart. (Check for changes in behavior, rashes, difference in sleep patterns, introduction or amplification of self-stimulatory behavior, or mood swings).

4. Buy small samples. Check to see if they work instead of acquiring large jars of supplements that you find out don't make a difference for you child.

5. Ask what supplements should be taken with food, not with other supplements, by themselves, or at night.
   * **Do not take digestive enzymes with a probiotic!** (The enzyme will digest the probiotic without any effect on your child's system!)

6. Sometimes, supplements—even in the smallest quantities—can overload a child's system. It is important to follow doctor's and supplement manufacturer's directions.

7. Supplement breaks: It is OK to take "supplement vacations." Take a break two or three times a year where you remove all supplements. Add one back in three days apart and take note of your child's reactions and behaviors each day.

8. A negative reaction to a supplement can be behavior that will pass or can be a truly negative reaction. As a parent, know the difference. Should you...
   • Stop the supplement immediately
   • Or wait to see how your child behaves with a smaller-dose adjustment
   The answer here is yours to discover.

9. KEEP IN MIND you should not just give random supplements to your child unless you are willing to stop them just as quickly. It has to be something that is done with careful thought and observation.

BOTTOM LINE: Go one step at a time. Use your doctor's advice and assistance. Trust yourself.

DAN (Defeat Autism Now)

The Autism Research Institute convened a group of about thirty carefully selected physicians and scientists in Dallas in January 1995 for the express purpose of sharing information and ideas toward defeating autism as quickly as possible. The participants, from the U.S. and Europe, represent the most advanced thinking by some of the best minds in the autism world. The participants continue to work together toward the goal of finding effective treatments.

You can go to the DAN website to find a list of physicians treating autism with biomedical options. Parents and physicians who do not regard psychotropic drugs as the best or only means of treating autistic patients will welcome this advanced manual on clinical assessment.

I am going to go out on a limb here and say that most of my clients do not like their DAN doctors. If you don't like your doctor look elsewhere. Do not waste time half listening; there is too much to learn.

Nonstandard Approaches to Autism

In trying to do everything possible to help their children, many parents are quick to try new treatments. I believe that every treatment has helped someone. However, before spending time and money and possibly slowing your child's progress, talk with experts, evaluate the findings of objective reviewers, and seek out referrals from other families.

Facilitated Communication is a method by which the child's arm is supported so that he can type on a keyboard. This method has been proved and disproved so many times that the majority of professionals just stay away from it. In the nineties, it was all over the news and quickly followed by a rash of sexual-assault accusations that were put down in court. For the most part, scientific studies showed that the typed messages actually reflected the thoughts of the person providing the support. So the method was dropped. However, many parents, thrilled to be communicating with their child, persevered and some of those individuals became independent typists. An example would be Sue Rubin, the extremely autistic award-winning writer of her own documentary "*Autism Is A World*. I think it is important to note that the majority of autistic individuals have some cerebellum dysfunction which can lead to an intention tremor (hands move away from intended object when it gets close to the item aimed for) and make typing unsupported next to impossible.

Holding Therapy is when the parent hugs the child for long periods of time, even if the child resists. Those who use this technique contend that it forges a bond between the parent and child. Some claim that it helps stimulate parts of the brain as the child senses the boundaries of her own body. I tried this technique with several children and still have no idea whether it was useful or not. There is no scientific evidence to support it.

Auditory Integration Training: Here, the child listens to a variety of sounds with the goal of improving language comprehension. Advocates of this method suggest that it helps people with autism receive more balanced sensory input from their environment. When tested using scientific procedures, the method was shown to be no more effective than listening to music. However, I have personally seen great benefits in many children and even in myself from this therapy. **My Story**: as a child I had pixilated vision which means I saw things in pieces like a puzzle. After five days of (Berard) auditory training my vision normalized and I realized I had very bad taste in clothes. (wink) I saw things, people, and myself intact from head to toe for the first time in thirty-five years.

Doman/Delacato Method, in which people are reborn and then made to crawl and move as they presumably did at each stage of early development in an attempt to learn missing skills. Again, no scientific studies support the effectiveness of the method and none of the families that I have met who tried this method saw results.

Fibroblast Growth Factor 2 FGF2 (Neuropro) is a bovine protein which stimulates the growth of new neural connections in the damaged areas of the brain. Dr. Luis Carlos Aguilar of the Research Institute of Neuroplasticity and Cellular Development in Guadalajara, Mexico, is the pioneer of its use in treating children with autism.

Treatment for the child can be administered at home by giving a solution containing FGF2 sublingually. Usually, a 1 ml. vial of Neuropro is applied with a dropper over a seven- to ten-day period (depending on the patient). Every six months the child is examined by Dr. Aguilar and the concentration and interval are adjusted. The entire treatment can last anywhere from three to five years, and the results depend on the age of the patient and the severity of the autism in the "spectrum." According to the Aguilar website, the best-case scenario is... close to full recovery from autism. According to my experience with various clients... only the ADHD girl benefited.

Hyperbaric Oxygen (HBOT) has been utilized to treat autism in many countries throughout the globe. The rationale behind using hyperbaric for autism is that the treatments increase cerebral blood flow and thus oxygen is delivered to areas of the brain, which are thought to be oxygen deficient. Greater amounts of blood and oxygen begin to stimulate cerebral tissues and aid in recovery of idling neurons. HBOT also reduces excess fluids and swelling of brain tissues which aid in neurological function and a less confused state in autistic individuals. Hyperbaric is also used as a complementary therapy for the treatment of heavy metal detox for such materials as mercury. Hyperbaric assists in the metabolism of heavy metal removal. It can help a patient counteract the effects of heavy metal poisoning and helps the body deal with toxins even as noxious as cyanide. It is often used in conjunction with chelation and other detox procedures to help support the body to deal with the impact commonly seen in the removal of heavy metals, mercury, toxins, and other contaminants.

Additional Therapies: Live cell and Stem cell Therapy, Respin A, Anti Fungal, Detoxing Heavy Metals, IV Immunoglobin, Cranio Sacral Therapy, Music Therapy, Handle, Drama Therapy…. and more.

What Autism Medications and Brain-Changing Technologies Are Available?

Brain-Changing Technologies: Neurofeedback (Bio-feedback for the Brain) is the most exciting, easily accessible technology available. While it can be cost prohibitive, there are ways to maximize on the situation by training with professional-grade equipment in your own home under the direct supervision of an experienced clinician. I stay with the family for several days treating and training everyone in order to more fully understand their brains, and then I help them learn how to do the treatments on their child and themselves—thus the entire family grows and changes—eliminating the dynamic created when all the focus is centered on the so-called sick one. I guide and communicate regularly with the parents by phone, returning several times over the year to oversee the changes. It is a true team approach wherein the parents quickly become more of an expert than me. N**eurofeedback** is the most wonderful aid I have ever offered families of autism. I have worked with and changed the fine-motor skills, emotional stability, and expressive language of autistic individuals regardless of age (even adults) with these techniques. People change and become comfortable in their own skin at a rate I have not witnessed with any other therapeutic approach.

Medications are largely ineffective for treating autism itself, though some of the symptoms have been reportedly helped through the use of anti-psychotic medications to treat severe behavioral problems; antidepressant medication to handle symptoms of anxiety, depression, or obsessive-compulsive disorder; and anticonvulsant drugs for seizures. Stimulant drugs, such as those used for children with attention deficit hyperactivity disorder (ADHD), are sometimes used effectively to help decrease impulsivity and hyperactivity. However, I must warn you that several of the children I have worked with lost skills, became depressed, exclusive, and hallucinatory on at least one of these drugs. **Please read the side effects and contraindications before agreeing to administer anything!** Here's an example of a possible, yet easy-to-make mistake: Adderall cannot be mixed with baking soda which is contained in the Alka Seltser that many parents give because it relieves stomach pain which many autistic children have. Everything is a part of your child's system!

New medicines being investigated are Risperidone (recently approved for autism) and Lamictal (which is meant to be used for seizures but is gaining some notoriety with autism clients, though again in my experience, the advantages seem small in comparison to neurofeedback). Supplements like Idebenone are occasionally prescribed as if they are medications. Medicate with care! I have seen a nice calming effect on the appropriate child using herbs to stimulante like Inositol and/or Theanine. However, still many of my clients have tried them and none of these clients were "markedly" helped while some were made more body defensive and hyperactive.

Other Therapies: There are a number of controversial therapies or interventions available for autistic children. Many are just plain quackery as the charlatans take advantage of the desperation of loving parents. However, lots of my families have had success with the most unusual discoveries (diet coke to help with focus), and I've heard of everything from drinking urine to riding horses. I myself have seen a great reduction in my son's thirst, constant state of wanting, and his gastric issues by treating him with a quarter teaspoon of plain old baking soda and an eight-ounce glass of water once a day five days a week. Since there is a scientific basis for most of the choices and none of them work for everyone, it is imperative that the therapy in question makes sense to both the disorder and the people implementing it. As my neuroanatomy professor always said, "The devil is in the details." So have faith in your instincts and get referrals from people you trust before engaging in the purchase of any promised quick-fix-miracle cures.

Following are some of the therapies I have witnessed as useful in some way for some children: DHA oil, Flax Seed oil (two of my clients stopped seizing once large doses of this were introduced), Flower of Sulpher, AIT (my son Cash left the fourth day of AIT talking up a storm after many years of slow painstaking speech. He was so excited that he kept interrupting himself and saying, "Can you hear how fast I'm talking?" Though his speech slowed down again he never fully returned to his previously tardy state), Cranial Sacral, Tomatis, Secretin, Baking Soda (used because Secritin was hard to get—healed my son's gut enough to put dairy back into his diet), B-12, Magnesium, Pancreatic Enzyme, SuperNu Thera, Omega 3 fatty acids, Calcium, Aloe Vera, Brushing, QX machine, Handel.

Chelation: this is a method of removing toxins like mercury from the system and it usually stirs up what is hidden in the body. This "stirring up" can increase the symptoms of autism, at least temporarily. Most of the children I work with regress and become sickly when their parents are chelating or cleansing them with prescribed medications. This being the case, and since all these children seem to improve at the same rate, when using neurofeedback, combined with play and family dynamics training, regardless of what biomeds, diets, or chelations they do, I've chosen to use only very gentle methods with my sons. These slow-working chelators include, but are not limited to, ionized footbaths, baking soda baths, Epsom salt baths, daily doses of garlic, and pure chlorella tablets. I have never been a hundred percent decided about chelation. I did strongly consider a more aggressive form of chelation for Dar and Rye: For Dar because of his numerous vaccinations and for Rye because of his numerous fillings containing traces of mercury. However, I was concerned that chelating with any of the stronger methods would leech the mercury from Rye's teeth into his brain, and I was equally as concerned that removing his fillings would have the same results. I was concerned because it happened to me. That's how I found out about the silver fillings /mercury connection: When my silver fillings were exchanged for white ones I got mercury poisoning. I was very sick, unable to focus, drive, or carry on a conversation. My thyroid was damaged and my immune system compromised. Eventually—with the help of the famous Dr. Atkins—I chelated the mercury out of my system. However, the cure was almost as bad as the curse. I was weak, my body hurt, my head ached, and I felt as if I would disappear. In fact, I was never fully better until I introduced my brain to neurofeedback. Thus I decided to not be so aggressive with my sons and have not tried any of the prescribed chelators, IV or otherwise, because they were improving steadily without it.

My sons' progress was evidence enough for me to feel confident in taking this more patient approach. However, given that Dar still has so far to go, the jury on this issue remains out. Especially in light of the fact that recently one of my clients had an IV chelation treatment and the effect was purely amazing. The communicative level of his speech tripled and his EEG waves balanced. His progress held long enough for us to build on it with neurofeedback and play, so though the chelation effect wore off he is still changing rapidly. Because of this child's changes in brain-wave activity, I am revisiting the concept and considering this therapy for Dar even as I write. (However, by the time I did the reedit I had decided against chelating in the traditional way. I am, however, investigating using Natural Peptide Clathration Therapy to get the toxins out. Trust me; there is always some new something (even when your child is no longer autistic) to try and help them with. (wink)

CHAPTER FOURTEEN

Selecting an Autism Treatment Program

Parents are often disappointed to learn that there is no single best treatment for all children with autism, possibly not even for any specific child given that most successful programs change their treatment approaches over and over again. Even after a child has been thoroughly tested and formally diagnosed, there is no clear "right" course of action. The diagnostic team may suggest treatment methods and service providers, but ultimately it is up to the parents to consider their child's unique needs, research the various options, and decide.

Above all, parents should consider valid their own intuitive sense of what will work for their child. Keeping in mind that autism takes many forms, parents might want to investigate whether a specific program has helped children like their own.

Can Social Skills and Behaviors Be Improved?

Yes! Yes! Yes! And Yes! A number of treatment approaches have evolved in the decades since autism was first identified. Some therapeutic programs focus on developing skills and replacing dysfunctional behaviors with more appropriate ones. Others focus on creating a stimulating learning environment tailored to the unique needs of children with autism.

Researchers have begun to identify factors that make certain treatment programs more effective in reducing—or reversing—the limitations imposed by autism. Treatment programs that seem to produce the greatest gains build on the child's interests, offer a (mostly) predictable schedule, teach tasks as a series of simple steps, actively engage the child's attention in highly structured activities, and provide regular reinforcement of behavior.

Parent involvement has also emerged as a major factor in treatment success. Parents work with teachers and therapists to identify the behaviors to be changed and the skills to be taught. Recognizing that parents are the child's earliest teachers, more programs are beginning to train parents to continue the therapy at home. Research is beginning to suggest that mothers and fathers who are trained to work with their child can be as effective as (if not more effective than) professional teachers and therapists.

Children Best Suited to ABA, Floortime, Son-Rise®, RDI

Not to be redundant but this is a personal decision made by the families and cannot be decided on by an outsider. Each one of these programs works to benefit the child in some way as long is it works stylistically with the family. Perhaps more important than what program you choose is who is working it. In many cases the true reasons for why a child did or didn't progress is immeasurable because it comes organically out of the intuition of the people involved. So how to choose? Know yourself first: Personally I would never run a data-driven, super-structured program because I am not motivated in this way and would likely set it up to fail. This is not because I don't love my children or the children I am hired to help, but because since I don't blossom in an environment like that, it is a hard one for me to believe in and employ. We are all different. Choose the program that suits your operating style and then ask yourself if living within the structure of this methodology will be a happy event or a stressful one. Choose the happy answer. For me that was Son-Rise® and neurofeedback; for you it may be ABA and homeopathy.

The Pros and Cons of ABA, Floortime, Son-Rise®, RDI

ABA has been around the longest and as such is much more supported by schools and practitioners alike. However, its main problem is that many of the children do not generalize their skills and often respond as a robot would rather than with the fluidity typical people use.

Floortime is gaining a lot of ground as the alternative therapy and some schools have been setup throughout the country. The children in these schools seem to be more "natural" and involved than with ABA. They also generalize better; however, there is not as much long-standing data.

Son-Rise® is a parent-driven program so there is no school to partner with, making you, the parent, expert and provider in search of techniques. You purchase consultations, take classes, and learn the methodologies. It's up to you. This is both a pro and a con. There are very few facilitators in the field.

RDI, like Son-Rise®, is a parent-based therapy founded on the theory of drawing the child out through social interaction. However, RDI uses more than one room within which to teach and is based more on hard science than warm psychology. Again, being parent-based while purchasing support is the pro and the con.

Choosing an ABA, Floortime, Son-Rise®, RDI Practitioner

Once you have chosen the style within which you wish to work and are searching for a practitioner in the field, you may be lost in the noise of multiple possibilities or desperate for any old person dependent upon your geographic location. My suggestion is that you choose no one rather than choose someone you are not comfortable with. Better to have only a loving mom to learn from than a whole team of distraught family members not fully following the advice of the professional they hired. Another way to guide yourself is to check on how your potential practitioners answers make you feel: informed and helped or stupid and confused. Go with informed. Often, when a professional is new to the field and doesn't actually know the answers you seek, they pretend and speak in a confusing manner just to safeguard their own ignorance. Regardless, even if the practitioner is well informed, you must be able to understand them well enough to follow their advice. So if you don't, keep looking.

In short: If a practitioner is not sharing with you his or her ideas, and reasons for those ideas, and respecting you as the expert on your child (because nobody knows your child like you do), then you need to find a new practitioner. Period.

Exploring Autism Treatment Options

While holding tight to your instincts you may find these questions help you get started when interviewing potential helpers and considering various treatment programs:

- What is the fundamental belief of your approach?
- What do you believe my child is capable of?
- How will you plan his/her activities, based on his choices or yours?
- Are the daily schedules and routines predictable or unpredictable and why?
- How is progress measured?
- Will my child's behavior be closely observed and recorded?
- Will my child be given tasks and rewards that are personally motivating and how will you choose them?
- How successful has this program been for other children?
- How many children have gone on to placement in a regular school and how have they performed?
- If you don't have the answers to these questions, why not?
- Do your staff members have training and experience in working with children and adolescents with autism?
- Is the environment designed to minimize distractions or stimulate neurons?
- Will the program prepare me to continue the therapy at home?
- What are the costs, time commitment, and location of the program?
- How much individual attention will my child receive?

Be aware that the above list is just to help you get started. Every family is different. Use these questions or create your own. The truth is that there is no perfect way to interview; it is all a process of discovery.

Developmental Approaches to Autism

Professionals have found that many children with autism learn best in an environment that builds on their skills and interests while accommodating their special needs. Programs employing a developmental approach provide consistency and structure along with appropriate levels of stimulation. For example, a predictable schedule of activities each day helps children with autism plan and organize their experiences. Using a certain area of the classroom for each activity helps students know what they are expected to do. For those with sensory problems, activities that sensitize or desensitize the child to certain kinds of stimulation may be especially helpful.

In one developmental preschool classroom, a typical session starts with a physical activity to help develop balance, coordination, and body awareness. Children string beads, piece puzzles together, paint, and participate in other structured activities. At snack time, the teacher encourages social interaction and models how to use language to ask for more juice. Later, the teacher stimulates creative play by prompting the children to pretend being a train. As in any classroom, the children learn by doing.

Although higher-functioning children may be able to handle academic work, they too need help to organize the task and avoid distractions. A student with autism might be assigned the same addition problems as her classmates. But instead of assigning several pages in the textbook, the teacher might give her one page at a time or make a list of specific tasks to be checked off as each is done.

Behaviorist Approaches to Autism

It has been observed that when people are rewarded for a certain behavior, they are more likely to repeat or continue that behavior. Behaviorist training approaches are based on this principle. Dr. O. Ivar Lovaas pioneered the use of behaviorist methods for children with autism more than twenty-five years ago. His methods involve time-intensive, highly structured, repetitive sequences in which a child is given a command and rewarded each time he responds correctly. For example, in teaching a young boy to sit still, a therapist might place him in front of a chair and tell him to sit. If the child doesn't respond, the therapist nudges him into the chair. Once seated, the child is immediately rewarded in some way. A reward might be a bit of chocolate, a sip of juice, a hug, or applause—whatever the child enjoys. The process is repeated many times. Eventually, it is hoped that the child will begin to respond without being nudged and sit for longer periods of time. The idea is that learning to sit still and follow directions provides a foundation for learning more complex behaviors. Using this approach for up to forty hours a week, some children may be brought to the point of near-normal behavior. Others are much less responsive to the treatment.

Dr. Lovaas' approach is an extremely challenging way to work with or raise children. Not only are the hours intensive but also the approach itself creates the mindset of the child being everyone's little problem to fix. This way of thinking can lead to codependency, which runs the risk of taking the humanity out of the program and its implementers. Such a group psychology is dangerous and inhibits the genuine pleasure that raising and teaching autistic individuals can offer. The premise of teaching in this manner also completely ignores the sensory challenges and stomach discomforts of the child while placing all the blame for their "self absorbed" behavior on attitudinal and cognitive challenges.

Some researchers and therapists believe that less intensive treatments, particularly those begun early in a child's life may be more efficient and just as effective. So, over the years, researchers sponsored by NIMH (National Institute of Mental Health) and other agencies have continued to study and modify the behaviorist approach. Today, some of these behaviorist treatment programs are more individualized and built around the child's own interests and capabilities. Many programs also involve parents or other non-autistic children in teaching the child. Instruction is no longer limited to a controlled environment but takes place in natural, everyday settings. Thus, a trip to the supermarket may be an opportunity to practice using words for size and shape. Although rewarding desired behavior is still a key element, the rewards are varied and appropriate to the situation. A child who makes eye contact may be rewarded with a smile, rather than candy. NIMH is funding several types of behaviorist treatment approaches to help determine the best time for treatment to start, the optimum treatment intensity and duration, and the most effective methods to reach both high- and low-functioning children.

CHAPTER FIFTEEN

Some Common Questions

Can It Be Cured? This is an interesting question. Since autism is diagnosed via a list of behavioral symptoms, the answer would have to be that if the symptoms recede enough to mean that the child or adult no longer meet the criteria, he or she has been cured. This being stated the answer is *yes*.

Can Autism Be Outgrown? I have never met a professional other than myself who would answer yes to this question. However, as I just said, I would answer yes. Why? Because while doing neurofeedback on autistic individuals I have observed some interesting parallels in brain wave function between autism and ADHD. So, since around twenty percent of ADHD children have been known to outgrow the disorder and since some sensory brain issues like synesthesia (seeing sound, tasting shapes) are often outgrown in childhood, my guess is there are many who would be diagnosable at one age and not at another.

How Do Families Learn to Cope with Autism? In my opinion just the idea that one must "cope" with autism is a setup for failure. The word *cope* brings to mind long periods of suffering, alleviated momentarily by groups of people getting together to share their pain, and then going out to get some more. This life is definitely available to you and your family. Call any of your local autism support groups located on the Internet. My suggestion is to bypass this thinking and go straight to adoring your autistic child and all the things you are about to learn because of him. I suggest getting neurofeedback for the whole family and then taking a class in Son-Rise® play techniques or in Floortime or call Brain and Body (www.brainbody.net) for Family Dynamics counseling. Every family has its own unique challenges; this is just yours. It may not be what you intended to be doing, but it is a great way to become wiser and learn new ways to parent all children. In the end—if embraced—autism can be your greatest motivation for change. Hint: When frustrated walk away, take a bath, call a supportive friend, start again, do it with gratitude, because it feels better and feeling better will change your approach to yourself and your child and that will change your lives. Don't cope; adore.

What Hope Does Research Offer for Autism? Researchers are looking at ways to replenish the deficient Oxytoxin (bonding hormone) in the brain and are in search of genetic links (already found some contributing chromosomes #7, #11, and #14) so that expectant mothers can be tested (something that is already available for potential RETTS babies). Researchers are studying ways to reduce the excessive inflammation in ASD individuals and studying several new (symptom relieving) medicines. Studies on how best to teach an ASD child and causal relationships with the environment and heredity are ongoing. For a more complete answer read under the sub heading *What Research is Being Done?* Section Two, Chapter II.

CHAPTER SIXTEEN

Growing Up with Autism

Autism and the Family

The most challenging aspect of raising one or even many autistic children was best summed up by one of the mom's I work with. She was expecting family to visit from out of town and feeling stressed. We were talking about her feelings, and she was explaining that even though she fully accepted and loved her daughter, that even though she was totally happy with all her treatment choices and could definitely see progress in her child, she felt stressed every time her extended family came for a visit because they always came with arms full of advice about other treatments and therapies. She threw up her hands and cried, " I am always being put in the position of defending my dissertation. I just want to be seen as a graduate with a degree and left to make my own choices." The best advice I could give her was to tell her to graduate herself. "You are the expert. Just think of it as a continuing education consultation."

Managing the Stress: Stress makes it more difficult to think clearly, to remain calm, and to cope with anxiety and the events in life that can exacerbate anxiety. One of the most exacerbating things you can do is to view your child as a problem full of broken pieces. Every child is unique, and every child requires special handling. Yours just has a label. If you see your child's unusual behaviors as the enemy and try to expunge them, you will always be at war with a member of your own family, because for each behavior you train away a new one will pop up to take its place. Instead, investigate and try to see what your child finds fun in the bizarre aspect of his/her chosen activity. Join your child in play; and after a while, vary the game. This way, you will not be trying to extinguish parts of your child by hating what she/he likes. Rather, you will be building upon his/her interests to normalize that activity into something more useful for learning and socialization. Actively admiring your child removes the stress. As for those often-repeated, hard-to-take repetitious sounds, try flinging a towel on doors that are constantly slammed, padding your tables, or buying plastic spoons instead of noisy metal ones. Having fun with it makes it easier to come up with good ideas.

Finally, reach for help. Psychotherapy, biofeedback, exercise (e.g., aerobic, yoga, Tai Chi) and meditation/prayer have been shown to be effective in decreasing stress.

Siblings of Autism: Children follow our lead even when they appear not to be. If you see the situation as a problem, so will your child. Instead, share a different vision. Praise constantly your non-autistic children for helping with their sib. Teach them about autism, not as if it is devastating, just as if it simply is. Involve everyone in the learnings you will have and share your excitement for how brilliant you will all be as you gain a greater understanding of how the brain inter-acts with its environment. Be creative, inclusive, and make little one-on-one dates with all of your people. This approach is not just for your child; it is also for you: when you share, when you lead with excitement and acceptance, that is also what you feel.

Grandparents of Autism: Grandparents can be your great-est resource when raising autistic children. However, should they feel too uncomfortable or physically incapable of keeping up with your child, assure them that they are still of value and appreciate what they can do. Imagine how wonderful it would be to have Grandma cook every Sunday, swing by with the meat loaf, and drop off some gluten-free cookies; or perhaps Grandpa is the cook and Grandma does your grocery shopping, or maybe your parents are just a wealth of home-remedy information. Whatever they have to offer, help them find it. Many grandparents are simply lost as to how and what to do. The greatest gift you can give yourself is to encourage help. Allowing grand-parents to participate in this way permits them the opportunity to be generous and experience your gratitude. This can be a very bonding scenario for all. (However, if the grandparents in question are—despite all your efforts—unable to be accepting and supportive, keep them at arm's length. Do not waste your energy trying to convert them and save it for your child.)

Home Safety: Home safety is a serious issue as many autistic kids are very gifted escape artists. Creating a safe environment requires knowing your child and understanding his or her motivations and abilities. It also requires staying a step ahead. Windows and doors can be secured with special locks, and if necessary windows can be screwed shut. The usual outlet covers and cupboard locks work for some children while others can climb to the top of any surface and handle any typical-child safety lock. Stoves can be turned off at breakers or unplugged and furnaces can be gated. Rest assured that for every danger zone your child chooses to perseverate on, there is a solution. In fact, most things have already been invented though you may have to add a little creativity.

The best safety is of course constant supervision, but every super person needs some sleep. So get comfortable laying down boundaries with the intention of helping him/her learn to become the guardian of his/her own safety.

Begin by explaining what you want and why. For example, "There are germs in the toilet that may make you sick. I want to keep you healthy; that's why I won't let you put your hands in the toilet." Now block him/her from the toilet. Your child will only know what you want if you tell her/him. Children with autism often have attention problems and slower mental processing speed. Therefore, be prepared to tell your child repeatedly. This is not a failure in your ability to teach; this is just the way he/she learns. Now, be OK if your child tantrums. Keep her/him safe if he/she flings herself/himself around. However, don't react with any emotion. If your child likes to destroy things, minimize the choices and keep nothing around that would upset you to have broken. If he/she simply pulls away and moves to engage in her/his repetitive behaviors, thank him/her for not putting her/his hands in the toilet and give him/her some time to process what you have said. If she/he listens and complies, respond with gusto, celebrating and telling him/her how amazing she/he is.

The idea here is to shape your child's behavior in the same way that you would encourage a plant to grow towards the light. Give no emotional response to the behaviors you wish to discourage (leave them in the dark) and give lots of joyous (sunny) delight for the things you want to help grow. Your child may not be motivated by the same socially acceptable things as you. So help your child find his/her way. Lay down the road map with very frequent positive reinforcements such as, "I love it when you look at me," "What a great voice you have" and "You're the nicest person; I'm so lucky to have you." Your child will respond even if at first she/he shies away. So explain everything, especially how incredible you think each of his/her accomplishments are.

Just because your child may not communicate normally, don't assume she/he doesn't understand. Many people push and pull autistic children while working under this assumption. Perhaps many of his/her outbursts are related to just such a world of having no control.

Educational Needs: As with all children the educational needs of your autistic child will shape and reshape themselves over the years. Some autistics attend college, others work in craft shops, many simply learn to vacuum for mom. You have many choices for your child's future, but don't worry about making future plans in the present. Working with autism requires handling things one step at a time. Start from where you are at and add something. If your child can talk but is filled with trepidation in new environments, start by making the old home environment new; have him help you redecorate; then get the new environment (for example, new teachers) to come to the home. Create a comfort level and then, choosing a small class, move him into it. The important thing here is to maintain the position of legal guardian and decider of his choices. You are the final say, so relax and be a partner.

Remember that, although you will be working with experts in mental health and education, you are the expert on your child. Choose professionals who recognize your expertise, greet you with respect, and thrive when partnering with parents. Helping your child takes congruency of approach, consistency in the environment, and a modeling of functional relationships. For optimal improvement, you must be part of the team. There is no mystery in what behaviorists do. Have them share their knowledge and then be excited to share yours. You will be richer as a result of the interplay between teaching your child, other professionals, and yourself. Life with autism truly can be a blessing.

Dealing with the Autistic Adolescent: As autistic individuals kick into the usual hormonal changes of adolescence, their personality can change from quiet and alone to frustrated and self-injurious. This is not, however, always or even most often true. What does seem to be prevalent in autistic adolescents is a fair amount of depression and sexual acting out. Many teens become inactive and unmotivated. Others become moody and experience outbursts of anger. This is often true of the young autistic individual as well; however, it is much less intimidating to watch a child tantrum than a full-grown, six-foot teenager. Some teens require meds during this period; however, in my experience neurofeedback and supportive speak will usually correct the imbalance in arousal levels and return the teen to a state of cooperativeness.

Managing Loss of Normalcy: As your child becomes more aware of his/her difference in the world, remember when you were first presented with the dilemma of autism. Remember how challenging it was to accept that your life would always be different now. Remember... that....

You may not have dreamed of or imagined raising a child or even children with autism. This may not be the way you pictured your life as a youngster playing Barbie dolls or GI Joe. The future that became your present may not have given you what you expected. However, it did give you a marvelous challenge full of excitement and joy once you learned to see it that way. You can lament what wasn't, or embrace what is.

So how would the lamenting choice look? Years and years of struggling, denying and dealing with shame and thoughts such as, "Why me?" until one day you realize that no one seems able to "fix" your child without some kind of coordinating effort by you. So you start, fifteen or twenty years later. Good for you for making the decision, if that's who you already are. However, if you are standing in the beginning part of this story, it's a lot easier and quicker to roll up your sleeves, fill yourself with gratitude for all you are about to learn, and get at it now.

Remember that the choice of "getting at loving it" all started because you were noticing some differences in your child and then help your child through the same process. Share your learnings; even if he/she doesn't express through speech, she/he may understand it, so, explain, explain, explain, that in many ways you are the same.

Using Interests to Boost Self-Esteem: Children with autism often have strange or rigid interests that others tease them for.

However, most often these same fascinations can be their saving grace. For example, a child who is into dates can be the keeper of the special events and birthdays' calendar. Or if its food she's into, meal preparation or just tossing salads can be her special gift. The child who cares about closing doors can be on safety patrol, and the one that likes rubber boots can line up and clean all the shoes. Self-esteem goes up when a person has a part to play in life and others value us, so value what your child does and watch his spirit soar.

Autism and Developing Sexuality: Autistic teens need clear comfortable precise explanations about how their body feels and what is and isn't acceptable. There is no room for shyness in this arena as any misunderstanding could lead to grave results in the public domain. There are some great sex books and videos that teach masturbation, though I have yet to discover any that combine this with clearly spelled social rules. Many children have to be taught not just the concept of privacy but also, since they are often too literal to generalize, they may need constant help with what that actually means (For example, my son was masturbating and moaning loudly in the bathroom of his sister's house while her in-laws were visiting. He believed he'd been private because he had closed the door. OOOPS!) The teachings continue and with a good sense of humor, some patience and persistence, the lessons are learned and the memories are a riot.

CHAPTER SEVENTEEN

Transitioning to Adulthood

By the time your child is an adult, his level of functioning has likely found its place and you will have a clearer idea of what is possible. Some can move out; some cannot. But independent or not, your child is no longer a child and his or her history means that he/she is a hybrid of both young and old. Be sensitive to this strange combination. Explain with simplicity but speak in a mature fashion to your autistic adult. Dress them for their age and encourage independence as much as possible.

Planning for Your Autistic Child's Future: There are many ways to envision your autistic child's future: group homes, family support, independence, institution, supported living, with a job, with an allowance, supported with trust fund money or Social Security or by and with you. Since nothing can be foreseen in the early years, setting up a trust fund is a good idea (as it always is for any of your children).

Finding the Right Living Arrangements: Once your child is grown and you all agree that it is time to move into a new situation, finding the right fit requires an open-eyed approach to your offspring's skill sets. If some kind of supported situation is needed, make sure you interview the caretakers of any program you are considering. If group living is a consideration, have your child meet the other residents and encourage them to share their feelings or view points. If your child is a poor communicator, observe any untoward changes in his/her attitude during your visits and try to ascertain if there is any way to make the transition easier. Do your best to bring comfortingly familiar bits of furniture from home. And if you feel uncomfortable with the arrangement, give yourself permission to change your mind.

Making the Leap from School to a Career or Job: The best scenario here is if the school program includes some job training and placement and the job happens even before school ends. Most programs for special individuals can be set up with this kind of transitional support. If this is not possible in your area, encourage your child to start with a part-time job. In fact, if your child is still young, start helping him find employment opportunities around the house and the neighborhood. I worked with one boy who began his independence on a household token system. He worked for his tokens doing odd jobs and paid for room and board every night with the earned tokens. The family slowly changed the system to a weekly pay and bill schedule. This boy is now fully self-supporting and living on his own.

Finding an Employment Fit: Helping adults with autism find the right employment follows the same principles as helping them grow and learn. Start with their interests; incorporate their hyperactivity level, their ability to attend, and their desire to work. Try to understand the picture they have for themselves (I worked with a girl who simply wanted to wear dresses and work in an office). Then search for a career that fits their image. For example, if she likes movie stars, sees herself as a night worker, and counts grocery items in the cupboard, she might work in the concession stand at the local theater.

Of course she may go through ten or twelve movie theater jobs, a couple video store jobs, and end up stocking shelves in the local grocery store. Great! Learning how to maintain a job requires experience, and learning that you don't want to be fired often is better accomplished by being fired. It's a beautiful learning curve as long as nobody sees being fired as synonymous with being a failure, because in fact being fired is only synonymous with learning how to not be.

CHAPTER EIGHTEEN

Some Helpful Hints

Strategies for Everyday Living: Teaching the autistic adult to handle the day-to-day realities of independence can be a challenge. Adults with autism go off track frequently and lose their focus. This struggle can lead to depression and withdrawal. Setting up schedules, to-do lists, computer reminders, and regularly phoning to go over plans is a good strategy. However, as with everything else, all of this is highly individualized. Everything, and I mean everything, with autism works most efficiently when it comes out of the autistic individual's own desires. So if they like their lists dated backwards, great, date them backwards. In my experience for the most part, where autistic adults are concerned, a busy yet only slightly demanding, very scheduled life, that includes lots of family support and contact, is the most successful.

Autism and Sleep: If your child suffers from sleep disturbances, as do many autistic children, make sure that his/her disturbances do not become yours. Inadequate sleep makes coping with life's challenges more difficult. Of course, there are many health store and over-the-counter sleeping pills that may help. However, taking excessive over-the-counter sleep aids is not a good answer; they can make things worse. Similarly, taking benzodiazepines (e.g., Xanax®) on a chronic basis is not recommended by many experts. For one thing, your sleep may be too heavy, and that may increase your anxiety as you worry about being available to your child. In addition, medication can make your sleep worse, at least temporarily, if you stop taking it. You may become dependent on benzodiazepines; and they can impair your cognition, memory, and reaction time. A published study has shown that average doses of alprazolam (Xanax®) can impair driving, attention, and reaction time. These are skills that you are going to need in order to properly supervise your autistic child. Sleep medication for your child is also a complicated decision and must always be done under the strict supervision of a qualified physician.

Even if you do try medication, many spectrum children do not respond well or even at all. Conversely, some are calmed significantly by the tried-and-true "ride in the car," lavender under the nose, or hemi-sync sleep music. Neurofeedback is also a great sleep regulator. However, if your child is still awake despite all your best efforts, do continue to investigate. But, investigate later; you need your sleep now. Therefore, create a safe environment in which he/she cannot hurt herself/himself whether awake or asleep, and go to bed. The only way to prioritize your child is to prioritize you.

Don't Romanticize the Disorder: Many people see an autistic child as a child in some other zone with special talents. They use terms such as "in his own world," "gifted," or "indigo child." They mystify the child's unusual ability to focus on the minute details of colors, smells, textures, or sounds. Because they can't understand it, they assume it to be magical. If people are telling you not to try and change your child because his/her special talents may be expunged, thank them for their concern; then walk away and get back to the business of reaching out to your child. The fact is, all parents teach. And so will you. The only difference is that you are going to be intentional and learned about it. Of course your child is special and unique. Even among the population of spectrum individuals, your child has her/his own special brand of beautiful. That is the marvelous aspect of this "build upon his interests" approach. We are not going to take away; we are going to add. We are going to help him/her and you become more, not less.

While You Play, Teach: Use music. Many autistic individuals respond positively to music. Some even speak only in song. Therefore, sing. If your child calms, gets excited, comes nearer, looks at you, or joins in, you have a means to communicate. Sing your instructions, sing your praise, sing your ideas, and sing your love.

Use numbers. As with music, numbers can be the delight of an autistic child. Bemoaning an obsession with numbers misses the opportunity to interact and to begin the bridge of bonding. Play with the numbers. Count how many drawers to the pajama drawer or how many steps to the toilet, subtract each tooth after adding the number of brush stokes, or lay out pictures of the family in ranges of ages and match the years in which they were born. Numbers, numbers, numbers. What a great opportunity to improve your math skills.

Use puzzles. Once again, here is an opportunity to teach and connect. Anything can be made into a puzzle: favorite Disney characters, pictures of favorite toys, or a pair of old coveralls. If she/he won't look at you, try puzzles of eyes or mask puzzles with the eyeholes cut out, which once put together can be put on. If he/she looks at you, say, "Thanks."

Use tickles, squeezes, and airplane rides. Many autistic kids respond to sensory and vestibular treatment modalities. They have challenges in this area. Your child may even be performing her/his own therapy by spinning or head banging. However, if you start giving rides, tickles, and squeezes, you become an integral part of your child's world while at the same time stimulating her/his proprioceptive, sensory, and vestibular nuclei.

More than with any other child, be prepared to do it again and again and again and again. As he/she asks for more, so do you: another sound, a whole word, a sentence, two sentences, etc. Then, because you appreciate her/his trying, give the ride whether he/she says the word or not.

I'm sure this sounds like a lot more playing than you had planned. Lucky you. Your child is about to help you reorganize your adult years and stay young.

Closing

WHEW!! That was a lot of information! It took a lot of living to gather it all, and I absolutely LOVE that I am able to share. But before I wrap this up, I want to slow down for a moment and share a few stories…

When my grandson Shay was four, he used to talk like this: "gunk, gunk, gunk." He played with sticky substances on the top of his lip and walked on his toes. He looked at our noses instead of our eyes and loved Thomas the Train to distraction. We never had him diagnosed but there wasn't much doubt he was autistic. I watched him and watched him and watched him and then it occurred to me that total communication was the way to cure his talking issues. Not because anybody told me but just something about him and that idea made sense. So my daughter and I made a plan. We'd learn sign language and do it in a really exciting way all around our faces to make talking fun and get him to copy us while keeping his fingers out of his mouth and attracting his eyes towards ours… It worked. He started to talk and was verbally age appropriate six months after we started. That experience with Shay reminded me of something that I think is possibly the most important thing I can share with other parents (over and over again): to trust my instincts and myself. Nobody knows your child like you.

Compared to his three brothers, my son Cash was pretty easy. He mostly stood at the window and stared at our car—often vomiting just for the warm sensation of it. He was soft and sweet and spent the whole first year of kindergarten mute. Cash was so amazing. When he was six he noticed that his brother Chance could hand over hand on the monkey bars while he could barely run because his arms and legs wobbled. I guess he didn't like being so uncoordinated because all that summer he got himself up and dressed by seven, ate breakfast, packed a sandwich, and went into the backyard for the day. He stayed out there trying and trying and trying to hold his own weight on the overhead bar that held up our swings. It was inspiring and painful to watch. I wanted to help but I didn't; it was hard but—I stayed out of it. He practiced every day for most of the summer. By the beginning of second grade he could hand over hand from one end of the monkey bars to the other. Cash made curing autism look easy because he did it himself. So if any of you are lucky enough to have a motivated child on the spectrum, just get out of the way and guide him/her in. Become a cheerleader, "Come on, use your words, a whole sentence; you can do it!" And let him/her figure it out on their own. The point here is that sometimes stepping aside is being proactive. Cash has been living independently and working on the pipelines since 1998.

So in closing, I want to say that I truly believe we are always doing the best we can with what we know. And you have taken a very wise and wonderful step toward empowering yourself with the knowledge you need to best help your child. In this book is the information, in your heart is the motivation, and every time you look into your child's eyes you will find inspiration. Now go love life with your wonderful child, and when you feel lost come back to the book for some direction…. After all, I already lived it so you get to start where I left off… Lucky you!!

Best,
Lynette Louise

Research and Resources

Books:

1. ***ADD: The 20-Hour Solution: Training minds to concentrate and self-regulate naturally without medication*** by Mark Steinberg, Ph.D. & Siegfried Othmer, Ph.D.
2. ***Biofeedback for the Brain*** by Paul G. Swingle
3. ***The Brain That Changes Itself*** by Norman Doidge
4. ***Change Your Brain Change Your*** by Life Daniel G. Amen
5. ***Dorlands Illustrated Medical Dictionary*** by Saunders
6. ***DSM-IV-TR***, published by the American Psychiatric Association
7. ***French's Index of Differential Diagnosis*** edited by Arthur H. Douthwaite
8. ***Getting Started With Neurofeedback*** by John N Demos
9. ***The Healing Power of Neurofeedback*** by Thom Hartmann
10. ***Healing Young Brains: The Neurofeedback Solution*** by Robert W. Hill, PhD & Eduardo Castro, MD
11. ***The History of Psychiatry*** by Alexander and Selesnick
12. ***An Introduction to Brain and Behavior*** by Bryan Kolb & Ian Q. Wilshaw
13. ***Mind Wide Open*** by Steven Johnson
14. ***The Open Focus Brain*** by Les Fehmi PhD and Jim Robbins
15. ***The Neurofeedback Book*** by Michael and Lynda Thompson
16. ***New Encyclopedia of Vitamins, Minerals, Supplements, & Herbs*** by Nicola Reavley
17. ***A Symphony In The Brain*** by Jim Robbins

Articles:

1. *Big Pharma and American Psychiatry: The Good the Bad and the Ugly* by S.S. Sharfstein, **Psychiatric News**
2. *The Dictionary of Disorder: How one man revolutionized psychiatry* by A. Spiegel, **The New Yorker**
3. *Madness explained: Why we must reject the Kraepelian paradigm and replace it with a 'complaint-oriented' approach to understanding mental illness* by R. Bentall, Medical Hypotheses
4. *Spectrum concepts in major mental disorders* by J. D. Maser & H. S. Akiskal, Psychiatric Clinics of North America

Studies:

I have read complete studies on the effectiveness of neurofeedback on the reactivity of autism and many synopsized studies on autism as well as other brain disorders and their influence from various modalities.

In addition to the above sources, all studies and therapies mentioned have also been investigated through the use of home pages and web searches.

All the rest came from my life, my very unique perspective, my notes, my teachers or my children's reports.

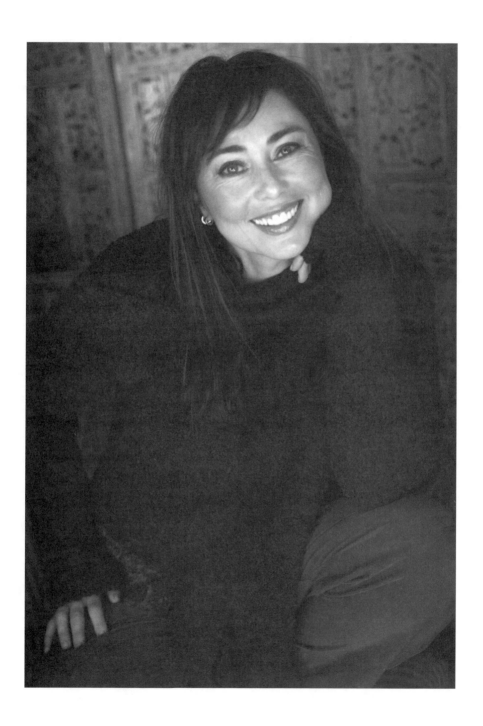

Lynette Louise, MS, NTC BCIA-EEG Board Certified in Neurofeedback PhD in MOM

Born in Calgary, Alberta (Canada) in 1957, Lynette Louise left school at fifteen, married, and had two children before turning twenty. By the time she was twenty-nine, she had adopted four toddlers, all boys with varying degrees of autism. "Having been a foster parent," says Lynette, "I couldn't stand that the kids would be bounced from home to home. I had to keep them!" Along the way, she added two troubled teenage girls to the mix, one with learning disabilities, completing the family with eight children in all. The story of how these children not only survived but also flourished is a testament to Lynette's persistence, unconventional approaches, and steadfast love.

A major turning point came when Lynette moved the family to a shelter after separating from her husband. Following this painful episode, Lynette worked an array of odd jobs—everything from mail carrier to advice columnist—in order to support the children as a single parent. But she kept returning to her first love: the theatre. Throughout the years, Lynette has performed stand-up (winning the title of Toronto's funniest comedian in 1990), landed parts in several movies, and even hosted a weekly television cooking show on *Canada's Life*

Network. She also independently produced comedy and music shows, turning the family into a traveling theatre troupe. In the early 1990's she wrote, produced, and performed Behind Bars, a musical show that toured prisons throughout Canada and the United States. Her first CD *Sing Me A Song…* please was released in 1994 while her first book *JEFF: a sexually realized spiritual odyssey of stepping into love* was published in 2003.

In the pursuit of helping her children, Lynette relocated to the United States in 1996. "America saved my life," she admits. "I had constant problems with the Canadian schools. Then when I moved to the States I discovered that in America the alternative of home-schooling was more accepted." Loading the brood into an RV, she spent a year and a half traveling around the country with her children. Traveling in this way allowed her to work closely with each of them. This period of "travel therapy" dovetailed perfectly with a new program Lynette had been introduced to: the Option Process, a treatment that stresses one-on-one play with the parent as therapist. She eventually received certification as an Option counselor.

Today as young-adults, all of Lynette's children function independently except for Dar (twenty-nine), who continues to live with her. Dar was the most severely challenged and abused of all her children when he came to her at age four after several years of being locked in a closet by his alcoholic mother. Lynette calls him a "slow moving miracle" who continues to make extraordinary progress, especially since beginning neurofeedback therapy several years ago.

Lynette became certified as a child facilitator by the Autism Treatment Center of America and as a neurofeedback practitioner, studying with leaders in the field, including Catherine Rule of Northampton, Massachusetts, and Dr. Harold Burke of Westlake, California. Her training and understanding of neurofeedback was greatly enhanced by the honors college degree in mainframe computer languages she earned during her twenties. Lynette has recently (2010) completed her Masters Degree in Social and Behavioral Science as well as becoming board certified (Nationally and Internationally) in Neurofeedback, Biofeedback-EEG.

In 2004 Lynette founded the Brain and Body Clinic, a treatment center for autism and other brain disorders using neurofeedback, a therapy that improves functioning by training individuals to control their own brainwave activity. Although originally based in Santa Monica, California, Lynette decided a clinical setting was counterproductive to the majority of her clients. She now works on site with clients and their families all over the world.

Lynette is simultaneously performing Internationally in her one-woman play, *THING TO THING TO THING—From Crazy To Sane With Biofeedback, Autism, And The Brain*. Full of funny, heartbreaking, and triumphant stories drawn from her life, the show is a composite of monologues, brain science, and music during which Lynette recounts her twenty-year search for ways to help her special-needs children develop into independent adults. The play was first performed in May of 2007 at Highways Performance Space in Santa Monica, California. Gaining popularity at public venues in Southern California, Lynette then took the show on the road to theatres in cities and towns across the United States. An abbreviated conference version of *THING TO THING TO THING* was performed and received a standing ovation at the annual conference of the International Society for Neurofeedback and Research in San Diego. Her new, more provocative show *CRAZY TO SANE* has been getting standing ovations nationally. In addition to these two live shows being presented as a singular experience Lynette also combines them with her motivational speeches into a seminar-length six-hour presentation, *SCIENCE, LIFE AND LEARNINGS,* for families and professionals throughout North America. Arrangements are underway for performances at other professional events, including many leading autism conferences.

On the horizon is a new autism-related TV show, the pilot for which was originally aired at the Autism One Conference in Chicago 2010.

Contact her via her website: www.lynettelouise.com.

Robert D. Reed Publishers Order Form

Call in your order for fast service and quantity discounts!
(541) 347- 9882

OR order on-line at **www.rdrpublishers.com** using PayPal.
OR order by FAX at **(541) 347-9883** OR by mail:
Make a copy of this form; enclose payment information:
Robert D. Reed Publishers
1380 Face Rock Drive, Bandon, OR 97411

Send indicated books to:

Name_____

Address_____

City_____ State _____ Zip _____

Phone: _____ Fax _____ Cell_____

E-Mail _____

Payment by check /_/ or credit card /_/ (All major credit cards are accepted.)

Name on card _____

Card Number _____

Exp. Date _____ Last 3-Digit number on back of card _____

	Quantity	Total Amount
Miracles Are Made: A Real-Life Guide to Autism by Lynette Louise, MS, NTC, BCIA-EEG Board Certified in Neurofeedback, PhD in MOM $17.95	_____	_____
ADD: The 20-Hour Solution: Training minds to concentrate and self-regulate naturally without medication by Mark Steinberg, Ph.D. & Siegfried Othmer, Ph.D. $14.95	_____	_____
Raindrops on Roman: Overcoming Autism: A Message of Hope by Elizabeth Scott $14.95	_____	_____
Autism Recovery Manual of Skills and Drills by Elizabeth Burton Scott, M.A. & Lynne Gillis, O.T. $16.95	_____	_____
California Squizine: Healthy Food That's Fast, Fun, and Squeezable For Kids by Malclm Kushner $11.95	_____	_____
Special Foods for Special Kids: Practical Solutions & Great Recipies for Children with FOOD ALLERGIES by Todd Adelman & Jodi Behrend $16.95	_____	_____
A Kid's Herb Book for children of all ages by Lesley Tierra, L.Ac., AHG $19.95	_____	_____

Quantity of books ordered: _____ Total amount for books: _____

Shipping is $3.50 1st book + $1 for each additional book: Plus postage: _____

FINAL TOTAL: _____